The Intersection of Food and Public Health

Current Policy Challenges and Solutions

Public Administration for Public Health
Nicolas A. Valcik, Central Washington University, USA

The Intersection of Food and Public Health
Current Policy Challenges and Solutions
Edited by A. Bryce Hoflund, John C. Jones and Michelle C. Pautz

Collaborative Healthcare Networks
Building Community among Local Partnerships Organizations
Theodore Aaron Wachhaus, Jr.

Gun Violence
Evaluating Perceptions, Causes, and Consequences
Nicolas A. Valcik, Marvin E. Letteer and Warren S. Eller

The Intersection of Food and Public Health

Current Policy Challenges and Solutions

Edited by
**A. Bryce Hoflund, John C. Jones, and
Michelle C. Pautz**

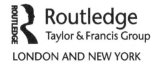

Routledge
Taylor & Francis Group

LONDON AND NEW YORK

First published 2018
by Routledge
4 Park Square, Milton Park, Abingdon, Oxon OX14 4RN
605 Third Avenue, New York, NY 10017

First issued in paperback 2023

Routledge is an imprint of the Taylor & Francis Group, an informa business

British Library Cataloguing-in-Publication Data
A catalogue record for this book is available from the British Library

ISBN: 978-1-03-256984-0 (pbk)
ISBN: 978-1-4987-5895-6 (hbk)
ISBN: 978-1-315-15309-4 (ebk)

DOI: 10.1201/9781315153094

Typeset in Times New Roman
by Nova Techset Private Limited, Bengaluru & Chennai, India

Publisher's Note
The publisher has gone to great lengths to ensure the quality of this reprint but
points out that some imperfections in the original copies may be apparent.

We dedicate this volume to all of those individuals working to understand and address food systems and food insecurity issues in their communities and around the world.

Contents

3 **Unintended consequences of nutritional assistance programs: Children's school meal participation and adults' food security**   33
TEJA PRISTAVEC

4 **The food environment and social determinants of food insufficiency and diet quality in rural households**   55
CHRISTIAN KING

PART V
Missing connections in food, nutrition, and health policy

PART VI
Changing food and health policy

List of Figures

List of Tables

Acknowledgments

This endeavor would not have been possible without the help of many individuals, including those whose names are included throughout this volume, as well as many others whose names are not. The centrality of food studies and systems is increasingly apparent to researchers and activists, and we are privileged to have the opportunity to continue these important conversations from a variety of disciplinary and multidisciplinary perspectives. We are grateful for the efforts of each of the authors included in this volume along with the commitment and dedication of the individuals who helped each of these research endeavors come to the page.

More specifically, we wish to acknowledge the help provided by B.J. Fletcher, who is a doctoral student in public administration at the University of Nebraska at Omaha. His dedication and attention to detail was essential in pulling this volume together. We are thrilled to be part of the Routledge Studies in Public Health series and appreciate the support of series editor, Grace McInness. Further, we would like to thank Nicolas A. Valcik for encouraging us to pursue this project and the editorial team at Routledge for their guidance.

A. Bryce Hoflund wants to thank her family, friends, colleagues, and coeditors for their love, support, and guidance throughout this process. In particular, she would like to thank her husband, David Bilek, and her dog, Jasper, for providing gentle support and encouragement over the years and especially as she worked on her first book project.

John C. Jones wants to thank his coeditors for their continued friendship and mentorship throughout this process. They continue to inspire him to struggle on through the dissertation process and to keep focused on the light at the end of the tunnel! Michelle C. Pautz wants to acknowledge the love and support of her family. Having an academic as a member of the family is never easy and her husband, Steven, and their three wonderful dogs, Emma, Sydney, and Victoria, know that all too well. Their ability to endure speaks volumes of their humanity. She is forever grateful for the love and support that they all give. Steven is an amazing source of support and quiet strength that she never knew she needed. Emma, Sydney, and Victoria, each, in their own ways, provide essential assistance. Emma shows me perseverance must be married with sass, Sydney is ever present ensuring fidelity to the task and the importance of a good squeaker, and Victoria always has a wagging tail just when it is needed most.

A. Bryce Hoflund
Omaha, Nebraska

John C. Jones
Dayton, Ohio

Michelle C. Pautz
Dayton, Ohio
November 2016

Contributors

Alicia Andry earned an MS in urban studies and is currently completing an MA in geography at the University of Nebraska at Omaha. Her research interests include sustainable food systems, cultural food landscapes, and urban geography. Outside of her immediate discipline, she is also interested in functional nutritional health, wellness, and longevity.

Tania Calvao is a senior attorney with a JD from Universidade Sta. Ursula (Rio de Janeiro, Brazil), LLM from University of Houston (Texas), and MBA and MSF from University of St. Thomas (Houston, Texas). Her research specializations include ethics, government policy and regulation at University of St. Thomas, and energy, environmental and natural resources law at University of Houston. She has advanced academic qualifications from the University of London, Queen Mary and Westfield College, Wharton Business School, University of Pennsylvania, and the Kennedy School of Government, Harvard University. Calvao has been a member of the Brazilian Bar Association, Rio de Janeiro Chapter since 1990 and has held memberships in the Association of International Petroleum Negotiators in the United States and the European Community Trademark Association. Calvao has practiced law in Brazil for 20 years and currently practices international corporate law in Houston with O. J. Lawal & Associates Law Firm. She also continues her research in Houston, Texas.

Diana Cuy Castellanos, PhD, RDN, is an assistant professor at the University of Dayton. She is a registered dietitian and works in community health. Her research interests include dietary acculturation in minority populations, community-based participatory research, and food security. She has published her work in multiple professional journals and textbooks.

Can Chen is an assistant professor in the Department of Public Administration, Steven J. Green School of International and Public Affairs, at Florida International University. His main research interests focus on state and local government budgeting and finance.

Joanne Christaldi, PhD, RDN, is an assistant professor of Nutrition and Didactic Program in Dietetics, Director at West Chester University in West Chester, Pennsylvania. Her research interests include hunger and food insecurity, chronic disease prevention, obesity prevention and treatment, and qualitative theory and methodology.

Carol Ebdon is the regents/foundation professor in the School of Public Administration at the University of Nebraska at Omaha. Her research, primarily relating to local government public budgeting and financial management, has been published in a variety of journals.

Angela L. Glover, PhD, is an online instructor for the University of Nebraska Omaha, Omaha, Nebraska and a literacy coach for Omaha Public Schools. Her research interests include creative non-fiction, food studies, and writing pedagogy.

Adele Hite is a PhD candidate in communication, rhetoric, and digital media at North Carolina State University, Raleigh, North Carolina, as well as a registered dietitian with a master's in public health nutrition. Her work encompasses the rhetorical and cultural studies of food politics, nutrition science, and public health; science-based policy controversy; and the ethics of dietary guidance.

A. Bryce Hoflund is an associate professor in the School of Public Administration at the University of Nebraska at Omaha. Her research focuses on food policy and food safety regulation, healthcare regulation and policy, network organizations, and network management and leadership. She has published her work in *Regulation & Governance, Administration & Society*, the *Journal of Health and Human Services Administration, Public Organization Review*, and *Food Studies: An Interdisciplinary Journal*, and *Political Science Quarterly*, and a book chapter in *Voices of Hunger: Food Insecurity in the United States*. She earned a PhD in public administration from Virginia Tech.

Georgia Jones is an associate professor and extension food specialist in the Department of Nutrition and Health Sciences at the University of Nebraska-Lincoln. She teaches scientific principles of food preparation and food safety and sanitation. She conducts extension programs in the area of food literacy.

John C. Jones is a doctoral candidate at the joint Urban Systems program hosted by Rutgers University and the New Jersey Institute of Technology. John's main research interests surround the intersection of the challenges that America's postindustrial cities face in a globalizing world and the development of urban food systems. His dissertation examines the potential of local food enterprises as a vehicle for economic development in the post-industrial cities of Newark, New Jersey and Dayton, Ohio.

Christian King is an assistant professor of health policy in the Department of Nutrition and Health Sciences at the University of Nebraska-Lincoln. His research interests are in health policy and social policy. Some of his recent work has examined food insecurity and some of its consequences for low-income families.

Emily C. Kohls is a registered dietitian and a food service director for the Department of Veterans Affairs. She earned her master's in public administration from the School of Public Administration at the University of Nebraska at Omaha. Her research interests include food insecurity, food deserts, and food policy.

Helena C. Lyson is a PhD candidate in sociology at the University of California, Berkeley, California. Her research focuses on community food systems, sustainable agriculture, health inequities, and social movement activism at the disciplinary nexus of sociology and political science.

Megan McGuffey is a doctoral student at the University of Nebraska at Omaha. Her central research interests include food policy, citizen participation and active citizenship, and local government management. McGuffey holds a bachelor of arts degree in political science from the University of Nebraska-Lincoln and a master of public administration from the University of Nebraska at Omaha.

Sabrina Neeley, PhD, MPH, is the director of population health curriculum in the Office of Medical Education at Wright State University's Boonshoft School of Medicine and is also an assistant professor in the Department of Population and Public Health Sciences. Her research is focused on understanding social determinants of health and how sociocultural, environmental, and individual factors influence health decision-making and behavior.

Michelle C. Pautz is an associate professor of political science and director of the MPA program at the University of Dayton. Her research focuses on the interactions between front-line regulators and the regulated community. Additional research interests include government food policy and regulation and film and politics. Her work has appeared in *Administration & Society, Administrative Theory & Praxis, Journal of Environmental Studies & Sciences, Policy Studies Journal, PS: Political Science & Politics, Public Voices,* and the *Review of Policy Research,* among others. She is the coauthor of *The Lilliputians of Environmental Regulation: The Perspective of State Regulators* and *US Environmental Policy in Action: Practice & Implementation.* She earned a PhD in public administration from Virginia Tech.

Teja Pristavec is a PhD student in the Sociology Department at Rutgers, The State University of New Jersey, New Brunswick, New Jersey. Her research interests include food, inequality, the life course, and quantitative methods.

Jennifer Geist Rutledge is an assistant professor of political science at John Jay College of Criminal Justice-CUNY, New York. Her research focuses on food and agricultural policy, comparative social policy, and human rights.

Timothy J. Shaffer is an assistant professor in the Department of Communication Studies and assistant director of the Institute for Civic Discourse and Democracy at Kansas State University, Manhattan, Kansas. He is also principal research specialist with the National Institute for Civil Discourse at the University of Arizona. Shaffer has published in the *National Civic Review, The Good Society,* the *Journal of Public Deliberation*, and is editor of *Deliberative Pedagogy: Teaching and Learning for Democratic Engagement*, forthcoming from Michigan State University Press. His research interests include deliberative politics in institutional and community settings as well as civic professionalism.

Bhavna Shamasunder is assistant professor in the Urban and Environmental Policy Department at Occidental College, Los Angeles, California. She teaches and conducts research on environmental health and justice with a focus on the disparate and cumulative burdens faced by communities of color and the poor. Her work also examines how social movements leverage science in campaigns for justice. Her current project addresses community-based participatory research on health impacts from neighborhood oil drilling in Los Angeles. She earned her doctorate at the University of California, Berkeley in the Department of Environmental Science, Policy, and Management. Previously, Bhavna developed and ran the Environmental Health Program at Urban Habitat, a Bay Area environmental justice organization.

Anthony Starke is a doctoral student at the University of Nebraska at Omaha. His research emphasizes the role of public policy and public institutions on the construction of identity (e.g., race, class, gender and sexual orientation, etc.). Starke holds bachelor of science degrees in psychology and human services from Old Dominion University (Norfolk, Virginia) as well as a graduate certificate in nonprofit management and master of public administration degree from Virginia Commonwealth University (Richmond, Virginia).

Courtney I. P. Thomas, visiting assistant professor (PhD, Virginia Tech, Blacksburg, Virginia, 2010). Professor Thomas's research interests include international political economy, food safety and security, genocide studies, and public policy. She currently teaches undergraduate courses in world politics, international political economy, and nations and nationalities. She has presented her research at conferences in Ljubljana, Slovenia; Salzburg, Austria; Baltimore, Maryland; Washington, DC; Urbana, Illinois; Austin, Texas; and Berkeley, California. Dr. Thomas's publications include: *In Food We Trust*, University of Nebraska Press, 2014; *Voices of Hunger* (ed.), Common Ground Publishing, 2014; *Political Culture and the Making of Modern Nation States,* Paradigm Press, 2014; *International Political Economy: Navigating the Logic Streams, an Introduction* (coauthored with Edward Weisband), Kendall Hunt, 2010; *The Biocorporeality of Evil: A Taxonomy* (coauthored with Edward Weisband) in *Inside & Outside of the Law: Perspectives on Evil, Law, and the State* (Shubhankar Dam and Jonathan Hall, eds.), Inter-Disciplinary Press, 2009; and *Big Blocks of Cheese and Other Lessons on American Government: 15 Weeks in the West Wing* (coauthored with Sandra E. Via) in *Teaching Matters: Strategy and Tactics to Engage Students in the Study of American Politics* (Daniel Shea, ed.), Prentice-Hall, 2010.

Introduction

Currently, ideas about food are in flux from a variety of sources. Examples of this evolution include recognizing the importance of food on health by public health and medical professionals; changing consumer desires around the production methods and components of their food, a greater focus on injustices within the national food system; evolving knowledge of how the food system impacts the environment; and shifting economic and technological realities that underpin where and how food is produced, distributed, and sold. These shifting ideas about food exist in contrast to the narrative of the highly functioning industrialized global food system that emerged in the second half of the twentieth century. Therefore, the nexus of food studies and politics and public health should be obvious, yet a text that successfully integrates the two topics is elusive. This edited volume fills that void by covering in an engaging and comprehensive way key topics in food studies and systems as they relate to public health. The volume comprises research that examines current problems in food studies and how various stakeholders are attempting to address problems in unique ways.

The intersection of food policy and public health has come into focus recently regarding how policy connects to larger public health concerns, including obesity, diabetes, nutrition, and food safety issues. The prevalence of adult and childhood obesity has become a major public health concern. According to the Centers for Disease Control (CDC), more than one third of adults are obese and approximately 12.5 million of children and adolescents aged 2–19 years are obese (Ogden et al. 2015). The estimated annual medical cost of obesity in the United States is approximately $147 billion (Finkelstein et al. 2009). Correspondingly, the CDC has consistently noted in recent years that dietary-related health morbidities (i.e., diabetes, hypertension, heart diseases, etc.) remain high (Centers for Disease Control 2016). Food safety is another public health concern. The CDC estimates that about 48 million people are sickened, 128,000 are hospitalized, and 3,000 die each year from foodborne illnesses, and foodborne illnesses have a significant societal cost associated with them (Scallan et al. 2011a,b). One study estimates that the nation spent between 51 and 77 billion dollars annually on medical expenses and lost productivity as a result of foodborne illnesses (Scharff 2012).

Social justice concerns, such as food insecurity, food deserts, and concerns for workers in factory farms, is another emerging area of food studies. In the first decade of this century, food insecurity rates rose in 41 states. In the other nine states, the numbers stayed flat. In 2015, the U.S. Department of Agriculture (USDA) estimated that 42.2 million people lived in food insecure households (Coleman-Jensen et al. 2016). Food deserts, areas where fresh fruits, veggies, and other healthy whole foods are not available, as well as food swamps, areas where food options are disproportionately higher in sugar, fat, or salt, are also a growing concern and are related to food insecurity. The USDA (2009) estimates that more than 23.5 million people live in food deserts, which exist simultaneously both in highly urban and highly rural spaces. Poverty is often the link between the two; more than half of individuals living in food deserts are low income.

Finally, the intersection of food policy and public health is related to environmental issues and building and maintaining sustainable communities. The agricultural industry has experienced dramatic changes over the past few decades. Coinciding with this, the growth of general awareness of environmental and sustainability concerns has also inspired many to become concerned with the sustainability of the food industry. Global competition and the national agricultural and trade policies that favor large-scale farms have hurt small farms. Furthermore, Pirog (2009) examined produce arrival data from the USDA's Marketing Service and estimated that fresh produce arriving in Chicago by truck had traveled over 1500 miles on average. The long-distance food travel leads to more energy consumption and pollution emission that contributes to global warming and lower air quality. Water, air, and soil quality can impact communities located near major agricultural centers.*

These are highlights of the ubiquitous nature of food studies topics and concerns. Given the inherent interdisciplinary nature of food studies, this volume has a broad scope that integrates a range of topics within food policy and public health from a wide range of perspectives. This volume is organized around the following questions as they relate to the U.S. food system and public health: What units of analysis are being used or have been used to study the food system? Are they appropriate? What is the role of the regulatory state in the U.S. food system? What are some understudied areas of the U.S. food system? What are some potential ways of addressing these issues? What are some of the current debates related to food production? What are some of the current challenges related to food distribution and how are they being addressed? What are the politics of food policy? What are the governance challenges associated with food policy? What role should social contexts play in the construction of knowledge and advocacy of food system reformers and researchers?

Accordingly, the goals for this book are threefold. Our first goal is to provide an overview of current challenges to the food system and present research that examines potential solutions to those challenges since there has been an

---

* An earlier version of the three reasons to study food policy appeared in the Winter 2016 School of Public Administration newsletter and was written by A. Bryce Hoflund and Megan McGuffey.

explosion in the interest in addressing challenges related to the U.S. food system. Research on food is rather unique as food is simultaneously experienced on an intensely personal level, but also on a level that is shared by every other human being. We deliberately cultivated a list of topics that cuts across a wide spectrum and hope that nearly every reader should find some element to interest them. This volume is broad in scope and covers a variety of issues and concerns at the intersection of public health and food at the national, state, and local levels.

Our second goal is to fill a gap in the public health and food policy literatures by beginning a conversation that addresses how food public and public health issues increasingly intersect with each other. Further, we hope this conversation underscores the interdisciplinary nature of food research. Over the past decade, many students and scholars have become interested in studying the U.S. food system and its challenges; however, the scholarship in this area remains relatively scarce. This volume fills this gap. We primarily selected topics that are in the initial stages of being studied by researchers and will be of interest to a wide variety of advanced undergraduate and graduate students, scholars, practitioners, and policymakers.

Our third goal is to shift the conversation of food, its production, distribution, and consumption, as well as the public policies that underpin it, into the twenty-first century. As we noted above, major shifts are underway surrounding how producers, consumers, regulators, planners, researchers, and healthcare professionals interface with the food system. However, as implied by many of the authors in this work, our current narratives about the food system and its functions are rooted in twentieth century realities and need updating.

This book is intended to serve as a supplementary, or secondary, text in undergraduate and graduate courses related to food systems, food policy, public policy studies, nutrition, and public health. Each contributor provides a review of the current research literature in a particular area and then explores and applies that discussion to a particular food systems issue. Each chapter offers an overview of a particular topic in food systems as well as offers lessons learned for scholars and practitioners by examining each proposed aspect of the food system.

In Part I, "Where the personal intersects with public policy," we open with a piece by Angela Glover that examines how personal food choices intersect with larger public health issues. This piece serves as a framing piece for this book in that it highlights and demonstrates that policy emerges from the personal. Glover uses an auto-ethnographic lens to demonstrate the very intimate, personal relationship we all have with food and how that very private relationship might in turn influence our interactions with the broader world. We choose this chapter as our starting point to encourage all readers to reflect about how their personal food space influences how they examine the broader food system.

In Part II, "Understanding food insecurity," explores the history, policies, and social and environmental determinants of food insecurity. In their chapter, Joanne Christaldi and Diana Cuy Castellanos discuss the history and context of food insecurity and the associated national and local food and nutrition policies. In Chapter 3, Teja Pristavec's rather paradoxical study of the impacts of children's school mean participation on adults' food security finds that those adults whose children participate in school meal programs are likely to be more food insecure than those whose children do not participate in school meal programs. In the next piece, Christian King uses data from the Behavioral Risk Factor Surveillance System (BRFSS) to study how food access affects the dietary intake (particularly fruit and vegetable consumption) and the food security of a sample of adults living in rural areas. Finally, Emily Kohls's case study of a rural food desert provides some much-needed insight into the programs and activities that exist to address food access in rural areas.

The chapters in Part III, "Exploring the regulation of food," address a variety of key issues in food safety regulation from functional foods to the role of school food service directors in the regulatory state. Courtney Thomas examines the proliferation of functional foods and questions of legitimacy, accountability, and regulatory challenges associated with the rise of these types of foods. Bhavna Shamasunder's piece on chlorpyrifos—one of the most widely used pesticides in the world—traces the history and controversies associated with its use and argues for food systems and a precautionary public health-based approach to regulatory decision-making over pesticides. In our contribution to this volume, we explore the role of food service directors in three metropolitan areas—Omaha, Nebraska, Dayton, Ohio, and Newark, New Jersey—as both local administrator of National School Lunch Program (NSLP) as well as the subject of federal regulation regarding NSLP. The final piece in this section by Tania Calvao discusses the different approaches taken by the United States and the European Union with regard to regulation of genetically modified organisms.

The two chapters in Part IV, "Considering local food systems," explore the changing nature of local food systems and the challenges they face in light of the twenty-first century changes to communities. Alicia Andry's chapter discusses the origins and evolution of the industrial food system, examines local alternatives that are used to replace the industrial system, and suggests some basic steps that can be taken by public health administrators to assist in this cultural food shift. John C. Jones's chapter applies the emerging ideas of partnership governance to the challenges of developing a local food system in postindustrial communities.

In Part V, "Missing connections in food, nutrition, and health policy," the chapters are concerned with the ethical dimensions of food policy, the changing tools used to improve health and develop, implement, and evaluate policy, and the importance of food literacy. Adele Hite discusses the ethical implications of public health nutrition guidelines and proposes ways to create a more ethically responsible public health nutrition policy. In her two contributions to the volume, Sabrina Neeley describes Health in All Policies as an emerging approach to policy development and explores the *One Health* framework as a means of understanding and improving the interconnections between the health of humans, animals, and the environment, and the resulting impact on food safety and food security. Finally, Georgia Jones discusses the increasingly important idea of food literacy and how it can empower consumers to make informed food choices that can positively impact their health.

Finally, in Part VI, "Changing food and health policy," the authors discuss a variety of ways in which the food policy landscape is changing and ways to affect change in food policy. Anthony Starke and Megan McGuffey's piece explores the development of the concept of food justice and argues for the importance of including food justice as a key consideration in any policy proposal impacting food issues. The next two chapters examine school food reform movements at the national and local levels, with Jennifer Geist Rutledge's piece focusing on the passage of the 2010 Child Nutrition Act and the political forces that brought about this major policy change, and Helena Lyson's piece focusing on how groundbreaking school reform occurred at a large urban school district in Northern California. Carol Ebdon and Can Chen also discuss school food reform, and focus on the movement toward privatization of school food services in Nebraska and Florida. Finally, Timothy Shaffer discusses how a little-known discussion-based adult education program designed by the USDA during the New Deal and subsequently implemented by Cooperative Extension Service agents at land-grant-based universities can engage citizens in understanding issues as well as having their experience and knowledge help shape local, state, regional, and national policy.

We hope these chapters help to engage deeper discussions about the changing nature of food in the twenty-first century and how public health actors, along with interdisciplinary allies, can play a role in improving the dietary health of all people. Further, we are optimistic that readers will become more adroit in tapping into notions about the changing food system, and its challenges that exist outside of their primary discipline. Building a better food system for all is complex work and will require many people, with many talents, across all sectors of society. We look forward to continuing to engage with our authors and our readers in the future on this topic.

A. Bryce Hoflund, John C. Jones, and Michelle C. Pautz

REFERENCES

Centers for Disease Control. 2016. *Chronic Diseases: The Leading Causes of Death and Disability in the United States*. Retrieved from https://www.cdc.gov/chronicdisease/overview/

Coleman-Jensen, A., M. P. Rabbitt, C. A. Gregory, and A. Singh. 2016. *Household food security in the United States in 2015*. ERR-215. U.S. Department of Agriculture, Economic Research Service.

Finkelstein, E.A., J. G. Trogdon, J. W. Cohen, and W. Dietz. 2009. Annual medical spending attributable to obesity: Payer- and service-specific estimates. *Health Affairs* 28(5):822–831.

Ogden, C. L., M. D. Carroll, C. D. Fryar, and K. M. Flegal. 2015. Prevalence of obesity among adults and youth: United States, 2011–2014. NCHS data brief, no. 219. National Center for Health Statistics.

Pirog, R. 2009. *Local Foods: Farm Fresh and Environmentally Friendly.* Ames, IA: Leopold Center for Sustainable Agriculture.

Scallan, E., R. M. Hoekstra, F. J. Angulo, R. V. Tauxe, M. Widdowson, S. L. Roy, and P. M. Griffin. 2011a. Foodborne illness acquired in the United States—Major pathogens. *Emerging Infectious Diseases* 17(1):7–15.

Scallan, E., P. M. Griffin, F. J. Angulo, R. V. Tauxe, and R. M. Hoekstra. 2011b. Foodborne illness acquired in the United States—Unspecified agents. *Emerging Infectious Diseases* 17(1):16–22.

Scharff, R. L. 2012. Economic burden from health losses due to foodborne illness in the United States. *Journal of Food Protection* 75(1):123–131.

United States Department of Agriculture Economic Research Service. 2009. Access to affordable and nutritious food: Measuring and understanding food deserts and their consequences.

Part I

Where the personal intersects with public policy

1 Why "you are what you eat" matters when talking about school lunch

A personal narrative

Angela L. Glover

My mother's parents, ranchers living in rural Western Nebraska, grew gardens, raised and butchered their own livestock, and prepared from scratch the majority of their own meals. Fried chicken, fresh buttered yeast rolls, and potatoes dug up from the garden slathered in white gravy preceded cherry pie with freshly tumbled ice cream. Conversely, my paternal grandparents living in Fort Collins, Colorado punched in at a factory at the County Clerk's office. They prepared meals consisting of a meat, a starch, and a vegetable at home with ingredients found on the shelves at the local grocer.

The meat and potatoes mentality was prevalent in both the country and city and at times I identified with the children's tale that addressed the intersected lives of the country and the city mice. Our meals at home were similar to those of my Colorado grandparents as we lived in the middle of the United States, where there was no question as to where the beef was; however, shortcuts and convenience food were part of weekly meal planning since my parents' life's work was not spent growing and preparing food. Oftentimes, meat came from Styrofoam trays, potatoes from a box, gravy from a jar, and pie from the bakery section of the supermarket. Sure my maternal grandfather would butcher a cow and send it home with us from time to time, and my grandma would load the back of the station wagon up with fruits and vegetables in jars and rolls wrapped in tea towels, but those only lasted so long. My mom gardened in the summer, but it was not so she could can or preserve food for the long upcoming winter; rather, it was a reenacted part of a blood memory tied to her childhood summers growing up in Western Nebraska. We would share the beefsteak tomatoes and plethora of green beans with our neighbors once harvest was complete, but rarely did my mom can the bounty in preparation for winter like my country grandma. There was no pressure cooker, a box of ball jars, or wax liners in our pantry, and there was no sense of urgency when foraging the garden for ripe fruits and vegetables like there was in Grandpa's garden. It did not matter if we were gone for a week on vacation; we trusted the neighbor kid to water for us unlike my grandfather whose second job in retirement was to water, water, and water again after tending cattle for a younger local rancher.

Occasionally, when we would visit my city grandparents on one of our family vacations, we would pick up "to go" food and I vaguely remember eating

Kentucky Fried Chicken from a bucket in the back of our station wagon and thinking it tasted good, but different from the meal prepared by my country grandparents. Yes, the biscuits were flaky and the coleslaw was cut up into smaller bites, but the butter in the packet tasted weird. My taste for homemade butter straight from the shaken jar or churn developed early. In "Food, Self and Identity," Claude Fischler (1998) states, "food is central to our sense of identity. The way any given human group eats helps it assert its diversity, hierarchy, and organization, but also, at the same time, both its oneness and the otherness" (p. 1). The food I ate and eat as the granddaughter of a rancher is quite different from what I ate at home as a child or choose to eat today, even though this cuisine was locally sourced and farm raised. The meals served at the country grandparent's home were quite diverse from what my mother prepared, regardless of the health factors. I identify with fried chicken and seek it out whenever I can in order to measure it to what I remember eating as a child. The food we ate at home in the city was usually chosen for convenience, unless it was for a holiday; the food eaten in the country was often the result of living in a food desert and the need for independence of individuals who live there. The experiences of eating in a rural environment are essential to how I identify as an individual eater today and sometimes provide a way to engage in certain eating communities.

This oneness and otherness provides the threshold between the habits of the country and the city food experiences I shared with my family. For example, this morning I started the day out with a green smoothie full of organic kale, spinach, blueberries, ginger, turmeric root, hemp seeds, coconut oil, pineapple, and cucumbers grown from my own garden but then my snack was a bag of Cheeto Puffs, Almond M&Ms, and a Coca-Cola from McDonalds. I know I need to eat vegetables and they need to be grown organically or purchased locally, but my memories of gas station eating with my city grandparents, and even my mom, conjure blood memories of the best kind. My understanding of myself as an eater was intuitive and influenced by the private sphere of my family with the occasional influence of the public sphere. As Ruth Reichl (1999) puts it in *Tender at the Bone*, "food could be a way of making sense of the world (back cover)." The way I ate when I was young made sense to me; it was diverse, had a range of options, and was often shared with others who were introducing and modeling ways of eating to me; however; my world was much smaller than that of the students who are eating in public schools.

Today, the public sphere is increasing its influence on individuals and it is making it harder to understand one's food identity, let alone what one should or should not eat. In addition to the traditional influences of one's family, culture, and geographical region, the influences of visual rhetoric, advertising, traditional media, social media, and social policy must be factored in to understand why we eat what we eat and who we are because of what we eat.

To back up, one's food identity can be explained by looking at one's human relationship to food, which combines at least two scopes. The first tracks the biological to the cultural and the second links the individual to the collective (Fischler 1998, p. 2). These two scopes create a liminal space. For example, my mom attempted to prepare meals based on her childhood eating patterns, food literacy, and known food identity. These meals included liver and onions, pork chops and apple sauce, biscuits and gravy, and as she ventured into a liminal space as an eater I grew up eating tacos with ketchup on them instead of hot sauce. Our cultural eating experiences were limited to Mexican and Italian. Interestingly, we often ate Italian at home, with the "I" being pronounced in the long vowel form, but Thai, Korean, and German cuisine were foreign to me until I moved away from home. The first time I ate Asian food was my freshman year of college. As my mom's food identity transitioned from living in the country to the city, our family adapted to the daily food rituals of place and by the time I was in college we mostly ate out in restaurants due to my parent's lifestyle.

The public craze for cooking shows had not graced our four-station network television set; however, convenience foods, microwaves, crockpots, and the golden arches were available and my mom capitalized on what they had to offer after she re-entered the workforce once I entered high school. *Good Housekeeping* and *Better Homes and Gardens* magazines showcased recipes with processed foods intended to make life easier and on Wednesday, the local paper's "Living Section" reviewed new restaurants inviting alternatives to those who lacked the time or interest to grow and prepare food. Yes, the tune from Hamburger Helper was sung in our home, but it did not give my mom a quick and easy way to serve a home-cooked meal even though the jingle "hamburger helper, helped her hamburger make… a great meal" made this promise. By eating out in restaurants, we were given choices and the opportunity to try new foods such as taco salad and fried ice cream. Sure Mom tried her hand at the crockpot and made roast in speckled pans on Sunday, but these foods were never well received. The food prepared by our country grandma was what we identified with when a home-cooked meal was mentioned. Eventually, my mom became the go-to person for the latest news on restaurant openings in town and we became the family that dined out on holidays as well. Others would talk of the home-cooked food they longed for and what their folks would have waiting for them upon arriving home for college breaks. I would look forward to ordering a meal off a menu. Bee Wilson (2015) asserts in *First Bite: How We Learn to Eat,* "what we learn about food happens as children sitting at the kitchen table. Every bite is a memory and the most powerful memories are the first ones. At this table we are given food and love" (p. 17). Today I'm married to a chef, and one of the first inklings of "it might be love" came when he prepared fried chicken for me. His coleslaw and chicken batter each had a kick to them and since spicy food was still on the "we don't eat" list for me, I was cautious, but I soon discovered I liked a little spice and started seeking out Southern fried chicken. In fact, my husband's chicken was a close second to my grandma's, so eventually I said "I do."

Wilson continues, "our tastes follow us around like a comforting shadow. They seem to tell us who we are" (Preface). Since how we learn to eat is influenced by our parents, families, cultures, and celebrations, our food identity is in a constant state of betwixt and between. "I like" and "I don't like" shift over time, and what and why we eat shifts as well and draws us into and out of community. A point of distinction here regarding food identity: there is a difference between recognizing that what we eat is *what* we are and that what we eat constructs *who* we are. We symbolically consume identity through our food choices and, more specifically, by what we do not eat; hence, the identity of the eater is often characterized in communities: the fast-food eater, the cultural eater—I am Italian, and therefore I am only the Italian food eater, the healthy eater, the gourmet, the organic eater, the vegetarian eater, the gluten-free eater, the dieting eater, and the school lunch eater. It is important to have ownership and an understanding of how and why we interact with food and how it shapes who we are within the various food communities in which we live and interact. Like the family celebrations of many of our neighbors, ours revolved around food.

As a child, choosing a flavor and shape of a birthday cake with coordinating napkins was a big deal. I liked white cake with chocolate frosting for many years, and the design and the candle had to match. In keeping with my need for consistency, I often had a cake in the shape of a dog, not to be confused with the ever-popular Peanuts canine, Snoopy. Again, my mom did not have the luxury of watching Rachel Ray or Cupcake Wars and nor did she own the fancy pans to bake exact replicas, so she had to use her geometry skills and bake circles and squares that she cut into shapes to configure the cake. There was no fondant. She used simple powdered sugar frosting and from what I remember of the few photos that were taken, it was a glorious cake. Often the cake was consumed by just our family, but as we grew older, we were allowed to invite friends over to share in our yearly treat and we were invited to their homes to share in their celebrations where we learned about cupcakes, bars, and buntinis. As our private sphere grew to include the influence of friends, so did our curiosity for other cuisine. Victor Turner (2002) offers that with liminality, "communitas tends to characterize relationships between those jointly undergoing ritual transition. These bonds are anti-structural in the sense that they are undifferentiated [...]. Communitas is spontaneous, immediate, concrete and not shaped by norms. Communitas does not merge identities, it liberates them from conformity to general norms" (p. 72). The current intersection of public health and food is disrupting the communitas once found in the development of one's food identity within a family by imposing too many rules on the options that are being offered.

The private sphere of eating has been impacted by a public interest in food, whether for personal health reasons or sheer entertainment. Consumers are increasingly food-literate and empowered to comment on and ask for what they believe to be the best, whether it be local, sustainable, organic, or merely personal preference, and the current foodie culture and diversity of foods available in the United States have made food a more democratic facet of our society. Movies, TV, public speakers, community awareness programs, fairs, festivals, and classrooms are influencing how eaters understand and interact with food. From "Bravo" to the "Food Network" to online recipe sharing on Instagram, Pinterest, and Facebook via Tasty videos, today's eaters are showing up and are curious, and these eaters include students. This chapter aims to offer insight into the challenges and opportunities that intersect the space between an individual's food identity and public health as well as how the information age and current political interest in food and public health has increased students' food literacy, while also creating issues for families and students subjected to school nutrition regulations.

In addition to one's food identity, one's food literacy shapes a way of being and living whether it be the connoisseur of onion rings, the biggest loser, or the gourmet who travels the globe to eat the next bizarre food item revealed on Andrew Zimmer's show found on The Travel Channel. "You are what you eat" has been more clearly defined in the past decade and what and where you eat it brings people together in community. Families plan summer vacations around where they will eat with many of the destinations appearing as episodes on "Diners Drive-Ins and Dives" and restaurants featured in books by Jane and Michael Stern who have written extensively about road food found across the United States. Instagram, Twitter, and Facebook have pages devoted to "food porn," dishes meant to entice an appetite; news regarding food issues; and opportunities for eaters to engage in conversations with one another. Yelp and Urban Spoon offer eaters the opportunity to make or break a restaurant with the ability to comment on or write a review about a recent dining experience, and the big screen offers controversial, thought-provoking films such as *Fast Food Nation* by Eric Schlosser, *Supersize Me* by Morgan Spurlock, *Fathead* by Tom Naughton, and *Food Revolution* by Jamie Oliver, which ask viewers to engage with and question current food practices in the United States. As a country, we have embraced and problematized the quest for our next meal whether it be healthy, or novel, or on the top 10 list of our favorite sports figure, Hollywood celebrity, or political leader. Americans are eating and talking about eating and worrying about what they eat more than ever.

Being eaters of food, not to be confused with foodies, along with the traditional vows found in a marriage ceremony, my husband and I pledged to eat at the top 100 burger joints in America. Our first anniversary found us at the Hamburg Inn in Iowa City where we noted the portraits on the wall featuring politicians both elected and merely moving through town while caucusing in the state. We also noted the quality of the burger and fries we consumed, but honestly, the reason this place was listed in George Motz's (2008) *Hamburger America: A State by State Guide to 100 Great Burger Joints* was undoubtedly as much about the political celebrity factor as it was the food, which was good, but not as good, in my opinion, as the burger served at Bobos in Topeka, Kansas, but I digress. This fever for political celebrity is not all that new, but it is more pronounced than it was a decade ago. The inclusion of branding an eatery with a celebrity name in addition to identifying the cuisine it serves now includes a list of where the ingredients are sourced and whether or not they are organic. Not only can you eat at Jimmy Buffet's Cheeseburger in Paradise while shopping at many upscale malls, you can read about farm-to-table, local, sustainable efforts, and in some cases, from where the lamb and heirloom tomatoes featured on the evening's menu were procured.

This current interest in food transcends age groups and ranges from toddlers to retirees and individuals from all fields are weighing in including but not limited to nutritionists, athletic trainers, physicians, marketing gurus, educators, and politicians. Juliann Michaels, trainer of the stars and former host of the "Biggest Loser," is selling workouts and menu plans and Nutri System has noted Marie Osmond to be one of their most successful spokesmodels. Rachel Ray has been serving up meals and stories along with her own line of cookware for over a decade, and the competition for Top Chef is offering food enthusiasts the opportunity to watch up-and-coming chefs from around the nation compete for valuable cash awards and experiences to cook for world acclaimed chefs and community celebrities in their hometowns. Anthony Bourdain gave voice to sous chefs and kitchen workers in *Kitchen Confidential* and continues to offer dining experiences via his hit TV show "No Reservations." The Travel Channel features not only places to visit, but also eateries that complement the experience of the country, and "The Food Network" has something for everyone. One can learn how to eat on 40 dollars a day, start a food truck, and specialize in cupcakes. Bar-b-que, Italian, and Southern fried chicken are brought straight to us in our homes. Recipes are available online as are cooking tutorials by world-renowned chefs. Websites for *Cooks Illustrated* and *Epicurious* complement the programming of Julia Child and Martha Stewart and are joined by *Cooking Light, Bon Appetite*, and *Gourmet* magazines. Food glorious food is available if only we tune in or log on.

Local communities which have offered seasonal festivals honoring traditions and customs are now advertised to families who are invited and encouraged to sample cultural foods while experiencing music, art, and dance. Increased revenues assist with board-sponsored projects, scholarships, and future events and public health officials sell permits and licenses. Libraries, community centers, and schools along with home shows, state fairs, and farmer's markets provide opportunities to dine on food plated on a stick and to try products being grown and produced by local artisans. There is no loss of opportunity for the public to learn about, interact with, or eat food. Also, there are no missed opportunities to generate revenue while eating. T-shirts, ball caps, and cookbooks are available in order to preserve the memory and promote the event or business. The intersection between food and public health and the current challenges and solutions with regard to policy and politics is great.

The current political administration, led by First Lady Michelle Obama (2016), is attempting to alter those that came before it. Political administrations have always had a voice in what children eat at school, but lately this voice has entered with greater vibrato regarding what public school-aged children should eat in order to address the childhood obesity epidemic currently underway in America. In addition, it appears that the "achievement gap," with regard to test score disparity, is not one of learning or even being able to read, but of public health: Students cannot learn if they do not have proper nutrition. This is a fact. Without a healthy breakfast, behavioral problems occur and it is difficult to concentrate. So the changes made by the School Nutrition Association have not only raised the awareness of parents and those who prepare the food for students, but also of those involved in the process of educating and supplying food, including local sustainable organic growers, food vendors, and distributors, chefs, dietitians, researchers, college professors, entrepreneurs, and community activists. In Marion Nestle's (2007) *The Politics of Food*, she discusses how the food industry influences what we eat and therefore our health by way of healthy dietary advice, government influence and influences on the government, corruption faced by children due to governmental and public policy, and the deregulation of dietary supplements. This book was published shortly after food study programs became known entities on college campuses. Circa 1990, both New York University and Boston College began offering food studies programs, and as of today this field of study is growing. Food studies currently include looking at the connections between food and

- Food insecurity
- Food deserts
- Economics
- Production
- World hunger
- Public health
- Narrative
- Holidays
- Communities
- Travel
- Culture
- History
- Politics
- Science
- Criticism
- Schools
- Public health

As this list shows, food is a vehicle with which to study the world we live in and one's food identity stretches way beyond what was eaten for Sunday dinner or at grandma's house. Interestingly, one of the first food experiences many children have where someone else controls what ends up on their plate is at school whether it be at a daycare, preschool, public or private school.

Chef Jamie Oliver has taken on childhood eating habits with his program "Food Revolution" as have half the hosts on TV food and online cooking shows. Eating healthy and portion control are parallel to the quality of the food we are eating. Alice Waters, owner of Chez Panisse, a Berkeley, California restaurant famous for its organic, locally grown ingredients and for pioneering California cuisine, shares, "Teaching kids how to feed themselves and how to live in a community responsibly is the center of an education." Moreover, Michael Pollan's (2006) voice speaks honestly about what and how we ate in *The Omnivore's Dilemma* when he offered "deciding what you should eat will inevitably stir anxiety" (p. 37). Even Sesame Street has an opinion on our country's healthy eating initiative, which impacts a student's food literacy. The "Let's Move Campaign," started by First Lady Michelle Obama, has been embraced by a host of TV personalities including Rachel Ray and Jimmy Fallon both during day and nighttime programming. As noted by First Lady Michelle Obama, "America's Move to Raise a Healthier Generation of Kids is vital for the success of our country. In the end, as First Lady, this is not just a policy issue for me. This is a passion. This is my mission. I am determined to work with folks across this country to change the way a generation of kids thinks about food and nutrition" (Let'sMove.org). The "Healthy Lunch Time Challenge" invites students across the country to create healthy lunch recipes for a chance to win a trip to Washington, DC, and the opportunity to attend the Kids' "State Dinner" at the White House. Everyone is cooking and eating and thinking about what goes on his or her fork, and this is good, but are we all equally able to discern what is best for someone else's family or child? Yes, nutrition labels matter; yes, some food tastes better because of where it was grown or prepared, but ownership of one's palate is equally important, and a voice in what is being offered and eaten is paramount to whether or not the said food will be consumed, digested, and put to good use in one's body and whether or not Communitas will be achieved.

Responses to the changes made to school lunch programs vary from full support to disgruntled depending on who is responding. The full impact and repercussion of the changes made to the national school lunch program is yet to be seen, but these changes are certainly being questioned by many and pose realistic challenges for those being asked to eat the lunches. Yes, the lunches may be deemed healthy, but if the food offered is not being eaten, are students any better off than they were when they had a choice of what to eat that was informed by family, culture, and a small dose of media? Or, more importantly, what they liked or knew? Yes, we are all in agreement that a tray of all brown food is not good for us, but unless there is ownership in what one eats, do those calories count? In "How School Lunch Became the Latest Political Battleground," Nicholas Confessore (2014) notes how the "Healthy, Hunger-Free Kids Act" was intended to impose strict new nutrition standards on all food sold in public schools. The idea was to convince "a generation raised on Lunchables and Pizza Hut to learn to love whole wheat pasta and roasted cauliflower" (p. 4). Not only did this initiative backfire, but the School Nutrition Association is now the most public critic of this Act. In addition to Lunch Ladies battling the new rules, students are reacting adversely to what and how much is being served (p. 1). In Ariana Eunjung Cha's (2015) article, "Research Shows Healthy School Lunch Program Leading to Wasted Vegetables," "Public Health Reports" researcher Sarah Amin revealed that since the United States Department of Agriculture's (USDA) new requirements mandating that children taking part in the federal lunch program choose either a fruit or vegetable with their meals went into effect in 2012, children's consumption of fruits and vegetables actually went down 13% and worse, schools were throwing away a distressing 56% more food than before (p. 1). Moreover, faculty, staff, families, and community members are concerned about how this experience is impacting the educational process, which involves both social and emotional ramifications for students. Social media coverage on Facebook found on "The Lunch Tray" and "Lunch and Recess Matter" shows that there is a need for an ongoing dialogue and modification to school lunch guidelines currently practiced in the United States (Facebook 2016a,b). Specifically, on the "Lunch and Recess Matter," parents and educators dialogue about the amount of time and encouragement students are given to consume their food and the need for physical movement after eating. "The Lunch Tray" is currently explaining the Smart Snack Standards put forward by the USDA, which feed into Nestle's ideas presented in Food Politics regarding influences and their intended purposes. The posts on these pages and interactions on these pages are smart, informed, and necessary for the mandates currently facing the lunch trays of students in the United States. The OTHER Lunch Lady, an online catering service I founded in 2015, offers students options for how to build a lunch of their choice and delivers to private schools. The mission of The OTHER Lunch Lady (LLC) is twofold: the first is to make eating lunch at school a positive, fun experience for children while providing a healthy, entertaining alternative to the lunch programs available in local schools; the second is to provide a convenience for those packing lunches. To date, this small business has been able to provide lunch for summer camps, but is unable to get past the necessary SNA guidelines and packaging require- ments for public schools. The idea of allowing students to have a say in what they eat has proven successful. Many students order the same meal every day, which pediatricians support as calories in and calories out. Parents and school adminis- trators alike have been supportive of the business noting the ownership students have when creating their lunches works. Addressing parental concerns is a high priority for many school officials working to meet the requirements, mandates, and guidelines set forward by the current political administration. The topic of public health and food permeates conversations with politicians, school officials, and pediatricians and parents.

In speaking with Erin Vik, director of Nutrition Services of Westside School District in Omaha, Nebraska, I learned that parents in his school district were looking for more nutritional info, calorie counts, and ingredients that contain potential allergens and ways to pass on healthy eating habits, which are all impor- tant for student success. An answer the district has found to meet this need is a new website menu powered by LunchTray and developed by Noah Kochanowicz (Vik, E. 2016, personal interview). The site is mobile-friendly and provides information many parents are looking for as they manage the health concerns currently surrounding school lunch menus. According to Vik, "It's kind of a one- stop shop for what we do, it's much more accessible and timely for parents, teach- ers and students, since we're in the age of the smartphone."

My parents went home for lunch or carried leftovers in a pail or sack; there was no hot lunch program at their schools, and as a child, I preferred the lunch my mother packed for me so much that I took my lunch from first grade until my senior year of high school. I would occasionally eat on the days the cafeteria offered pizzawiches or chilli and cinnamon rolls. I knew the worst morning could be turned around if my lunch included a turkey sandwich with Miracle Whip on white bread cut on a diagonal, Lays potato chips, green grapes, and a Hostess Ho Ho, not to be confused with a Little Debbie. If there was a seasonal napkin and a note from my mom, I was assured I could make it through the rest of the school day. I had input and choice on what I was eating. Some of it was healthy, but not always. I understood that food was part fuel and part love. I intuitively knew eating was an act of community and that harm came from excess, and I wonder if we can change the way a country eats simply by looking at calories, fat content, and "healthy" choices. Yes, we need to move on and be aware of what we are putting in our bodies, but taking the joy and fun out of eating is not working. Knowing who we are as eaters and our food identity is paramount to understanding how public health and food will intersect in the future. Wilson ponders the question of how we learn to eat—both individually and collectively, "[how we learn to eat] is the key to how food, for so many people has gone so badly wrong. The greatest public health problem of modern times is how to persuade people to make better food choices" (p. 7). She simply identifies that "we have been looking for answers in the wrong places," and although I feel the process of addressing obesity and healthy eating practices for public schools is important, it is just as important to understand where an eater is coming from before the said changes are imposed. The conversation of which foods are being served in schools and why needs to be considered. The efforts to modify school nutrition and provide healthier options for those eating school lunches may be well motivated, but mandates rarely offer successful programs. A balance between who we are and what we eat needs to be addressed before we see this intersection of public health and food policy shift to a place where we as a nation should feel successful with what we are offering our children.

REFERENCES

Cha Eunjung, A. 2015. Research shows healthy school lunch program leading to wasted vegetables. *The Washington Post* 27 August.

Confessore, N. 2014. How school lunch became the last political battleground. *New York Times* 7 October.

FB Page. 2016a. Lunch and Recess Matter.

FB Page. 2016b. The Lunch Tray.

Fischler, C. 1998. Food, self and identity. *Social Science Information* 27: 275–93.

Motz, G. 2008. *Hamburger America: A State by State Guide to 100 Great Burger Joints.* Philadelphia, PA: Running Press.

Nestle, M. 2007. *Food Politics.* California, CA: University of California Press.

Obama, M. 2016. Let's Move. http://www.letsmove.gov/about

Pollan, M. 2006. *The Omnivoire's Dilema.* New York, NY: Penguin.

Reichl, R. 1999. *Tender at the Bone.* New York, NY: Broadway Books.

Turner, V. and Schechner, R. 2002. *Performance Studies: An Introduction, Second edition.* New York, NY: Routledge.

Wilson, B. 2015. *First Bite How We Learn to Eat.* New York, NY: Basic Books.

Part II
Understanding food insecurity

2 Child and adult food insecurity in the United States

Joanne Christaldi and Diana Cuy Castellanos

Introduction

In this chapter, a discussion of food security and related national and local food and nutrition policy is presented. First, a definition of food security, its history, and how it is measured within the context of the United States are discussed. Second, the authors present an outline of different social and environmental factors associated with food insecurity and its consequences on overall individual and community well-being. Finally, the authors close this chapter with an overview of federal and local food and nutrition policies and a discussion of the shortfalls within the food security policy, program, and research realms. The purpose of this chapter is (1) to provide readers foundational knowledge regarding food insecurity in the United States, (2) to review the research literature to determine the effectiveness of food and nutrition policies and initiatives in decreasing food insecurity, and (3) to discuss where future policy and research may need to focus to appropriately address this issue plaguing the U.S. society. Furthermore, sufficient information is provided for readers to draw their own conclusions regarding national and local food and nutrition policy and potential needed changes to address and impact food insecurity. In the context of this book, this chapter is meant to provide readers a perspective of yet another current food policy topic within the United States and to further grasp its complexity. In this chapter, questions proposed to readers include: Does the current USDA food security measurement truly measure food security as defined as "access by all people at all times to enough food for an active, healthy life, and includes, at a minimum: (a) the ready availability of nutritionally adequate and safe foods and (b) an assured ability to acquire acceptable foods in socially acceptable ways (e.g., without resorting to emergency food supplies, scavenging, stealing, or other coping strategies)" (Anderson 1990, p. 1575). What aspects of current national and local food and nutrition policy are effective and which are not effective? Finally, how should food and nutrition policy change at the national and local levels to become more effective?

Definitions of food security/insecurity

The issues of hunger and undernutrition in the United States have been examined informally since the early 1900s. However, it has taken many decades for a formalized definition and system of measurement to be created. The definition of food security has evolved over the past few decades with the origin of the definition occurring in the mid-1970s. Given the issues of poverty, hunger, and famine globally, the initial interest focused on the limitations within the food supply, limited access to enough food, and food price stability. Following the World Food Conference in 1974, modifying views developed regarding food security. Questions arose around vulnerable populations and evidence that the Green Revolution, which dramatically increased agricultural production worldwide through the use of high-yielding cereal grains, did not lead to reductions in poverty or undernutrition (Food and Agriculture Organization of the United Nations 2003). In the 1980s, The Task Force on Food Assistance created by President Reagan recognized the varied and complex terminology used to describe food security and created two working definitions of "hunger" as (1) "the actual physiological effects of extended nutritional deprivations" and (2) "the inability, even occasionally, to obtain adequate food and nourishment. In this sense of the term, hunger can be said to be present even when there are no clinical symptoms of deprivation." In 1990, official definitions of food security, food insecurity, and hunger were created by the Life Sciences Research Office of the Federation of American Societies for Experimental Biology and are as follows: (Anderson 1990, pp. 1575–1576, 1598):

- *Food security* was defined as "access by all people at all times to enough food for an active, healthy life, and includes, at a minimum: (a) the ready availability of nutritionally adequate and safe foods and (b) an assured ability to acquire acceptable foods in socially acceptable ways (e.g., without resorting to emergency food supplies, scavenging, stealing, or other coping strategies)."
- *Food insecurity* exists whenever there is "limited or uncertain availability of nutritionally adequate and safe foods or limited or uncertain ability to acquire acceptable foods in socially acceptable ways."
- *Hunger* in its meaning of "the uneasy or painful sensation caused by a lack of food" is in this definition "a potential, although not necessary, a consequence of food insecurity."

Current definitions set in 2006 by the U.S. Department of Agriculture (USDA 2015a) are consistent with the 1990 definitions, which, however, now include new language and four distinct levels of food security and insecurity. These definitions are as follows:

- *High food security*: No reported indications of food-access problems or limitations.
- *Marginal food security*: One or two reported indications—typically of anxiety over food sufficiency or shortage of food in the house. Little or no indication of changes in diets or food intake.

- *Low food security*: Reports of reduced quality, variety, or desirability of diet. Little or no indication of reduced food intake.
- *Very low food security*: Reports of multiple indications of disrupted eating patterns and reduced food intake.

History of hunger and food insecurity in the United States

Hunger in the United States became increasingly apparent with the transition from an agrarian to an industrial society and the great depression. With the great depression came federal programs to address the issue of hunger and economic downfall. The Federal Emergency Relief Administration (FERA) and Federal Surplus Relief Corporation (FSRC) were part of the "New Deal" in the 1930s under Franklin D. Roosevelt. At the end of the 1930s, the Food Stamp Program was implemented to help increase food purchasing power and decrease hunger. With this, farmers were paid for excess crop, and the food was then allocated to different states for distribution to the people. Hunger became a national security issue when about 40% of potential draftees were rejected due to malnutrition. In the early 1950s, the issue of hunger in the United States went dormant along with many of the federal programs implemented during the 1930s.

Hunger became a public issue in the United States in the late 1960s after John F. Kennedy witnessed it among children living in West Virginia and called for food assistance policy reform. In 1964 under Johnson, the Food Stamp Act was passed. Moreover, there was greater societal recognition of hunger when Senators Joseph Clark (D-PA) and Robert Kennedy (D-NY) saw people living with hunger in the Mississippi Delta and began to draw attention to the issue. Around this time, CBS broadcasted a series called "Hunger in America" that drew the Nation's attention to the issue of hunger. Furthermore, during the 1960s, many food assistance programs went through major reform or were started as a means to combat hunger. Such programs included the School Breakfast Program, Summer Food Service Program, and the Child and Adult Care Food Program.

During the 1970s, federal attention to hunger in the United States continued. During this decade, the Food Stamp Program was further reformed and the Special Supplemental Program for Women, Infants and Children began. In the early 1980s under Ronald Reagan and during the economic downturn, the Temporary Emergency Food Assistance Program was developed which provided commodity assistance to citizens. Fifteen food assistance programs were active at this time, and the "Task Force for Food Assistance" was created. However, as the economy rebounded, the food assistance programs experienced a decrease in funding and weakened. In the early 1990s, there was a rebound within the programs, but then came another decline with the implementation of the Temporary Assistance to Needy Families in 1996. An increased use of community food relief programs such as food pantries and soup kitchens was experienced potentially due to the decline in food assistance programs, specifically the Food Stamp Program. However, later in 2002, the Food Stamp program was re-established (O'Brien et al. 2004).

Measurements

Throughout this era of hunger and food assistance program development and transition, measurements of hunger were inconsistent. Hunger was measured through proxies such as dietary intake data, food assistance use, observation, and poverty statistics (Eisinger 1996, 1998).

The conversation around measuring hunger began in the 1980s with the afore-mentioned Task Force for Food Insecurity. The task force was charged with examining hunger throughout the United States and concluded that the need to measure hunger was crucial to policy formation and understanding national hunger. The lack of an operational definition and direct measure limited the ability to develop an informed policy that effectively targeted factors relating to hunger. Moving forward, the Food Research and Action Center (FRAC) in the mid-1980s was charged with developing a measure for hunger. The FRAC first attracted researchers and advocates to the table to develop an evidence-based measure targeting child hunger. The questionnaire was tested during the mid-1980s in two states and then further expanded to seven more states by the end of the 1980s. This project was termed the Community Childhood Hunger Identification Project (CCHIP). The measure was included in the 1990 National Nutrition Monitoring and Related Research Act. In the mid-1990s, it expanded to nine more states. In the early 1990s, data from the CCHIP showed that about one in eight children in these states were experiencing hunger (Wehler et al. 1991). In 1994, the Economic Research Service of the USDA, Food and Consumer Service, the Center for Disease Control and Prevention, and the Department of Health and Human Services in the U.S. collaboratively developed questionnaires to measure food security in the U.S. population that continue to be utilized today. The questionnaires were implemented as part of the Current Population Survey adminis-tered by the U.S. Census Bureau in 1995 to monitor food security among the U.S. population (FRAC 2015). The main questionnaire, the household food security questionnaire, consists of 18 items related to the anxiety of having sufficient food, adaptations used if the desired food is unaffordable, perceptions regarding qual-ity and quantity of food, and experiences of hunger or food scarcity and reduced food intake. The questionnaire addresses adults and children in the household, whereas the other questionnaires that can be used target only adults or only chil-dren (USDA 2015b).

In the United States, considerable time has been spent examining and alter-ing the definitions of food security and insecurity to better measure the extent of the problem, although the measurement has not changed significantly in the past 20 years. Operationally, the measurement addresses most of the constructs within the definition of food security. However, it does not directly measure dietary quality, therefore failing to determine if the family is able to consume a nutritionally sound diet leading to an "active, healthy life." It only addresses the perception of whether foods desired can be obtained.

Moreover, in regard to prevalence of food insecurity in the United States, statistics have shifted upward and downward over the past 20 years but have not been on a continual decline. Therefore, food insecurity has been a primary focus of nutrition assistance policy and programs. However, there continues to be a significant issue of food insecurity in the United States despite the efforts to reduce the problem. Additional research is needed and necessary to examine this public health issue more closely and to determine successful solutions that can be implemented in society to reduce the problem. Recommendations for such research are discussed at the end of this chapter.

Food insecurity prevalence in the United States

In 1995, food insecurity, as measured by the USDA Food Security Questionnaire, showed that about 12% of the U.S. population experienced food insecurity. From 1995 to 2007, food insecurity rates fluctuated between 10% and 12% but began to increase above 12% at the beginning of the economic downturn in 2008. Food insecurity reached its highest prevalence in 2011 at 14.9% and since has slowly been decreasing. In 2014, food insecurity in the United States was 14.3% with great differences between states. For example, between 2012 and 2014, the average rate of food insecurity was about 8.4% in North Dakota but 22% in Mississippi (Coleman-Jensen et al. 2015).

Associations and consequences of food insecurity

Consequences of food insecurity are detrimental to individuals as well as society as a whole. Therefore, it is important to identify and implement policies and programs that address associating factors in an attempt to decrease food insecurity.

Associating factors

There are multiple psychosocial, behavioral, and environmental factors associated with food insecurity leading to negative consequences on the individual and societal levels. Various psychosocial factors negatively associated with food security include income, education, social disorder, financial burden (debt, taxation, medical expenses, utility costs, housing cost), immigration, depression, anxiety, physical and mental disability, and single-parent households (Institute of Medicine and National Research Council 2013). Positively associated psychosocial factors include social cohesion and capital, family ties, and continuous employment. Furthermore, a sense of pride decreases individual participation in food assistance programs. Physical activity, cooking skill, food procurement, and financial budgeting are all positively related to food security, whereas behaviors such as gambling and drug use are negatively associated. Finally, multiple environmental factors correlated to food security include number of people in a household, household food storage and preparation facilities, food cost, transportation, store location, food availability, viable land availability, and media pressure (Bhargava et al. 2008; Carter et al. 2010; Coleman-Jensen et al. 2015). Food insecure individuals utilize coping mechanisms to attempt to ensure adequate food. This could include not paying utility bills, obtaining food in socially unaccepted ways, withholding food from self to provide for children, and purchasing energy-dense, low-cost foods that have minimal nutrient value (Holben 2010). Interestingly, food insecurity has not been linked to a lower caloric intake but has been associated with poorer dietary quality (Zizza et al. 2008).

Consequences of food insecurity

There are both psychosocial and health effects experienced by food insecure individuals. Studies show that people who are worried about feeding themselves and/or families adequately experience stress, anxiety, and depression (Carter et al. 2010). In children, food insecurity is associated with poorer academic performance, higher absenteeism, and altered social skills (Jyoti et al. 2005). Furthermore, Bernal and colleagues (2014) reported that children who were food insecure were more likely to have more household responsibilities such as cooking, taking care of younger siblings, and doing certain chores. In terms of health effects, research suggests that food insecure adults are more likely to be overweight, lack sleep, suffer from a chronic disease and experience a lower quality of life (Carter et al. 2010). Furthermore, owing to health failure, this may inhibit their capacity to work and contribute to continuous food insecurity. Pregnant woman have higher rates of gestational diabetes and excessive weight gain (Laraia et al. 2010). Food insecure older adults have higher rates of mental and physical deterioration compared to their food secure counterparts (Lee et al. 2010). Finally, children experience more growth stunting, obesity, and micronutrient deficiencies such as iron-deficient anemia (Skalicky et al. 2006; Carter et al. 2010). Many of the consequences are interrelated. For instance, high stress may be related to obtaining and preparing adequate food for self and family, which can affect metabolism and contribute to weight gain (Jyoti et al. 2005; Skalicky et al. 2006; Lee et al. 2010; Metallinos-Katsaras et al. 2012; Gundersen 2015).

Nutrition policy and nutrition assistance programs

National policy related to reducing the levels of food insecurity in the United States has been in existence for many decades with the passage of the Agricultural Adjustment Act of 1933 being at the forefront of agricultural policy. Furthermore, national food assistance programs have been in existence since the 1930s and were developed to (1) improve the nutritional status and food security of targeted segments of the population and (2) encourage the consumption of domestic agricultural commodities and other foods. Notable nutrition policies that work to increase food availability and accessibility to Americans and therefore have an impact on reducing food insecurity are as follows:

1. The National School Lunch Act of 1945 created the National School Lunch Program which provides free or reduced price lunches to qualifying students through government subsidies.
2. The Older Americans Act of 1965 includes several programs with one being support for nutrition programs including congregate and home-delivered meals.
3. The Child Nutrition Act of 1966 established the School Breakfast Program which provides free or reduced price breakfasts to qualifying children in schools and child care institutions.
4. The American Recovery and Reinvestment Act of 2009 raised the maximum SNAP benefit by 13.6%, allowing for increased food purchasing power.
5. The Healthy Hunger Free Kids Act of 2010, which funds child nutrition programs and free lunch programs in schools. In addition, the bill sets new nutrition standards for schools including wellness policies.
6. The Agricultural Act of 2014 includes The Farm Bill that enables the USDA to expand markets for agricultural products, create new opportunities for local and regional foods systems, and ensure access to safe and nutrition foods for all Americans, among other things.

The development of nutrition policy is directly linked to nutrition assistance programs which are used to support vulnerable populations to have increased access to food and can lead to improved food security. The three largest nutrition assistance programs include the Supplemental Nutrition Assistance Program (SNAP), the National School Lunch Program (NSLP), and the Special Supplemental Nutrition Program for Women, Infants, and Children (WIC). Evaluation and research regarding these programs have shown mixed results in terms of their benefits and limitations (Coleman-Jensen et al. 2015).

SNAP, which is the largest food assistance program in the United States, provides monthly benefits to eligible households to purchase approved food items at authorized food stores. Most SNAP recipients are children, working parents, the elderly, and people with disabilities. In 2014, SNAP provided benefits to 46.5 million on average per month, increasing the purchasing power of food insecure households (Coleman-Jensen et al. 2015). Approximately 53.7% of households that receive SNAP benefits are food insecure. Research examining the benefits of SNAP has shown considerable benefits in supporting vulnerable populations, reducing poverty and food insecurity, reduced low-birth-weight infants, reduced chronic disease, and increased access to food (Executive Office of the President of the United States 2015). Research investigating diet quality of SNAP participants has shown overall lower diet quality including inadequate intakes of whole grains, fruits, vegetables, fish, and nuts/seeds/legumes as well as excessive intakes of processed meats, sweets, bakery desserts, and sugar-sweetened beverages (Leung et al. 2012; Gregory et al. 2013). Furthermore, research has investigated SNAP participants and income-eligible nonparticipants in the prevalence of adequate diets (Condon et al. 2015). For children, research has shown that approximately 97% had adequate intakes of protein and carbohydrate, but nearly 20% consumed more energy from fat and roughly 80% consumed more saturated fat than recommended (Condon et al. 2015). Finally, 44% of adult SNAP participants are considered obese, which is greater than income-eligible or higher-income nonparticipants at 32% and 30%, respectively. Furthermore, 24% of child SNAP participants are considered obese, which is greater than income-eligible or higher-income nonparticipants at 20% and 13%, respectively (Condon et al. 2015).

The SNAP-Ed component of the SNAP program works to help ensure that SNAP participants are making healthy food and lifestyle choices to reduce their risk of obesity. The most current information for approved SNAP-Ed funding from 2009 indicated that $341 million federal dollars were spent covering half the total amount spent by each state. The Food and Nutrition Service encourages states to consider three behavioral outcomes for SNAP participants—make half your plate fruits and vegetables, increase physical activity, and maintain appropriate calorie balance. Therefore, education provided revolves around these three outcomes. State participation in SNAP-Ed is voluntary and requires the state to include matching resources, a budget, and an implementation plan (USDA 2015c). Research investing the success of SNAP-Ed curriculums has shown positive benefits in attitudes toward fruit and vegetable consumption, fruit and vegetable intakes, and improved self-efficacy toward preparing and consuming fruits and vegetables through farmers' markets based nutrition education and cooking classes and nutrition education series classes (Least 2014; Dannefer et al. 2015). Research has also shown positive benefits for interactive nutrition education lessons with children resulting in increased nutrition knowledge, eating more fruits and vegetables and drinking more water, and eating a healthy breakfast (Hecht et al. 2013). Finally, research suggests that SNAP-Ed interventions geared at the point of purchase sales in grocery stores leads to increased purchasing of vegetables (Scott 2014).

The NSLP operates in over 100,000 schools and childcare institutions. In 2014, the NSLP provided meals to approximately 30.4 million children every school day. Approximately 47.5% of households that receive NSLP benefits are food insecure. After the enactment of the Healthy Hunger Free Kids Act in 2010, school nutrition standards were changed to have school meals line up with the Dietary Guidelines for Americans. Lunches were changed to increase vegetables, fruits, and whole grains; establishing calorie ranges, and decreasing sodium and trans fats (Woo Baidal and Taveras 2014). However, some research has shown that these dietary changes have led to increased food waste, decreased participation, and increased operating costs.

WIC provides grants to states to support distribution of supplemental foods, health care referrals, and nutrition education to pregnant and breastfeeding women and children up to the age of five. In 2014, WIC served approximately 8.3 million participants per month. Approximately 41.1% of households that receive WIC benefits are food insecure. In 2007, the USDA introduced a new set of food packages for WIC participants. The changes to the food packages have helped them better align with the recommendations of the Dietary Guidelines for Americans and the American Academy of Pediatrics (USDA 2015d). Research has shown that WIC participants have increased intakes of key nutrients such as iron, vitamin C, and niacin without an increase in energy intake or a negative effect on fat and cholesterol intakes. Furthermore, it has been shown to be more effective than other nutrition assistance programs on improving nutrient intakes in preschoolers. Finally, WIC participation has been indicated as one of the reasons for a decline in the rates of iron deficiency anemia (USDA 2013).

The WIC program is the only nutrition assistance program with legislative and regulatory requirements to provide nutrition education to participants as specified by the Child Nutrition Act. Federal regulations mandate that the nutrition education being provided at no cost be easy to understand and include considerations such as the participant's nutrient needs and cultural preferences. According to the USDA, "the goals of WIC nutrition education are to (1) emphasize the relationship between nutrition, physical activity, and health with special emphasis on the nutritional needs of pregnant, postpartum, and breastfeeding women, infants and children under five years of age and (2) assist the individual who is at nutritional risk in achieving a positive change in dietary and physical activity habits, resulting in improved nutritional status and in the prevention of nutrition-related problems through optimal use of the WIC supplemental foods and other nutritious foods (USDA 2006)." Research studies focusing on WIC nutrition education have been limited but have shown increased consumption of fruits and whole grains and replacement of whole milk with lower fat milk (Ritchie et al. 2010). Research geared toward children has also shown positive outcomes with decreased TV screen time and increased fruit consumption (Whaley et al. 2010).

In addition, participation in nutrition assistance programs by eligible households is limited. According to the USDA in 2014, approximately 60% of eligible households participated in one of the three largest nutrition assistance programs during the past 30 days. This emphasizes the need for improved outreach and marketing to those who are eligible but do not participate (Coleman-Jensen et al. 2015). See Table 2.1 for details.

Local policy and grassroots movements addressing food insecurity

Policies implemented at the state and local governance levels are attempting to address food insecurity within communities. Many local and state governments are working to sustainably address food insecurity in their communities. For food production, local policies to increase land usage and decrease taxation are used to promote food production in urban areas. For example, many cities such as Cincinnati, Ohio; Trenton, NJ; and Syracuse, NY have vacant to vibrant programs where city land is sold for a below market price to individuals who will utilize the land for food production. Furthermore, some cities are providing tax

Table 2.1 Participation in Nutrition Assistance Programs by Eligible Households

Program	Share of Food Insecure Households that Participated in the Program during the Previous 30 Days	Share of Households with Very Low Food Security that Participated in the Program during the Previous 30 Days
SNAP	44.0	48.5
Free or reduced price lunch	32.2	27.6
WIC	10.4	7.6
Any of these programs	60.5	60.6
None of these programs	39.5	39.4

Source: Coleman-Jensen, A., M. P. Rabbitt, C. Gregory, and A. Singh. 2015. United States Department of Agriculture Economic Research Service. Household Food Security in the United States in 2014. http://www.ers.usda.gov/publications/err-economic-research-report/err194.aspx

deductions on land used for food production or assisting with providing water sources on local urban gardens and farms. In terms of distribution, cities are providing more user-friendly and accessible transportation to help local residents access local food markets. In addition, cities are providing support to food distributors and providing city space for farmers' markets, food hubs, food coops, and mobile markets, thereby increasing food distribution avenues. Finally, local policies are addressing food access and promoting healthy food access. For instance, Minneapolis implemented a policy where all grocery stores and specialty food stores had to provide a certain amount of perishable fruits, vegetables, meats, breads/cereals, and dairy items. The idea of the policy is to increase access to fresh foods throughout the city. Pennsylvania had implemented tax deductions for grocers who opened stores in areas of limited fresh food access. Zoning ordinances restricting the availability and access to fast food is increasing throughout the United States. For example, Westwood Village, CA has restricted the number of fast food restaurants allowed on a street and the city of Arden Hills, MN restricts fast food restaurants from being a certain distance from other community entities such as schools and churches (Community Health Councils 2009). Philadelphia, PA has implemented several initiatives since 2010 to increase food access to low-income residents including a SNAP double bucks incentive program, a Healthy Corner Store initiative, and promoting an increase in farmers' markets (Department of Public Health Philadelphia).

Many changes occurring within local food systems may be due to a strong food policy council. Food policy councils play a role in local food system policy and change. They are unique and specific to each area community and usually consist of representation from various community entities. Their purpose usually includes but is not limited to working to influence local political capital and policy to encourage a strong local food system.

Local grass-root movements are becoming more common throughout the United States and are often called the "alternative" food or community security food initiatives (CSFI). These initiatives are often aimed at increasing affordable healthy foods to all individuals and addressing local food deserts through increasing food production, distribution, and access. Many times these initiatives work with a local food policy council and/or utilize local policy to move the initiatives forward. Such initiatives include community/urban gardens, farmers' markets and food stands, community-supported agriculture and food banks (Martinez et al. 2010). There was a substantial increase in these initiatives throughout the 2000s (Vogel 2016). Historically, though, the "alternative" or "local" food movement has been connected with a White, middle to upper class population (Colasanti, Conner and Smalley 2010). However, more recently, there are more CSFIs placed in low-income areas and/or in areas with a diverse population to increase fresh food access and change the overall food system to be more locally based and positively impacting food insecurity (Baker et al. 2006; Allen 2010). Many CSFIs utilize local policies and food assistance programs as a resource to assist in increasing food access. For example, CSFIs may utilize the vibrant to vacant program to obtain land for food production (Cuy Castellanos et al. [unpublished]). Furthermore, CSFIs may accept electronic benefits transfers from SNAP recipients, and vouchers from other federal food programs— such as the Senior Farmers' Market Nutrition Program, and Women, Infants, and Children (WIC) farmer's market vouchers—thereby increasing food access to low-income citizens (Oberholtzer, Dimitri, and Schumacher 2012; McGuirt et al. 2015; Dimitri and Oberholtzer 2015). Also, recently, a USDA report indicated that more customers are using SNAP benefits at local farmers' markets (Low et al. 2015). Again, the idea of CSFIs and certain food policies to address food security mainly addresses the issue of food access.

Empowering local cities and counties with more autonomy in addressing food insecurity in their communities may prove to be efficient and effective. Many of the programs and policies around food insecurity are made or administered at the federal and state levels. About 89% of the funding for the Farm Bill is used to support nutrition programs such as SNAP, WIC, and the School Lunch Program. Some of these programs, such as WIC, are funded at the federal level and administered at the state level. Furthermore, policies addressing food insecurity could be connected to agricultural policy, since often food insecurity is connected to food access. Much of agricultural policy in the United States addresses the production of commodity crops for food export or processing or for nonfood uses such as biofuels. Local food growth is minimally supported at the federal level (USDA 2015).

Allowing cities or counties to have more control over how programs are run or funds are allocated can allow funds to be used to address specific food insecurity contributing factors. One way to do this is through a strong local food policy council. Concurrently, strong food policy councils can encourage necessary collaboration to identify social and environmental factors affecting food insecurity within the community and develop a community-wide food security plan. Community members from different sectors of the community such as public, civic, and private can provide different views that allow for a holistic view of food insecurity and its local contributing factors. The councils can be integral in promoting policy reform, program development and implementation, community-wide collaboration and funding allocation encouraging communities to care for their own (Schiff 2008) through food production and distribution and nutrition program development and implementation.

Research gaps

Different initiatives and policies are being developed in an attempt to address food insecurity. As seen over the past 20 years, there have been fluctuations in the prevalence of food insecurity in the United States, which greatly mimic the economic fluctuations during times of recession and inflation. Further, there are various programs, policies, and initiatives in place to address food access specifically and therefore food insecurity. For example, within the past two decades, there has been a substantial increase in farmers' markets, community, and urban gardens, federal programs increasing local food purchasing power and local and state policies to increase food production and access throughout populations (Martinez et al. 2010). However, there is limited empirical research indicating the impact of these initiatives in truly addressing food security directly. Several studies show that an increase in alternative food initiatives such as farmers' markets, CSAs, and food hubs, particularly those initiatives accepting SNAP benefits and other federal assistance vouchers, in low-income areas does increase food access through providing available and affordable produce (Flaccavento 2011; Barham et al. 2012; Sitaker et al. 2014). Although small studies, some have shown such initiatives that address food access do lead to a direct increase in fresh food intake in participants (McCormack et al. 2010; Miewald, Holben, and Hall 2012; Ruelas et al. 2012; Sitaker et al. 2014). However, with this said, others suggest that increasing accessibility is only one aspect of food consumption and policies and initiatives around food insecurity cannot ignore factors such as the psychosocial influences of food consumption (Pearson et al. 2005; Cuy Castellanos et al. in press). Future research, policies, and initiatives may need to address multiple factors of food insecurity and not solely focus on food access. Nutrition programs that increase nutrition knowledge and skill and initiatives addressing food access need to be connected.

To encourage responsible spending, empirical research needs to examine the effectiveness of current federal, state and local programs in decreasing food insecurity and improving dietary behavior. In terms of federal programs and policies, research suggests an increase in purchasing power, but there is still the question of whether the programs promote healthy dietary behavior defined by the Dietary Guidelines for Americans (Cole and Fox 2008; Davis and You 2010). Nutrition education within the programs may lead to improved dietary outcomes. Research has focused on the inclusion on nutrition education with federal nutrition assistance programs. Only the WIC program mandates that recipients participate in nutrition education. Research has shown that nutrition education has had a significant impact on attitudes, knowledge, and behavior related to consumption and preparation on healthy foods. However, there appear to be wide variations in the delivery characteristics that lead to success and programs need to include a well-designed and delivered program evaluation plan in order to draw conclusions regarding the best practices.

For local policies, as already seen, many cities are implementing programs and policies to develop a local, equitable food system; however, data showing the impact of such programs and policies are limited. The intent of many food insecurity programs and policies is to increase food access. Studies examining food insecurity and dietary behavior prior to implementation and following each through time can provide insight on the impact of such programs and policies. Furthermore, comparing the effectiveness of each can be determined by comparing rates between city subpopulations or similar cities that have implemented different programs or policies.

Another aspect that needs to be further examined is the current way food security is measured. The measurement was developed over 20 years ago and assesses an individual or household's social and environmental factors relating to food access. The definition of food security is the "access by all people at all times to enough food for an active, healthy life, and includes, at a minimum: (a) the ready availability of nutritionally adequate and safe foods and (b) an assured ability to acquire acceptable foods in socially acceptable ways (e.g., without resorting to emergency food supplies, scavenging, stealing, or other coping strategies)." However, the measurement does not determine dietary quality; the measurement is limited to examining access to foods respondents prefer. Food preference does not equal quality and healthy food. Therefore, an argument could be made that the measurement does not adequately measure food security. Another issue with the screener is with its execution. The measurement is part of the Current Population Survey. The survey is provided in English and Spanish. However, there are many population groups in the United States, many of whom do not speak either English or Spanish. Furthermore, low literacy or illiterate populations may not be able to accurately complete the survey. Therefore, representation of many vulnerable population groups may be lacking in the data.

REFERENCES

Allen, P. 2010. Realizing justice in local food systems. *Cambridge Journal of Regions, Economy and Society* 3:295–308. doi: 10.1093/cjres/rsq015.

Anderson, S. A. 1990. Core indicators of nutritional state for difficult-to-sample populations. *Journal of Nutrition* 120:1555–1600.

Baker, E. A., Schootman, M., Barnidge, E., and Kelly, C. 2006. The role of race and poverty in access to foods that enable individuals to adhere to dietary guidelines. *Preventing Chronic Disease* 3:A76–87.

Barham, J., Tropp, D., Enterline, K., Farbman, J., Fisk, J., and Kiraly, S. 2012. *Regional Food Hub Resource Guide*. Washington, DC: U.S. Department of Agriculture, Agricultural Marketing Service. http://dx.doi.org/10.9752/MS046.04-2012

Bernal, J., Frongillo, E. A., Herrera, H. A., and Rivera, J. A. 2014. Food insecurity in children but not in their mothers is associated with altered activities, school absenteeism, and stunting. *Journal of Nutrition* 144:1619–26.

Bhargava, A., Jolliffe, D., and Howard, L. L. 2008. Socio-economic, behavioural and environmental factors predicted body weights and household food insecurity scores in the early childhood longitudinal study-kindergarten. *British Journal of Nutrition* 100:438–444.

Carter, K. N., Lanumata, T., Kruse, K., and Gorton, D. 2010. What are the determinants of food insecurity in New Zealand and does this differ for males and females? *Australian and New Zealand Journal of Public Health* 34:602–608.

Colasanti, K. J. A., Conner, D., and Smalley, K. 2010. Understanding barriers to farmers' market patronage in Michigan: Perspectives from marginalized populations. *Journal of Hunger and Environmental Nutrition* 5:316–338. doi: 10.1080/19320248.2010.504097.

Cole, N. and Fox, M. K. 2008. *Diet Quality of American by Food Stamp Participation Status: Data from the National Health and Nutrition Examination Survey, 1999–2004.* FNP Report No. FSP-08-NH. Washington DC.

Coleman-Jensen, A., Rabbitt, M. P., Gregory, C., and Singh, A. 2015. United States Department of Agriculture Economic Research Service. Household Food Security in the United States in 2014. http://www.ers.usda.gov/publications/err-economic-research-report/err194.aspx (accessed February 20, 2016).

Community Health Councils. 2009. *Zoning in on Healthy Fast Food.* Retrieved from http://www.chc-inc.org/downloads/NFW%20Fast%20Food%20Fact%20Sheet.pdf

Condon, E., Drilea, S., Jowers, K., Carolyn, L., Mabli, J., Madden, E., and Niland, K. 2015. *Diet Quality of Americans by SNAP Participation Status: Data from the National Health and Nutrition Examination Survey, 2007–2010.* United States Department of Agriculture, Food and Nutrition Service. http://www.fns.usda.gov/diet-quality-americans-snap-participation-status-data-national-health-and-nutrition-examination

Castellanos, D., Keller, J., and Majchrak, E. Exploring the connection between community food security initiatives and social-cognitive factors on dietary intake. *Journal of Food Systems, Agriculture and Community Development* 7(1):21–31.

Dannefer, R., Abrami, A., Rapoport, R., Sriphanlop, P., Sacks, R., and Johns, M. 2015. A mixed-methods evaluation of a SNAP-Ed farmers' market-based nutrition education program. *Journal of Nutrition Education and Behavior* 47:516–525.

Davis, G. and You, W. 2010. The thrifty food plan is not thrifty when labor cost is considered. *Journal of Nutrition* 140:854–857.

Dimitri, C. and Oberholtzer, L. 2015. Potential national economic benefits of food insecurity and nutrition incentives program of the U.S. agricultural act of 2014. *Journal of Agriculture, Food Systems, and Community Development* 5:49–61.

Eisinger, P. 1996. Toward a national hunger count. *Journal of Social Service Review* 70:214–234.

Eisinger, P. 1998. *Toward an End to Hunger in America.* Washington, DC: Brookings Institution Press.

Executive Office of the President of the United States. 2015. *Long-Term Benefits of the Supplemental Nutrition Assistance Program.* Retrieved from https://www.whitehouse.gov/blog/2015/12/08/new-cea-report-finds-snap-benefits-are-crucial-families-sometimes-inadequate

Flaccavento, A. 2011. *Is Local Food Affordable for Ordinary Folks? A Comparison of Farmers' Markets and Supermarkets in Nineteen Communities in the Southeast.* Charlottesville, VA: Scale, Incorporated. Retrieved from http://www.ruralscale.com/resources/downloads/farmers-market-study.pdf

Food and Agriculture Organization of the United Nations. 2003. *Trade Reforms and Food Security: Conceptualizing the Linkages.* Retrieved from http://www.fao.org/docrep/005/y4671e/y4671e00.htm

Food Research and Action Center. 2015. *A History of Food Insecurity Measure*. Retrieved from http://frac.org/reports-and-resources/hunger-and-poverty/a-history-of-the-food-insecurity-measure/

Gregory, C., Ver Ploeg, M., Andrews, M., and Coleman-Jensen, A. 2013. *United States Department of Agriculture Economic Research Service. Supplemental Nutrition Assistance Program (SNAP) Participation Leads to Modest Changes in Diet Quality.* Retrieved from http://www.ers.usda.gov/publications/err-economic-research-report/errl47.aspx

Gundersen, C. 2015. Food insecurity and poor sleep: Another consequence of food insecurity in the United States. *Journal of Nutrition* 145:391–392.

Hecht, L., Wass, J., Kelly, L., Clevenger-Firley, E., and Dunn, C. 2013. SNAP-Ed steps to health inspires third graders to eat smart and move more. *Journal of Nutrition Education and Behavior* 45:800–802.

Holben, D., Position of the American Dietetic Association. 2010. Food insecurity in the United States. *Journal of the American Dietetic Association* 110:1368–1377.

IOM (Institute of Medicine) and NRC (National Research Council). 2013. *Supplemental Nutrition Assistance Program: Examining the Evidence to Define Benefit Adequacy.* Washington, DC: The National Academies Press.

Jyoti, D. F., Frongillo, E. A., and Jones, S. J. 2005. Food insecurity affects school children's academic performance, weight gain, and social skills. *Journal of Nutrition* 135:2831–2839.

Laraia, B., Siega-Riz, A. M., and Gundersen, C. 2010. Household food insecurity is associated with self-reported pregravid weight status, gestational weight gain, and pregnancy complications. *Journal of the American Dietetic Association* 110:692–701.

Least, C. 2014. Pennsylvania SNAP-Ed exploratory study shows significant increases in fruit and vegetable intake. *Journal of Nutrition Education and Behavior* 46:S154.

Lee, J. S., Fischer, J., and Johnson, M. A. 2010. Food insecurity, food and nutrition programs, and aging: Experiences from Georgia. *Journal of Nutrition for the Elderly* 29:116–149.

Leung, C. W., Ding, E. L., Catalano, P. L., Villamor, E., Rimm, E. B., and Willett, W. C. 2012. Dietary intake and dietary quality of low-income adults in the supplemental nutrition assistance program. *American Journal of Clinical Nutrition* 96:977–88.

Low, S. A., Adalja, A., Beaulieu, E., Key, N., Martinez, S., Melton, A., Perez, A., Ralston, K., Stewart, H., Suttles, S., Vogel, S., and Jablonski, B. B. R. 2015. *Trends in U.S. Local and Regional Food Systems*. AP-068, U.S. Department of Agriculture, Economic Research Service. January.

Martinez, S., Hand, M., Da Pra, M., Pollack, S., Ralston, K., Smith, T., Vogel, S., Clark, S., Lohr, L., Low, S., and Newman, C. 2010. *Local Food Systems, Concepts, Impacts, and Issues*. Technical report. U.S. Department of Agriculture, Economic Research Report Number 97.

McCormack, L. A., Laska, M. N., Larson, N. I., and Story, M. 2010. Review of the nutritional implications of farmers' markets and community gardens: A call for evaluation and research efforts. *Journal of the American Dietetic Association* 110:399–408.

McGuirt, J. T., Ward, R., Elliot, N., Bullock, S. L., and Pitts, S. J. 2015. Factors influencing local food procurement among women of reproductive age in rural eastern and western North Carolina (USA). *Journal of Agriculture, Food Systems, and Community Development* 4:143–154.

Metallinos-Katsaras, E., Must, A., and Gorman, K. 2012. A longitudinal study of food insecurity on obesity in preschool children. *Journal of the Academy of Nutrition and Dietetics* 112:1949–1958.

Miewald, C., Holben, D., and Hall, P. 2012. Role of a food box program in fruit and vegetable consumption and food security. *Canadian Journal of Dietetic Practice and Research* 73:59–65.

Oberholtzer, L., Dimitri, C., and Schumacher, G. 2012. Linking farmers, healthy foods, and underserved consumers: Exploring the impact of nutrition incentive programs on farmers and farmers' markets. *Journal of Agriculture, Food Systems, and Community Development* 2:63–77.

O'Brien, D., Aldeen, H. T., Uchima, S., and Staley, E. 2004. Hunger in America: The Definitions, Scope, Causes, History and Status of the Problem of Hunger in the United States. *The UPS Foundation and the Congressional Hunger Center 2004 Hunger Forum Discussion Paper.* Retrieved from http://www.hungercenter.org/wp-content/uploads/2012/10/Hunger-in America-Americas-Second-Harvest.pdf

Pearson, T., Russell, J., Campbell, M. J., and Barker, M. E. 2005. Do 'food deserts' influence fruit and vegetable consumption? A cross-sectional study. *Appetite* 45:195–7.

Ritchie, L. D., Whaley, S. E., Spector, P., Gomez, J., and Crawford, P. B. 2010. Favorable impact of nutrition education on California WIC families. *Journal of Nutrition Education and Behavior* 42:S2–S10.

Ruelas, V., Iverson, E., Kiekel, P., and Peters, A. 2012. The role of farmers' markets in two low income, urban communities. *Journal of Community Health* 37:554–562.

Schiff, R. 2008. The role of food policy councils in developing sustainable food systems. *Journal of Hunger and Environmental Nutrition* 3:206–228.

Scott, M. 2014. A three-year develop-pilot-revise process produces effective and enjoyable behavior-based nutrition lessons. *Journal of Nutrition Education and Behavior* 46:S156.

Sitaker, M., Kolodinsky, J., Jilcott Pitts, S. B., and Seguin, R. A. 2014. Do entrepreneurial food systems innovations impact rural economies and health? Evidence and gaps. *American Journal of Entrepreneurship* 7:3–12.

Skalicky, A., Meyers, A., Adams, W., Yang, Z., Cook, J., and Frank, D. 2006. Child food insecurity and iron deficiency anemia in low-income infants and toddlers in the United States. *Maternal and Child Health Journal* 10:177–185.

United States Department of Agriculture, Food and Nutrition Service. 2013. Women, Infants and Children (WIC), About WIC-How WIC Helps. Retrieved from http://www.fns.usda.gov/wic/about-wic-how-wic-helps

United States Department of Agriculture. 2015. The Farm Bill. Last modified July 13. Retrieved from http://www.usda.gov/wps/portal/usda/usdahome?navid=farmbill

United States Department of Agriculture, Economic Research Service. 2015a. Definitions of Food Security. Last modified September 8. Retrieved from http://www.ers.usda.gov/topics/food-nutrition-assistance/food-security-in-the-us/definitions-of-food-security.aspx

United States Department of Agriculture, Economic Research Service. 2015b. Food Security Data Access and Documentation Downloads. Last modified September 9. Retrieved from http://www.ers.usda.gov/data-products/food-security-in-the-united-states.aspx

United States Department of Agriculture, Economic Research Service. 2015c. Supplemental Nutrition Assistance Program (SNAP). Last modified May 22. Retrieved from http://www.ers.usda.gov/topics/food-nutrition-assistance/supplemental-nutrition-assistance-program-%28snap%29/nutrition-education.aspx#reports

United States Department of Agriculture, Food and Nutrition Service. 2015d. *Special Supplemental Nutrition Program for Women, Infants, and Children (WIC) Food Packages Policy Options Study II (Summary).* Retrieved from http://www.fns.usda.gov/wic-food-package-policy-options-ii

United States Department of Agriculture, WIC Works Resource System. 2006. *WIC Program Nutrition Education Guidance.* Retrieved from https://wicworks.fns.usda. gov/nutrition-education

Vogel, S. 2016. *Number of US Farmers' Markets Continue to Rise.* https://www.ers.usda. gov/data-products/chart-gallery/gallery/chart-detail/?chartid=77600

Whaley, S. E., McGregor, S., Jiang, L., Gomez, J., Harrison, G., and Jenks, E. 2010. A WIC-based intervention to prevent early childhood overweight. *Journal of Nutrition Education and Behavior* 42:S47–S51.

Wehler, C. A. et al. 1991. *Survey of Childhood Hunger in the United States. Community Childhood Hunger Identification Project.* Food Research and Action Center, Washington, DC.

Woo Baidal, J. A. and Taveras, E. M. 2014. Protecting progress against childhood obesity—The National School Lunch Program. *New England Journal of Medicine* 371:1862–1865.

Zizza, C., Duffy, P., and Gerrior, S. 2008. Food insecurity is not associated with lower energy intakes. *Obesity* 16:1908–1913.

3 Unintended consequences of nutritional assistance programs

Children's school meal participation and adults' food security

Teja Pristavec

Introduction

In 2012, 33 million adults and 15 million children were living in the 17.6 million American households classified as food insecure (Coleman-Jensen et al. 2013), or without "access [...] at all times to enough food including at a minimum: a) the ready availability of nutritionally adequate and safe foods, and b) the assured ability to acquire acceptable foods in socially acceptable ways (e.g., without resorting to emergency food supplies, scavenging, stealing, and other coping strategies)" (Anderson 1990, p. 1575). Food insecurity puts both children and adults at higher risk for negative physical and mental health outcomes (Bhattacharya et al. 2004; Kaiser and Townsend 2005; Martin and Lippert 2012; McLaughlin et al. 2012). However, the condition is unequally distributed within households, with adults more frequently food insecure than children (Nord and Parker 2010). One explanation for this uneven distribution is adult buffering, in which adults allocate resources to prioritize children's needs (Maxwell 1996; Ahluwalia et al. 1998; Nord and Parker 2010; Carney 2012).

The U.S. Department of Agriculture's (USDA) Food and Nutrition Service (FNS) runs several nutritional assistance programs addressing food insecurity, with the National School Lunch Program (NSLP) and the School Breakfast Program (SBP) targeted specifically at children. While previous research links school meal programs to children's educational (Belot and James 2011), dietary (Clark and Fox 2009), and behavioral (Mann 2012) outcomes, it does not examine the possibility that they may, by providing a substantial amount of calories to children, have the unintended benefit of reducing adult buffering and addressing adult food insecurity. School meals providing consistent access to nutritious food for children may allow for a reallocation of household food resources and therefore be an indirect means of increasing adults' food security.

In this chapter, I examine whether children's participation in school meal programs is associated with adults' food security. Previous studies examined the link between nutritional assistance programs and food insecurity for children (Campbell et al. 2011; Howard and Prakash 2012), but few considered their implications for adults (Bhattacharya et al. 2004; Arteaga and Heflin 2014). While the assumption that the benefits of food assistance programs extend beyond their intended individual recipients and benefit entire households is accepted in the international development literature (Beaton and Ghassemi 1982), it is not well examined in the U.S. context. Calls were made for research on protective adult behaviors in food insecure families (Bhattacharya et al. 2006), of which food buffering is one example. This study considers a possible association between participation in child nutritional assistance programs and adult food security in the same families.

To explore the relationship between children's school meal participation and adult food security, I use combined 2007–2010 National Health and Nutrition Examination Survey (NHANES) data (CDC 2010). I address the following research questions:

1. Is children's school meal participation associated with adults' food security in the same households?
2. How does the association between children's school meal participation and adults' food security vary by program participation (NSLP only, both SBP and NSLP), subsidy level (reduced price and free), and meal receipt frequency (1–5 times per week)?

Background

Food insecurity is associated with a range of negative child and adult outcomes

Food security refers to having consistent access to sufficient food that is readily available, nutritionally adequate, and safe, while being able to acquire it in socially acceptable ways (Anderson 1990). In 2012, 17.6 million U.S. households (14.5%) representing 33 million adults and 15 million children were food insecure (Coleman-Jensen et al. 2013). About 60% of households experience food insecurity as recurring, and about 20% experience it as chronic (Nord et al. 2002).

At an individual level, the experience of household food insecurity consists of uncertainty and worry, inadequate food quality, inadequate food quantity, and social unacceptability (Coates et al. 2006). Through decreased quality and quantity of food, disruption in eating patterns, malnutrition, and psychological distress (Nord and Parker 2010), food insecurity is associated with several negative outcomes for children and adults. For children, food insecurity is associated with physical and growth impairment (Kaiser and Townsend 2005), being overweight (Larson and Story 2011), problem behaviors (Mann 2012), poor mental health (McLaughlin et al. 2012), and impaired academic performance (Jyoti et al. 2005). For adults, food insecurity is associated with reduced diet quality, nutrient inadequacy, and obesity (Adams et al. 2003; Bhattacharya et al. 2004). Food insecure adults are at greater risk of diabetes (Meng et al. 2014), chronic disease (Gowda et al. 2012), and mental illness (Whitaker et al. 2006).

Adults may buffer children from food insecurity within the household

Individual-level food insecurity is therefore associated with detrimental outcomes for both adults and children. At the household level, particularly households with children have higher rates of food insecurity (Coleman-Jensen et al. 2013). However, research shows that within households, children are protected from the condition. Fewer children than adults have very low food security (Nord and Parker 2010). Very low food security is about six times higher for adults than for children in food insecure households (Nord and Hopwood 2007).

Adult buffering, in which adult caretakers compromise their well-being to provide for children, may explain the differences in food security status for individuals within the same household. Adult caring and protective behaviors act as a buffer shielding children from unfavorable outcomes. In food-related adult buffering, buffering refers to "the practice of [a mother] deliberately limiting [her] own intake in order to ensure that children [...] get enough to eat" (Maxwell 1996, p. 295). Mothers deprive themselves of food to feed their dependents (Carney 2012), have lower quality food intake (McIntyre et al. 2003), and worse health outcomes than others within food insecure households (Tarasuk 2005). Mothers, but not their children, decrease frequency of fruit and vegetable consumption and experience eating pattern disruption as their food insecurity status worsens (Kendall et al. 1996). Adults other than mothers may also engage in such food-related protective behavior (Ahluwalia et al. 1998; Bhattacharya et al. 2004; Martin and Lippert 2012), as poverty is frequently predictive of adults' but not children's dietary outcomes (Bhattacharya et al. 2006). Parents likely put children's food needs before their own due to societal expectations regarding caretaking (Slater et al. 2012), possible child neglect sanctions (Administration for Children and Families 2014), and concern about the impact of inadequate nutrition on child development (Fiese et al. 2011). Adults may, therefore, adopt buffering behaviors when household food resources are scarce.

Child nutritional assistance programs may offset adult buffering

The institutional provision of meals for children may reduce the need for adult buffering, as it provides a proportion of children's daily or weekly meals outside the home. Child nutritional assistance programs may represent an indirect means of increasing adults' food security.

The FNS runs several nutritional assistance programs that adults may use to cope with food insecurity, five of which are aimed specifically at children. This analysis focuses on the NSLP and the SBP for two reasons. First, they represent the largest U.S. federal child nutrition assistance programs, with the NSLP costing $11.6 billion, and the SBP costing $3.3 billion in 2012 (FNS 2013a,b). Second, in contrast with other assistance programs, they are available to all children in participating institutions and are designed to provide full meals, contributing substantially to children's daily food intake.

Both the NSLP and the SBP provide low-cost or free meals to enrolled children attending public schools and nonprofit private schools. The NSLP is available at virtually all public schools and in over 80% of private schools (Currie 2003), with the program available nationally to over 90% of all students (Burghardt et al. 1995). In the 2009–2010 school year, a total of 86,816 institutions served school breakfast and 99,685 served school lunch, with 87% of participating institutions serving both (Food Research and Action Center 2011, p. 19). Meals served must meet federal requirements and follow the nutrition standards established in the Dietary Guidelines for Americans.

The level of a family's financial contribution depends on household income (income eligibility) and family circumstance (categorical eligibility). Income eligibility qualifies children under a certain threshold of the federal poverty level to receive subsidized meals. Children from families with incomes over 185% of the federal poverty level pay full price, with local school food authorities setting the prices while still operating the service as a nonprofit program. Children from families with incomes between 130% and 185% of the federal poverty level are eligible for reduced-price meals, with the maximum charge of $0.40 per meal in the NSLP and $0.30 per meal in the SBP (Department of Agriculture 2012, p. 93). Children from families with incomes at or below 130% of the federal poverty level qualify for free meals. Categorically eligible children are those also considered income-eligible based on their family's participation in other nutrition assistance programs, as well as homeless, migrant, Head Start, and runaway children. U.S. citizenship or legal documentation status is not a condition for NSLP and SBP participation. Once certified, children are eligible to receive free or reduced-price school meals for the entire school year and for up to 30 operating days of the new school year. In fiscal year 2009, over 31 million children participated in the NSLP, and over 11 million participated in the SBP, with 63% of all lunches and 82% of all breakfasts served free or at a reduced price. Both children's participation and the proportion of subsidized meals served increased in 2010 (FNS 2014), continuing a trend beginning at the programs' inception.

School meals provide a substantial number of calories to children

Reliance on nutritional assistance programs is one coping strategy adults have at their disposal when dealing with food insecurity. School breakfasts and lunches represent alternate means of securing food for children. By providing meals adults would otherwise have to supply, freed-up household resources may reduce the need for adult buffering and be reallocated to increase adults' food security.

The FNS considered the need to provide an adequate number of calories for children from food insecure households (Department of Agriculture 2012) in its NSLP and SPB meal standards. The nutritional guidelines specify that school breakfasts must provide 350–500 kcal for children in grades K–5; 400–500 kcal in grades 6–8; and 450–600 kcal in grades 9–12, while school lunches must provide 550–650 kcal for children in grades K–5; 600–700 kcal in grades 6–8; and 750–850 kcal in grades 9–12 (Byker et al. 2013).

These amounts represent over a third of children's average daily intake. On average, children consume 35% of their typical daily intake at school, and the rest at home or at other locations (Briefel et al. 2009). For NSLP-only participants, the percentage is higher at 40%, and at 51% of total daily intake consumed at school for children participating in both the NSLP and SPB. Research indicates that children participating in the NSLP consume more calories (Gleason and Suitor 2003) and a higher quantity of foods during school lunch than their non-participating counterparts (Campbell et al. 2011). Participating secondary school students consume almost 300 kcal more than nonparticipants, for an average of 808 kcal per student (Briefel et al. 2009).

School meals are particularly important as a source of daily intake for food insecure children. Children from food insecure and marginally food secure households obtain a higher proportion of their daily food intake at school than their food secure peers, and participation rates only partially explain this difference (Potamites and Gordon 2010). Compared to those paying for school lunches, children receiving them for free or at a reduced price consume more servings, with the effect stronger for those fully subsidized (Howard and Prakash 2012). Further, children as young as nine are already aware of household food insecurity and participate in adults' coping strategies (Fram et al. 2011). The age of 11 to 16-year-olds describe eating more when food is available and taking maximum advantage of school lunches (Connell et al. 2005). Children's decisions to maximize caloric intake at school may also decrease the overall burden on the household food supply.

Resource reallocation and link to adult food security

Spillover studies, expenditure studies, and resource reallocation studies offer further support for the expectation that children's school meal participation may reduce the need for adult food buffering and increase adult food security. First, school meal programs have spillover effects extending beyond the individuals at whom they were originally targeted. For example, preschool children's participation in the SBP is associated with an improvement in children's as well as adults' diets (Bhattacharya et al. 2004). Similarly, as an unintended benefit of school meal programs, relaxing household food resource constraints may improve not only adult diet but also adult food security.

Second, the literature examining the effects of nutrition assistance programs on food expenditures finds that such programs improve the ability to increase spending on food items (Hoynes and Schanzenbach 2009). Even when providing monetary vouchers not tied to food purchases, low-income households used them on food (Smith et al. 2012). Studies focusing on school meal programs indicate that the NSLP and the SBP supplement food expenditures (West and Price 1976; Long 1991). This suggests that the resources school meal participation free up are reallocated to food purchases, providing households with additional meals, and may thus reduce food insecurity (Schmidt et al. 2013).

Finally, resources are scarcer in food insecure households than in food secure ones. Greater scarcity may imply a greater need for efficient allocation, and food insecure households may be more likely to redistribute newly available resources between its members. Food expenditures vary across income groups; compared to high-income households, low-income ones spend a larger proportion of their income on food (Nord 2009). Previous research examining the link between school meals and intrahousehold reallocation of calories finds that families with higher incomes do not decrease the amount of food otherwise offered to children with receipt of greater school meal benefits, but families with lower income are likely to do so (Jacoby 2002).

In summary, spillover effects of nutritional assistance programs for other household members indicate that the retained resources may be used on additional food, and show that the redistribution is more likely to happen in low-income households. This suggests that the provision of school meal programs to children may operate in a similar way and have the unintended benefit of alleviating adult food insecurity. However, no previous research supports this proposition. I explore the question empirically.

Data and methods

To assess the question of whether children's participation in school meal programs is associated with adults' food security, I combine waves 2007–2008 and 2009–2010 of the NHANES (CDC 2010). NHANES is a cross-sectional, continuous, nationally representative survey of the U.S. population that collects data about disease conditions, risk behaviors, and diet and nutrition. It surveys the civilian, noninstitutionalized population of all ages, using a stratified multistage probability sample (CDC 2010). It is one of five nationally representative surveys that include the USDA Household Food Security Survey Module (HFSSM).

Compared to related datasets, NHANES contains more detailed information about children's school meal participation, including data about the availability, receipt, type, and frequency of school meals. NHANES also collects data about adult food security at both the household and individual level and includes the full version of the USDA's HFSSM. Additionally, NHANES oversamples minority populations more at risk of food insecurity, and reflects the population of school meal program participants (Ralston et al. 2008), making it suitable to address my research questions.

Sample

I limit the sample to households with children attending kindergarten through high school during the school year. I further delimit it to students whose institutions offer at least the NSLP, as it is likely that nonparticipating schools differ in unobserved characteristics from those offering the program. Additionally, I restrict the sample to those below 185% of the federal poverty line, or those who are income-eligible for free or reduced-price meals, as individuals in households above the poverty line do not qualify for subsidized meals and are unlikely to be food insecure (Coleman-Jensen et al. 2013). Since missing data did not exceed

5% on any variables, I use list wise deletion to drop cases missing data for any of the variables used in the analysis. The final analytic sample includes 2449 children attending schools that offer at least the NSLP and those who live in households with adults and below 185% of the federal poverty line. For analyses focusing on the NSLP, the sample size is 2316 cases due to missing values on the lunch subsidy level and receipt frequency.

Dependent variable: Adult food security

I base the dependent variable, adult food security, on the HFSSM included in NHANES. The HFSSM includes 18 questions concerning ways of providing sufficient food and coping with food scarcity (Bickel et al. 2000). For adults and households without children, scores are calculated using 10 question items. Children's scores are calculated using an additional eight questions and added together in the household measure. The categories refer to a 12-month period, classifying adults, children, and households into one of four categories: full food security (no food insecurity conditions); marginal food security (one to two food insecurity conditions); low food security (three to five food insecurity conditions); or very low food security (six to ten food insecurity conditions) (Current Population Survey Food Security Supplement 2012).

I operationalize adult food security by calculating a food security score from the 10 adult-related questions of the HFSSM that were collected in the household interview and released on each household member's record. I compute the number of affirmative responses to food security items per USDA guidelines and reverse-code for an increasing score to indicate higher food security. I use the dependent variable as a continuous measure; as a categorical measure recoded into the four food security categories of very low, low, marginal, and full adult food security; and as a dichotomous measure collapsing very low and low food security into adult food insecurity, and marginal and full food security into adult food security (Bickel et al. 2000).

In addition to predicting overall adult food security, I use individual HFSSM questions relating to adult experience in the household as dependent variables to examine whether children's school meal participation improves particular adult food security outcomes. I dichotomize the items measuring frequency of food insecurity occurrence into food insecurity (happened every month or some months but not all) and food security (never happened).

Key independent variable: Children's school meal participation

I operationalize children's school meal program participation using three questions. I use a dichotomous measure of whether or not the school offers the NSLP and the SBP ("Does your school serve school lunches/breakfasts/? These are complete lunches/breakfasts/that cost the same every day.") to measure the type of meal received. I use a continuous variable (1× per week to 5× per week) to measure the frequency of meal receipt ("During the school year, about how many times a week do you get a complete school lunch/breakfast/?"). I use a three-category variable (free, reduced price, and full price) to measure the level of benefits ("Do you get these lunches/breakfasts/free, at a reduced price, or do you pay full price?").

Control variables

I include a series of individual- and household-level controls* in the final models to examine whether associations persist or are explained away after controlling for other factors linked to food security. At the individual level, I control for the child's gender. I further control for the child's race, as food insecurity is higher than the national average in minority households (Coleman-Jensen et al. 2013), and minority children represent a large portion of school meal program participants (Ralston et al. 2008). Additionally, I control for the child's age, as adult buffering occurs less frequently for older children (Potamites and Gordon 2010). At the household level, I control for factors associated with increased household food insecurity that may prevent adult buffering efforts. I construct a dummy variable indicating whether the household included at least one employed adult, as households with unemployed adults are more likely to be food insecure (Nord and Parker 2010). I control for household size, with food insecurity more prevalent in larger households (Coleman-Jensen et al. 2013), and include a dummy variable indicating whether the household had income under or at and above $20,000. Further, I control for emergency food, SNAP, and state or county cash assistance as other types of assistance received that may alleviate the condition (Schmidt et al. 2013).

Analytic plan

To examine whether children's school meal program participation is associated with adults' food security, I predict adult food security as a continuous score in an OLS regression in Model 1.† I compare adults in households with eligible nonparticipants to those in households with NSLP recipients only and NSLP-plus-SBP recipients.‡ Additionally, I run a series of logistic regressions predicting each of the 10 adult-related HFSSM items that comprise the adult food security measure.

I estimate a series of models to examine how the association between children's school meal participation and adults' food security varies by the level of program

---

* Individual-level controls refer to the child, as NHANES does not allow for linking children to particular adults, and I therefore cannot control for adult characteristics.
† In a sensitivity analysis, I also predict adult food security as a binary measure in a logistic regression, and as a categorical measure in an ordered logistic regression. While I use food security operationalized in these three ways in all the following analyses, I display results using only adult food security score as a continuous measure. Coefficients obtained using adult food security as a categorical or a binary measure did not differ in direction or degree of magnitude from those obtained using a continuous measure.
‡ The cell size for SBP-only participants was too small to allow for analysis. In addition, SBP-only participants are likely to differ from other participants by unobserved school-level characteristics, as the SBP is a program smaller than NSLP and usually offered in conjunction with, rather than separately from, the NSLP.

participation, subsidy level, and meal receipt frequency. In Model 2, I predict the adult food security score examining subsidy level differences by comparing those receiving NSLP meals at full price to those receiving them at a reduced price or for free. Finally, in Model 3, I predict adult food security to examine differences by meal receipt frequency by comparing adults in households with NSLP participants by the number of times per week the children receive school lunch.

I run all analyses using probability weights for the combined 2007–2008 and 2009–2010 waves of NHANES, adjusting for its stratified multistage probability sampling. I display coefficients for OLS regression results and odds ratios for logistic regression results. No interaction terms were statistically significant. Multicollinearity did not pose a problem for the present analysis. The correlation matrix at the bivariate level did not show high correlations between pairs of independent variables, and regressing each independent variable on all other independent variables did not produce high coefficients of determination.

Results

Descriptive statistics

Table 3.1 shows descriptive statistics for the unweighted analytic sample ($n = 2449$). The sample was gender-balanced, with a mean age of 10.5 years (SD = 3.90), and predominantly Hispanic (46%) due to oversampling. The children resided in households with an average of five members (SD = 1.46), a combined household income over $20,000 (61%), and at least one employed adult (88%). One-half of children (51%) came from households that have received food stamps in the past year, while fewer received emergency food (18%) or state or county cash assistance (12%) during the same time period.

Seven percent of children were eligible nonparticipants in school meal programs, and the majority of the sample (93%) consisted of children participating in at least one. Most (59%) participated in both the NSLP and the SBP. The subsample of children receiving at least the NSLP ($n = 2316$) on average received the school meal every day of the week (SD = 0.82), and the majority received it for free (81%).

Adults within these households had a mean food security score of 7.77 (SD = 2.69) on a scale with a minimum of 0 (food insecure) and a maximum of 10 (food secure). Following the USDA scoring guidelines, most were highly food secure (42%), followed by those with marginal food security (22%), those with low food security (21%), and those with very low food security (16%).

Regression analyses

Is children's school meal program participation associated with adults' food security? How does the association change after controlling for individual- and household-level factors?

To examine whether children's school meal program participation is associated with adults' food security and how it changes after controlling for individual- and

Table 3.1 Unweighted Sample Descriptive Statistics ($n = 2449$)

Variable	%	Mean	Std. Dev.	Min.	Max.
Dependent Variable					
Food security score		7.77	2.69	0 (insecure)	10 (secure)
Food security binary/categorical					
Food insecure					
Very low food security	15.56				
Low food security	20.58				
Food secure					
Marginal food security	21.52				
High food security	42.34				
Key Independent Variables					
Program participation					
Neither	6.70				
NSLP only	34.46				
NSLP and SBP	58.84				
NSLP frequency/week ($n = 2316$)		4.72	0.82	1	5
NSLP subsidy level ($n = 2316$)					
Full price	9.46				
Reduced price	9.20				
Free	81.35				
Control Variables					
Child level					
Gender					
Male	50.88				
Female	49.12				
Age		10.51	3.90	4	19
Race					
White	22.70				
Black	26.09				
Hispanic	46.06				
Other	5.14				
Household level					
Household size		4.83	1.46	1	7
Household income					
Below $20,000	39.36				
At/above $20,000	60.64				
Employed adult in household (1 = yes)	87.51				
Food stamp receipt 12 months (1 = yes)	51.37				
Emergency food receipt 12 months (1 = yes)	18.21				
Cash assistance receipt 12 months (1 = yes)	11.80				

household-level factors, I first run OLS regressions predicting the adult food security score as a continuous variable (Table 3.2, Model 1), and then predict individual adult HFSSM items using logistic regressions to examine the adult food security status in detail (Table 3.3). Table 3.2 shows OLS regression results predicting the adult food security score based on the child's school meal participation level.

Model 1 ($R^2 = 0.20$) shows the association between adult food security and the number of school meal programs in which the child participates. The food security score of adults in households with a child only participating in the NSLP does not differ from those in households with eligible nonparticipants. However, adults in households with a child participating in both the NSLP and the SBP are expected to have a food security score 0.6 points lower (SE = 0.25; $p < 0.05$), on the scale from very low food security (0) to full food security (10), than those with income-eligible children participating in neither program. Additionally, adults in households with a Hispanic schoolchild ($b = -0.43$; SE = 0.19; $p < 0.01$) and households receiving emergency food assistance ($b = -2.76$; SE = 0.22; $p < 0.001$) are less food secure than those in households with a white schoolchild or in households not receiving emergency food, respectively. Similarly, the adult food security score is negatively associated with household size. For every additional household member, an adult's food security score is expected to decrease by 0.2 of a point (SE = 0.06; $p < 0.05$). In sum, I find that children's greater school meal program participation is associated with lower adult food security.

For a detailed examination of adult food security status based on a child's school meal participation, Table 3.3 shows results from a series of binary logistic regression models predicting individual HFSSM items that concern adult behaviors. Each row represents a separate logistic regression model. I run two models for each of the eight adult status HFSSM items, one without controls and one fully adjusted (presented in the row below the unadjusted model). For each of the eight regressions, I display the odds ratios representing the association between children's school meal program participation and the particular adult-related HFSSM item. The table only displays the odds ratios associated with children's school meal participation, omitting coefficients obtained on control variables.

Unadjusted logistic regression results show that adults in households with a child participating in a school meal program have 41% lower odds than adults in households with a nonparticipant child to eat as much as usual, 54% lower odds to avoid hunger, 80% lower odds to avoid losing weight, and 86% lower odds to avoid going hungry all day because there was no money for food. Not controlling for other factors, adult food security is, therefore, more common in households where eligible children do not participate in school meal programs. In adjusted models, the association persists for two of the conditions. Adults in households with a child participant have 87% lower odds of having eaten every day, relative to adults in households with income-eligible children who did not participate in the program, and 77% lower odds of not losing weight.

Taken together, the results show that even net of controls, adult food insecurity (both overall and by individual indicators) is higher in households where children

Table 3.2 Regression Results Predicting Adult Food Security Score by Child's School Meal Program Participation Level, Subsidy Level, and Meal Receipt Frequency

	Model 1: Participation Level (n = 2449)		Model 2: Subsidy Level (n = 2316)		Model 3: Receipt Frequency (n = 2316)	
	b	Std. Err.	b	Std. Err.	b	Std. Err.
Key Independent Variables						
Program participation (ref = no)						
NSLP only	−0.15	0.20				
NSLP and SBP	−0.62*	0.25				
Subsidy level (ref = full price)						
Reduced price			−0.22	0.32		
Free			−0.97**	0.30		
Receipt frequency (1–5×)					−0.02	0.09
Control variables						
Gender (ref = male)	0.08	0.12	0.03	0.13	0.06	0.14
Age (4–19)	−0.03	0.02	−0.03	0.02	−0.03	0.02
Race (ref = white)						
Black	−0.10	0.19	0.01	0.23	−0.11	0.22
Hispanic	−0.43**	0.19	−0.21	0.23	−0.36	0.20
Other	−0.20	0.62	−0.15	0.69	−0.22	0.72
HH size (2–7)	−0.15*	0.06	−0.15*	0.06	−0.18**	0.06
HH income at/above 20k (ref = below 20k)	0.37	0.20	0.35	0.21	0.44	0.21
Employed adult (ref = no)	0.16	0.17	0.16	0.18	0.20	0.18
Food stamps (ref = no)	−0.18	0.20	−0.01	0.23	−0.22	0.20
Emergency food (ref = no)	−2.76***	0.22	−2.89***	0.24	−2.93***	0.25
Cash assistance (ref = no)	−0.09	0.24	0.09	0.21	0.10	0.22
Constant	9.70***		9.91***		9.47***	
R^2	0.20		0.22		0.21	
F	$F_{(13, 20)}$ 20.24***		$F_{(13, 20)}$ 13.39***		$F_{(12, 21)}$ 15.53***	
Design Df	32		32		32	

*$p < 0.05$, **$p < 0.01$, and ***$p < 0.001$

Table 3.3 Odds Ratios from Binary Logistic Regressions Predicting Individual HFSSM Items Based on Children's School Meal Program Participation ($n = 2449$)

Dependent Variable	OR	95% CI	F	Df
Not Worried Food Run Out				
Model 1: No controls	0.61	0.33–1.10	2.95	(1,32)
Model 2: Full controls	0.76	0.45–1.29	9.45***	(12,21)
Food Lasted				
No controls	0.61	0.35–1.05	3.45	(1,32)
Full controls	0.76	0.45–1.26	20.09***	(12,21)
Can Afford Food				
No controls	0.65	0.36–1.15	2.38	(1,32)
Full controls	0.76	0.44–1.30	11.56***	(12,21)
Did Not Cut Meal Size				
No controls	0.70	0.43–1.13	2.32	(1,32)
Full controls	0.82	0.51–1.32	8.37***	(12,21)
Ate as Much as Usual				
No controls	0.59*	0.36–0.99	4.27*	(1,32)
Full controls	0.71	0.42–1.19	6.96***	(12,21)
Was Not Hungry				
No controls	0.46*	0.22–0.96	4.64*	(1,32)
Full controls	0.53	0.24–1.17	9.92***	(12,21)
Did Not Lose Weight				
No controls	0.20**	0.06–0.67	7.40**	(1,32)
Full controls	0.23**	0.07–0.83	9.44***	(12,21)
Ate Every Day				
No controls	0.14*	0.03–0.69	6.34*	(1,32)
Full controls	0.13*	0.02–0.73	4.69***	(12,21)

Note: In all the full controls models, I control for gender, age, and race at the child level; and household size, income, adult employment, food stamp receipt, emergency food receipt, and cash assistance receipt at the household level.

*$p < 0.05$, **$p < 0.01$, and ***$p < 0.001$

participate in school meal programs than in households where income-eligible children do not participate.

How does the association between children's school meal participation and adults' food security change by subsidy level and receipt frequency?

To examine how the association between children's school meal participation and adults' food security changes by subsidy level and meal receipt frequency, I run a series of OLS regressions predicting the adult food security score and display results in Table 3.2, Models 2 and 3.

Model 2 ($R^2 = 0.22$) shows the association between subsidy level for children participating in the NSLP and the food security of adults within the same household. Results indicate that the food security score for adults in households with a child receiving a reduced-price school lunch does not differ from those in households with a child receiving full-price meals. However, adults in households with a child receiving free lunches are expected to have a food security score one point lower (SE = 0.30; $p < 0.01$) than those in households with a child paying the full price. The score for those with a child receiving reduced-price meals does not differ from those paying the full price. Additionally, the model shows that adults in households receiving emergency food assistance are expected to have a food security score three points lower (SE = 0.24, $p < 0.001$) than those in households not receiving it. Further, for every additional household member, an adult's score is expected to decrease by 0.2 of a point (SE = 0.06, $p < 0.05$). In regard to subsidy level, I therefore find that adults in households with a child receiving free school lunches are more likely to be food insecure than those in households with a child paying the full price for the meals.

Model 3 ($R^2 = 0.21$) shows the association between a child's school lunch receipt frequency and the food security of adults within the same household. Results indicate no relationship between the number of school lunches a child receives per week and the food security score of an adult within the same household. However, for every one person increase in household size, an adult's food security score is expected to decrease by 0.2 of a point (SE = 0.06; $p < 0.05$). Further, adults in households receiving emergency food assistance are expected to have a food security score three points (SE = 0.25; $p < 0.001$) lower compared to those in households not receiving it. In summary, I do not find a relationship between a child's school lunch receipt frequency and adult food security status.

Discussion

This chapter examines the association between children's school meal program participation and adult food security. Although previous research on food security and nutritional assistance programs suggests that school meals provide a substantial amount of calories to children and may allow for intrahousehold food resource reallocation, reducing adult buffering and alleviating adult food insecurity, the results of the present analysis do not support this conclusion. In contrast, I find that children's school meal participation is negatively associated with adult food security, and is stronger when children receive higher levels of benefits.

Examining whether the association between children's school meal program participation is associated with adult food security, and how it varies by program participation level, subsidy level, and receipt frequency, I find that the factors are negatively associated. Parental buffering behavior does not appear responsive to a child's school meal program participation as the argument initially assumed. Additional analyses show that having lost weight and not eating all day are two adults' food security behaviors associated with children's school meal participation. The inverse association between children's school meal participation and adult food security is strengthened where benefit receipt is greater, with adults with children participating in more programs and receiving a higher level of subsidy having lower food security scores. The association is partially explained after controlling for individual- and household-level factors. For adults in households with a child who participates in both school meal programs as compared to one, and with a child receiving NSLP benefits at maximum subsidy level as compared to one receiving no subsidy, the negative association with food security scores persists. These results, showing that adults in child participant households are more likely to be food insecure than their counterparts with nonparticipant children, do not support the assertion that consistent access to food for children through school meal programs allows for sufficient reallocation of household resources to lower adult food insecurity. The presence of multiple hardships and the problem of sample self-selection may help explain the results obtained.

The findings may indicate the presence of multiple hardships in the households examined, all under the 185% of the federal poverty line, that prevent them from reallocating the freed-up resources to meal provision for adults. Studies show that winter cooling and summer heating costs represent a substantial burden for these households and seasonally exacerbate their food insecurity, with families having to choose between food and paying for utilities in "heat or eat" and "cool or eat" dilemmas (Bhattacharya et al. 2003). Low-income families shift their resources towards utilities and decrease their food intake in the winter, but this is not the case in high-income households. (Nord and Kantor 2006). Other research shows that school breakfast participation only reduces the risk of marginal but not low food insecurity (Bartfeld and Ahn 2011), indicating that program benefits only have spillover effects at a relatively high threshold. When freed up through school meal programs, additional resources may, therefore, be allocated to addressing other hardships, not to addressing adult buffering, or the benefits may not be sufficiently high to increase adults' food security.

In regard to benefit level, self-selection may explain the stronger and persistent negative association between greater levels of children's school meal participation and adult food security. Sample self-selection is a recognized federal assistance program evaluation issue (Nord and Golla 2009) that complicates assessments of whether meal programs lower the rate of food insecurity (Kaiser and Townsend 2005; Nord and Parker 2010, p. 1179). Estimates using NHANES show that over 60% of free lunch recipients come from households with an annual income below 130% of the poverty line (Ralston et al. 2008), and food insecurity rates are higher for households near and below the federal poverty line (Coleman-Jensen et al. 2013). This is despite the fact that school meal programs were not primarily intended to address food insecurity (Dillard 2009; Poppendieck 2010). Additionally, the cross-sectional nature of the data may exacerbate the self-selection problem: the data only offer a snapshot in time, but household food security status changes throughout the year. The snapshot may reflect either the program's benefits or the household's hardship.

The child's Hispanic ethnicity, household size, and emergency food receipt as control variables found to be associated with lower adult food security scores lend support to the self-selection explanation for the results obtained. Hispanic children participate in school meal programs at higher levels than white children (Ralston et al. 2008), and Hispanic households have both higher rates of food insecurity and a higher prevalence of very low food security than the national average (Coleman-Jensen et al. 2013). Further, food resource redistribution to address adult food insecurity may be more difficult in larger households with more children, children not attending school, or elderly members. Additionally, emergency food receipt is indicative of an extreme level of food hardship at which school meal provision may have no discernible positive association with adult food security scores. Consistent with this explanation, the association between household emergency food receipt and lower adult food security scores was significant at the highest threshold, with adults in such households having food security scores 3 points lower than those in nonrecipient households, sufficient to move an individual to a lower food security category.

In sum, in considering the implications of children's school meal programs for adults, I do not find evidence for spillover effects of the nutritional assistance programs. Instead, I detect sample self-selection indicating that school meal programs serve a significant population of children in households with food insecure adults. At its inception, the NSLP was not primarily intended as a welfare program addressing food insecurity. Rather, it was a response to overproduction and agricultural surplus (Dillard 2009) and a means of controlling food prices (Poppendieck 2010). Historically, it grew most significantly during the war on hunger and was rebranded from a general to a welfare program during the war on poverty; at the time, it aligned ideologically with compulsory schooling and the need to provide adequate nutrition for children in light of research showing that hunger is linked to reduced concentration, irritability, and disruptive behaviors, and that poor health may result in school absenteeism (Levine 2008). As a result, the program maintained a broad focus on all schoolchildren and not only those from food insecure households. While the programs were therefore primarily developed to control food prices and support domestic food production, and not to address food insecurity, the present result suggests that households may be using them to address this hardship. These findings may, therefore, indicate that school meal programs have a significant class component and are now primarily reaching households coping with food insecurity, rather than supporting the educational experience and providing nutritious meals for all children, as originally intended.

Limitations and future research

Dataset and sample issues limit the present study. First, NHANES' cross-sectional design precludes causal inferences, as it is not possible to distinguish between the effects of children's school meal participation on adults' food security from the effect of other correlates. While I find the presence of an association, I cannot disentangle the temporal ordering of the two factors or eliminate the possibility that a factor unaccounted for is driving the relationship. The periodicity of food insecurity further complicates the issue: for most households, food insecurity is recurrent, but not chronic (Coleman-Jensen et al. 2013). Within a year, the condition arises in three or more months for over 60% of households, and for 20% it arises almost every month (Nord et al. 2002). A measure with a more precisely delimited time period is necessary to address this temporal mismatch between children's school meal program participation and adults' food security.

Second, NHANES was not designed for assessing food insecurity or program policy issues and does not make publicly available information on urbanicity, region, and state factors (Coleman-Jensen et al. 2013). Average wages, housing costs, assistance program accessibility, and tax policies account are state-level factors associated with differences in food insecurity prevalence(Bartfeld et al. 2006). Additionally, macroeconomic conditions affect program participation (Hanson and Oliveira 2012), and states may have additional school meal program regulations in place. An improved analysis would include state- and school-level controls to more accurately establish eligibility and control for school characteristics.

Third, sample characteristics may have impacted the results obtained. Self-selection may partially account for the presence of a negative association between children's school meal program participation and adult food security. Previous research used the instrumental variables strategy and a difference-in-differences design to address the issue, neither of which is possible with NHANES due to its limited economic data collection. Certification error and undercoverage are two other sample-related factors warranting caution. While there are no direct ways to address the latter two, the issue of eligibility determination may be alleviated in datasets with more individual- and household-level economic information. Future research using longitudinal data and datasets containing more demographic and household information could determine with greater certainty the extent to which nutritional assistance program spillover effects occur within the household and the extent to which self-selection poses a problem in program evaluation.

REFERENCES

Adams, Elizabeth J., Laurence, Grummer–Strawn, and Gilberto Chavez. 2003. Food insecurity is associated with increased risk of obesity in California women. *Journal of Nutrition* 133(4):1070–1074.

Administration for Children and Families. 2014. *Child Abuse and Neglect*. Children's Bureau. Accessed May 23, 2016. http://www.acf.hhs.gov/programs/cb/focus–areas/child–abuse–neglect.

Ahluwalia, Indu B., Janice M. Dodds, and Magda Baligh. 1998. Social support and coping behaviors of low-income families experiencing food insufficiency in North Carolina. *Health Education and Behavior* 25(5):599–612. doi: 10.1177/109019819802500507.

Anderson, S. A. 1990. Core indicators of nutritional state for difficult to sample populations. *Journal of Nutrition* 120(11):1557–1600.

Arteaga, Irma, and Colleen Heflin. 2014. Participation in the National School Lunch Program and Food Security:An analysis of transitions into kindergarten. *Children and Youth Services Review* 47:224–230. doi: 10.1016/j.childyouth.2014.09.014.

Bartfeld, Judi, Rachel Dunifon, Mark Nord and Steven Carlson. 2006. *What Factors Account for State-to-State Differences in Food Security?* Economic Information Bulletin Number 20. Washington, DC: USDA Economic Research Service. Accessed May 23, 2016. http://www.ers.usda.gov/media/860374/eib20_002.pdf

Bartfeld, Judith S. and Hong-Min Ahn. 2011. The School Breakfast Program strengthens household food security among low-income households with elementary school children. *Journal of Nutrition* 141(3):470–475. doi: 10.3945/jn.110.130823.

Beaton, George H. and Hossein Ghassemi. 1982. Supplementary feeding programs for young children in developing countries. *American Journal of Clinical Nutrition* 35(4):864–916.

Belot, Michèle, and Jonathan James. 2011. Healthy school meals and educational outcomes. *Journal of Health Economics* 30(3):489–504. doi: 10.1016/J. Jhealeco.2011.02.003.

Bhattacharya, Jayanta, Janet Currie, and Steven Haider. 2004. Poverty, food insecurity, and nutritional outcomes in children and adults. *Journal of Health Economics* 23(4):839–862. doi: 10.1016/j.jhealeco.2003.12.008.

Bhattacharya, Jayanta, Janet Currie, and Steven Haider. 2006. Breakfast of champions? The School Breakfast Program and the nutrition of children and families. *Journal of Human Resources* 41(3):445–466. doi: 10.3368/jhr.xli.3.445.

Bhattacharya, Jayanta, Thomas Deleire, Steven Haider, and Janet Currie. 2003. Heat or eat? Cold-weather shocks and nutrition in poor American families. *American Journal of Public Health* 93(7):1149–1154. doi: 10.2105/ajph.93.7.1149.

Bickel, Gary, Mark Nord, Cristofer Price, William Hamilton, and John Cook. 2000. *Guide to Measuring Household Food Security, Revised.* Alexandria, VA: USDA Food and Nutrition Service.

Briefel, Ronette R., Ander Wilson, and Philip M. Gleason. 2009. Consumption of low-nutrient, energy-dense foods and beverages at school, home, and other locations among school lunch participants and nonparticipants. *Journal of the American Dietetic Association* 109(2):S79–S90. doi: 10.1016/j.jada.2008.10.064.

Burghardt, John A., Anne R. Gordon, and Thomas M. Fraker. 1995. Meals offered in the National School Lunch Program and the School Breakfast Program. *American Journal of Clinical Nutrition* 61(1S):187–198.

Byker, Carmen J., Courtney A. Pinard, Amy L. Yaroch, and Elena L. Serrano. 2013. Viewpoint: New NSLP guidelines: Challenges and opportunities for nutrition education practitioners and researchers. *Journal of Nutrition Education and Behavior* 45(6):683–689. doi: 10.1016/j.jneb.2013.06.004.

Campbell, Benjamin L., Rodolfo M. Nayga, John L. Park, and Andres Silva. 2011. Does the National School Lunch Program improve children's dietary outcomes? *American Journal of Agricultural Economics* 93(4):1099–1130. doi: 10.1093/ajae/aar031.

Carney, Megan. 2012. Compounding crises of economic recession and food insecurity: A comparative study of three low-income communities in Santa Barbara County. *Agriculture and Human Values* 29(2):185–201. doi: 10.1007/s10460-011-9333-y.

Centers for Disease Control and Prevention. 2010. *National Health and Nutrition Examination Survey Data.* Hyattsville, MD: U.S. Department of Health and Human Services, Centers for Disease Control and Prevention. 2009–2010. Accessed May 23, 2016. http://wwwn.cdc.gov/nchs/nhanes/search/nhanes09_10.aspx

Clark, Melissa A. and Mary Kay Fox. 2009. Nutritional quality of the diets of US Public school children and the role of the school meal programs. *Journal of the American Dietetic Association* 109(2):S44–S56. doi: 10.1016/j.jada.2008.10.060.

Coates, Jennifer, Edward A. Frongillo, Beatrice Lorge Rogers, Patrick Webb, Parke E. Wilde and Robert Houser. 2006. Commonalities in the experience of household food insecurity across cultures: What are measures missing? *Journal of Nutrition* 136(5):S1438–S1448.

Coleman-Jensen, A., Nord, M., and Singh, A. 2013. *Household Food Security in the United States in 2012.* Economic Research Report-155. Alexandria, VA: USDA Economic Research Service.

Connell, Carol L., Kristi L. Lofton, Kathy Yadrick, and Timothy A. Rehner. 2005. Children's experiences of food insecurity can assist in understanding its effect on their well-being. *Journal of Nutrition* 135(7):1683–1690.

Current Population Survey Food Security Supplement. 2012. *Technical Documentation.* Washington: U.S. Census Bureau. Accessed May 25, 2014. http://www.census.gov/prod/techdoc/cps/cpsdec12.pdf

Currie, J. 2003. US Food and Nutrition Programs. In *Means-Tested Transfer Programs in the United States*, edited by R. A. Moffit. Chicago, IL: University of Chicago Press, pp. 199–290.

Department of Agriculture. 2012. Nutrition Standards in the National School Lunch and School Breakfast Programs. Final Rule, RIN 0584–AD59. Federal Register 77(17). Accessed May 23, 2016. https://www.regulations.gov/#!documentDetail;D=FNS-2007-0038-64676

Dillard, A. J. 2009. Sloppy Joe, slop, sloppy Joe: How USDA commodities dumping ruined the National School Lunch Program. *Oregon Law Review* 87(2):221–259.

Fiese, Barbara H., Craig Gundersen, Brenda Koester, and Latesha Washington. 2011. Household food insecurity: Serious concerns for child development. *Society for Research in Child Development, Social Policy Report* 25(3):3–19.

Food and Nutrition Service. 2013a. National School Lunch Program Fact Sheet. Accessed March 25, 2014. http://www.fns.usda.gov/sites/default/files/nslpfactsheet.pdf

Food and Nutrition Service. 2013b. School Breakfast Program Fact Sheet. Accessed March 25, 2014. http://www.fns.usda.gov/sites/default/files/sbpfactsheet.pdf

Food and Nutrition Service. 2014. Food Distribution Programs. Accessed March 25, 2014. http://www.fns.usda.gov/fdd/food–distribution–programs

Food Research and Action Center. 2011. School Breakfast Program Scorecard 2009–2010. Accessed March 25, 2014. http://frac.org/wp–content/uploads/2011/01/

Fram, Maryah Stella, Edward A. Frongillo, Sonya J. Jones, Roger C. Williams, Michael P. Burke, Kendra P. Deloach, and Christine E. Blake. 2011. Children are aware of food insecurity and take responsibility for managing food resources. *Journal of Nutrition* 141(6):1114–1119. doi: 10.3945/jn.110.135988.

Gleason, Philip M. and Carol W. Suitor. 2003. Eating at school: How the National School Lunch Program Affects Children's Diets. *American Journal of Agricultural Economics* 85(4):1047–1061. doi: 10.1111/1467-8276.00507.

Gowda, Charitha, Craig Hadley, and Allison E. Aiello. 2012. The association between food insecurity and inflammation in the US Adult Population. *American Journal of Public Health* 102(8):1579–1586. doi: 10.2105/ajph.2011.300551.

Hanson, Kenneth and Victor Oliveira. 2012. *How Economic Conditions Affect Participation in USDA Nutrition Assistance Programs.* Economic Information Bulletin Number 100 (EIB-100). Alexandria, VA: Economic Research Service.

Howard, Larry L. and Nishith Prakash. 2012. Do school lunch subsidies change the dietary patterns of children from low-income households? *Contemporary Economic Policy* 30(3):362–381. doi: 10.1111/j.1465-7287.2011.00264.x.

Hoynes, Hilary W. and Diane Whitmore Schanzenbach. 2009. Consumption responses to in–kind transfers: Evidence from the introduction of the food stamp program. *American Economic Journal: Applied Economics* 1(4):109–139. doi: 10.1257/app.1.4.109.

Jacoby, Hanan G. 2002. Is there an intra household fly paper effect? Evidence from a School Feeding Programme. *Economic Journal* 112(476):196–221. doi: 10.1111/1468-0297.0j679.

Jyoti, Diana F., Edward A. Frongillo, and Sonya J. Jones. 2005. Food insecurity affects school children's academic performance, weight gain, and social skills. *Journal of Nutrition* 135(12):2831–2839.

Kaiser, Lucia L. and Marilyn S. Townsend. 2005. Food insecurity among US children: Implications for nutrition and health. *Topics in Clinical Nutrition* 20(2):313–320. doi: 10.1097/00008486-200510000-00004.

Kendall, Anne, Christine M. Olson and Edward A. Frongillo. 1996. Relationship of hunger and food insecurity to food availability and consumption. *Journal of the American Dietetic Association* 96(19):1019–1024. doi: 10.1016/s0002-8223(96)00271-4.

Larson, Nicole I. and Mary T. Story. 2011. Food insecurity and weight status among U.S. children and families: Are view of the literature. *American Journal of Preventive Medicine* 40(2):166–173. doi: 10.1016/j.amepre.2010.10.028.

Levine, Susan. 2008. *School Lunch Politics: The Surprising History of America's Favorite Welfare Program.* Princeton, NJ: Princeton University Press. doi: 10.1515/9781400841486.

Long, Sharon K. 1991. Do the School Nutrition Programs supplement household food expenditures? *Journal of Human Resources* 26(4):654–678. doi: 10.2307/145979.

Mann, HyungHur. 2012. The Public School Lunch Program and its contribution to the alleviation of problem behaviors. *International Journal of Business and Social Science* 3(18):142–150.

Martin, Molly A. and Adam M. Lippert. 2012. Feeding her children, but risking her health: The intersection of gender, household food insecurity and obesity. *Social Science and Medicine* 74(11):1754–1764. doi: 10.1016/j.socscimed.2011.11.013.

Maxwell, Daniel G. 1996. Measuring food insecurity: The frequency and severity of "coping strategies." *Food Policy* 21(3):291–303. doi: 10.1016/0306-9192(96)00005-X.

McIntyre, Lynn, N. Theresa Glanville, Kim D. Raine, Jutta B. Dayle, Bonnie Anderson, and Noreen Battaglia. 2003. Do low-income lone mothers compromise their nutrition to feed their children? *Canadian Medical Association Journal* 168(6):686–691.

McLaughlin, Katie A., Jennifer Greif Green, Margarita Alegría, E. Jane Costello, Michael J. Gruber, Nancy A. Sampson, and Ronald C. Kessler. 2012. Food insecurity and mental disorders in a national sample of U.S. adolescents. *Journal of the American Academy of Child and Adolescent Psychiatry* 51(12):1293–1303. doi: 10.1016/j.jaac.2012.09.009.

Meng, Ding, Norbert W. Wilson, Kimberly B. Garza, and Claire A. Zizza. 2014. Undiagnosed prediabetes among food insecure adults. *American Journal of Health Behavior* 38(2):225–233. doi: 10.5993/ajhb.38.2.8.

Nord, Mark. 2009. *Food Spending Declined and Food Insecurity Increased for Middle-Income and Low-Income Households from 2000 to 2007.* Economic Information Bulletin Number 61. Alexandria, VA: Economic Research Service.

Nord, Mark, Margaret Andrews, and Joshua Winicki. 2002. Frequency and duration of food insecurity and hunger in US Households. *Journal of Nutrition Education and Behavior* 34(4):194–201. doi: 10.1016/s1499-4046(06)60093-6.

Nord, Mark and Anne Marie Golla. 2009. *Does SNAP Decrease Food Insecurity? Untangling the Self-Selection Effect.* USDA Economic Research Report Number 85. Alexandria, VA: Economic Research Service.

Nord, Mark and Heather Hopwood. 2007. Recent advances provide improved tools for measuring children's food security. *Journal of Nutrition* 137(3):533–536.

Nord, Mark and Linda S. Kantor. 2006. Seasonal variation in food insecurity is associated with heating and cooling costs among low-income elderly Americans. *Journal of Nutrition* 136(11):2939–2944.

Nord, Mark and Lynn Parker. 2010. How adequately are food needs of children in low-income households being met? *Children and Youth Services Review* 32(9):1175–1185. doi: 10.1016/j.childyouth.2010.03.005.

Poppendieck, J. 2010. *Free for All: Fixing School Food in America.* Berkeley, CA: University of California Press.

Potamites, Elizabeth and Anne Gordon. 2010. *Children's Food Security and Intakes from School Meals: Final Report.* Report Number 61. Princeton, NJ: Mathematica Policy Research.

Ralston, Katherine, Constance Newman, Annette Clauson, Joanne Guthrie, and Jean Buzby. 2008. *The National School Lunch Program: Background, Trends, and Issues.* Economic Research Report Number 61. Alexandria, VA: Economic Research Service.

Schmidt, Lucie, Lara Shore-Sheppard, and Tara Watson. 2013. The Effect of Safety Net Programs on Food Insecurity. NBER Working Paper No. 19558. Accessed March 27, 2014. http://www.nber.org/papers/w19558

Slater, Joyce, Gustaaf Sevenhuysen, Barry Edginton, and John O'Neil. 2012. 'Trying to make it all come together': Structuration and employed mothers experience of family food provisioning in Canada. *Health Promotion International* 27(3):405–415. doi: 10.1093/heapro/dar037.

Smith, C, Parnell, W, Brown, R, and Gray, A. 2012. Providing additional money to food-insecure households and its effect on food expenditure: A randomized controlled trial. *Public Health Nutrition* 16(8):1507–15. doi: 10.1017/S1368980012003680.

Tarasuk, Valerie. 2005. Household food insecurity in Canada. *Topics in Clinical Nutrition* 20(4):299–312. doi: 10.1097/00008486-200510000-00003.

West, Donald A. and David W. Price. 1976. The effects of income, assets, food programs, and household size on food consumption. *American Journal of Agricultural Economics* 58(4):725–730. doi: 10.2307/1238816.

Whitaker, Robert C., Shannon M. Phillips, and Sean M. Orzol. 2006. Food insecurity and the risks of depression and anxiety in mothers and behavior problems in their preschool-aged children. *Pediatrics* 118(3):859–868. doi: 10.1542/peds.2006-0239.

4 The food environment and social determinants of food insufficiency and diet quality in rural households

Christian King

In 2014, 14% of households (or 48 million people) in the United States experienced food insecurity, a disruption in eating patterns or reduction in food consumption, preventing them from maintaining a healthy and active life (Coleman-Jensen et al. 2015). Trends in food insecurity in the United States have remained at around 14% since 2008. Food insecurity, which includes the inability to eat a healthy diet (malnutrition) and food deprivation, is associated with several micronutrient deficiencies, notably in vitamin B_{12} and folate (Alpert and Fava 1997; Reynolds 2002; Tiemeier et al. 2002). These deficiencies could help explain why food insecurity has many negative consequences. For example, food insecurity is associated with diabetes (Seligman et al. 2007), chronic disease (Seligman et al. 2010), maternal depression (Heflin et al. 2005; Whitaker et al. 2006), poor oral health (Muirhead et al. 2009), housing instability (King 2016), and other health problems (Gundersen and Ziliak 2015). These negative outcomes could have substantial direct and indirect costs through the healthcare costs resulting from poor health, chronic disease, and the loss of productivity or inability to work (Lee 2013; Phipps et al. 2016).

Several factors contribute to food insecurity, and low income is an important one (Coleman-Jensen et al. 2015; Gundersen and Ziliak 2015). As a result, institutional support through public assistance programs such as the Supplemental Nutrition Assistance Program (SNAP) has been found to be effective in reducing the risk of experiencing food insecurity (Ziliak 2015). However, the provision of institutional support is not a one-size-fits-all solution and is not always effective in all settings such as in rural communities (Garasky et al. 2006; Morton et al. 2005).

Although rural populations in the United States declined over time, rural residents still represented 15% of the total population spread across 72% of the land area nationwide in 2015 (United States Department of Agriculture 2016). Other than income, access to food is also a strong determinant of food security and dietary intake (United States Department of Agriculture 2009). There is no formal definition of the food environment and empirical studies typically use various measures relating to the availability, accessibility, and affordability of healthy foods (e.g., Morland et al. 2002; Kubik et al. 2003; Moore et al. 2008a,b). Rural communities tend to have a poorer food environment than urban communities because food sources are not evenly distributed and there is a lack of small grocery stores partly due to their consolidation into larger stores. Furthermore, rural communities typically face higher transportation costs, higher food prices, and have access to lower quality foods (Powell et al. 2007; Sharkey 2009). As a result, food insecurity and diet quality is a more severe issue for rural residents (Dean and Sharkey 2011; Coleman-Jensen et al. 2015).

Some evidence from the literature shows that the social context of rural communities could mitigate some of the negative impacts of poor food access and improve dietary intake (Morton et al. 2005; Garasky et al. 2006; Smith and Morton 2009; Smith and Miller 2011). However, these studies focus on case studies of one or a handful of rural communities. It is then difficult to determine the generalizability of these findings.

The first question this chapter examines is "(1) How do the type and number of stores affect food insecurity and diet quality in rural households?" While the studies on food access in rural areas document negative impacts of the food environment on dietary intake, these studies have limitations relating to their generalizability. This chapter uses a sample of rural residents from the Centers for Disease Control and Prevention's (CDC) Behavioral Risk Factor Surveillance System (BRFSS), which has the advantage of having a large number of respondents (the most recent years have about 400,000) and being administered in every state. As a result, when survey weights are used, the BRFSS is representative of the civilian noninstitutionalized adult population in the United States. The second question this chapter examines is "(2) How does the relationship between the number of stores available to rural residents and their dietary quality change when examining informal social support?" Some studies show that social capital and informal support networks reduce the risk of food insecurity for households in some rural communities (Garasky et al. 2006; Dean and Sharkey 2011; Dean et al. 2011). The last question this chapter examines is "(3) Can health behaviors explain some of the relationships between food access and dietary intake?"

Some studies have shown that the food environment is associated with health behaviors (e.g., Sallis and Glanz 2009), health behaviors are known to affect dietary quality (Pearson and Biddle 2011). However, whether individual health behaviors can overcome some of the negative impacts of food access is not well understood. The analysis in this chapter uses ordinary least squares regressions to examine food insecurity and diet quality. I conclude this chapter by discussing the potential policy implications of the findings.

Literature review

This section provides a review of the relevant literature. First, I explain how food deserts are commonly understood and how they relate to food access. I review studies examining the relationship between food access and dietary intake. I then review the literature examining how the social context and health behaviors affect dietary intake.

Food access and food deserts

According to the USDA, food access is commonly understood as the travel time to shop for groceries and the availability of healthy foods from food retailers. There are two commonly used measures in the literature to measure food access and the food environment: food stores density and store proximity (Charreire et al. 2010). Store density is a measure that estimates the number of stores in a geographical area. The proximity measure calculates the distance or travel time to stores. Food deserts refer to low-income households living far away from a grocery store.

Households live in food deserts if their income is below the federal poverty guidelines and the closest supermarket is greater than a mile away in urban areas and greater than 10 miles away in rural communities (United States Department of Agriculture 2012a,b). Food deserts tend to have higher poverty rates, a higher proportion of racial minority populations, higher population decreases, lower levels of education, and higher unemployment (United States Department of Agriculture 2012a,b). Rural residents face greater challenges in food access as there are fewer food store outlets in rural areas than in urban areas (Powell et al. 2007). Often, rural households need to travel greater distances than urban residents to buy groceries, with few to no walkable options available.

Food access and dietary intake

The availability and accessibility of food is a strong determinant of consumption. Grocery stores tend to have higher quality foods than convenience stores (Glanz et al. 2007). In addition, proximity and easy access to supermarkets is linked with greater fruit intake and food security (Rose and Richards 2004; Bartfeld et al. 2010). In a review of the literature, Larson et al. (2009) cite evidence showing that neighborhoods with better access to supermarkets and limited access to convenience stores tend to have healthier diets. While the evidence from the literature suggests that store density and proximity have a direct influence on food insecurity and diet quality, the few studies that examine rural settings are mainly based on case studies or geographically restricted samples.

Both store density and proximity are more problematic for rural households. Rural communities are not as well served by public transit as urban areas (Stommes and Brown 2002). As a result, rural residents are more reliant on cars as their main mode of transportation, which exacerbates the mobility issues of groups such as elderly people (Rosenbloom 2004). In addition, there are generally fewer grocery stores in rural areas than in urban areas (Powell et al. 2007). This means that rural households have fewer stores to shop for groceries and they have to travel larger distances to do their shopping (Sharkey 2009). These higher transportation costs could affect the type of foods rural households decide to purchase. Not only is fresh food more expensive than processed (or unhealthy) food (Monsivais and Drewnowski 2007; Monsivais et al. 2010), but also it does not last as long. Therefore, unless rural households are shopping more frequently, poor food access would likely lead them to purchase more processed foods that can last longer.

Dean and Sharkey (2011) show that greater distance to supermarkets is associated with lower consumption of fruits and vegetables in rural settings but not in urban settings. Rural neighborhoods tend to have poorer access to supermarkets and consume unhealthier foods. Gantner et al. (2011) examine an 8700-square-mile area in upstate New York and find that most food retail stores have unhealthy foods and less than half have fresh produce. In addition, these residents tend to live further away from fresh produce than processed foods such as soda and chips. Hendrickson et al. (2006) examine food access and food cost in four communities (two urban and two rural) in food deserts in Minnesota. They find that the major barriers to accessing healthy foods in these communities were cost, quality of food, and the limited choices available. In addition, two studies of rural communities in Iowa find that the lack of grocery stores increases the risk of food insecurity (Morton et al. 2005; Smith and Morton 2009).

Social context and dietary intake

The social environment, typically referred to as any informal type of social support or social capital, may also play a role in affecting diet quality and food insecurity. Households could receive assistance from friends and family in their social network, which would improve their diet quality and food security. For example, individuals might directly receive food from their network or improve their food access through transportation or better nutritional knowledge (Swanson et al. 2008; De Marco and Thorburn 2009).

Several studies have shown that social capital has protective factors against food insecurity (Walker et al. 2007; Kirkpatrick and Tarasuk 2010; dos Santos Interlenghi and Salles-Costa 2015). Households with stronger social and informal networks, and those are able to use them when in need, are less likely to experience food insecurity. On the other hand, De Marco and Thorburn (2009) find that social support does not have an association with food insecurity for a sample of households in Oregon. It may be that social support is relevant only in rural communities (Garasky et al. 2006; Morton et al. 2008), where they are relied upon more than in urban settings (Smith and Miller 2011).

Social support could mediate and overcome some of the food access and transportation issues. For example, rural residents with transportation issues—owing to cost or physical mobility—could rely on social support from friends and family to shop for groceries. Two studies examined rural communities in Central Texas and found that those with low social capital were more likely to be food insecure (Dean and Sharkey 2011; Dean et al. 2011). Smith and Morton (2009) find that the social environment and civic engagement can improve food access and food security in rural food deserts in Minnesota and Iowa. Garasky et al. (2006) argue that informal support networks could counteract the negative impacts of the poor food environment in rural households in two rural counties in Iowa. In addition, Morton et al. (2008) show that informal organizations such as food banks could benefit rural neighborhoods. Comparing between low-income urban and rural neighborhoods, the study also finds that the rural neighborhoods were more likely to engage in reciprocal nonmarket food exchanges by donating and receiving foods to friends and families.

Health behaviors and dietary intake

Aside from the physical and social environment, health behaviors also affect dietary intake. A review of the literature on sedentary behaviors and dietary intake concludes that there is an association with health behaviors and dietary intake (Pearson and Biddle 2011). In addition, one study focusing on children shows that sedentary behaviors such as lack of physical activity, television screening time, and poor sleep habits are strongly associated with food insecurity (Canter et al. 2016). Sallis and Glanz (2009) explain that the food environment could be conducive to active recreation and active transportation. This would imply that the food environment in rural communities would be less conducive to healthy behaviors due to the impracticality of walking to the grocery store. However, social support may mitigate some of the negative impacts of the food environment on health behaviors and dietary intake. For example, there is abundant evidence showing that social support is associated with health behaviors (Berkman et al. 2000). Individuals who have higher levels of social support are more likely to engage in healthier behaviors. Allgöwer et al. (2001) show that low social support is associated with unhealthy behaviors such as alcohol consumption, low physical activity, poor sleep, and risky behaviors such as not wearing a seat belt. As a result, social support and health behaviors could reduce some of the negative impacts of the food environment on food insecurity and diet quality.

In summary, despite findings on the physical and informal social environment on food consumption, research on their interaction is limited, especially in rural communities. In addition, it is unclear how generalizable the findings from previous studies on rural communities are.

Methods

This chapter examines the following questions: (1) How does the number of stores affect food insecurity and diet quality in rural households? (2) How does this relationship change when examining informal social support? (3) Can health behaviors explain some of these relationships?

Data for this chapter come from the CDC BRFSS, a telephone survey administered in all 50 states, which collects health-related information. The CDC explains that the survey has "become a powerful tool for targeting and building health promotion activities." The survey, which interviews about 400,000 randomly selected adults, has been administered annually in all 50 states since 1984. When survey weights are used, the BRFSS is representative of the civilian noninstitutionalized adult population in the United States.

The BRFSS survey has a core questionnaire standardized across all states, which compiles information about individual risk behaviors and preventive health practices that could affect their health status. Each state is encouraged to add additional optional modules and questions.

This chapter uses data from the 2009 to 2012 surveys and restricts the sample to nonelderly adults (less than 65 years old) in households living in metropolitan statistical areas (MSA) that have no center city or not living in MSA. The BRFSS provides information about the state and county each respondent lives in. I exclude from the sample adults with missing values on the county identifier. Observations with missing data on food insecurity and fruits and vegetables consumption are excluded from the sample. The analytical sample includes 60,174 adults living in rural households.

The analysis uses two outcome variables: food insecurity and the number of times a day a person consumes fruits and vegetables. Food insecurity is a binary variable measured using the following question: "How often in the past 12 months would you say you were worried or stressed about having enough money to buy nutrition meals?" Respondents who answered "always," "usually," or "sometimes" were considered food insecure. The standard measure of food insecurity is the U.S. Department of Agriculture Food Security Module (FSM), which is used in the Current Population Survey (CPS). The module asks a series of 10 or 18 questions for households without or with children and categorizes them as food secure or food insecure depending on the number of affirmative responses provided to these questions. The stress-related food security question was validated against the FSM and considered acceptable to measure food insecurity ($r = 0.71, p < 0.001$) (Irving et al. 2014). The food insecurity questionnaire was an optional module, which was not part of the core questions administered by all states. Only the following 13 states administered this module: Alabama, Delaware, Hawaii, Illinois, Indiana, Louisiana, Michigan, Nebraska, North Carolina, Oklahoma, South Carolina, Tennessee, and Wisconsin.

To measure fruits and vegetable consumption, I use five questions that ask how many times a day the respondent consumed different types of fruits and vegetables. I sum these responses and construct a measure indicating how many fruits and vegetables were consumed daily. The standard measure of diet quality is the Healthy Eating Index (HEI). The original measure was developed in 1995 by the United State Department of Agriculture's Center for Nutrition Policy and Promotion (CNPP). The measure has been refined every 5 or 10 years. The HEI-1995 was refined into the HEI-2005, which was refined into the HEI-2010. The CNPP is planning to update the HEI-2005. The HEI is composed of several food items, and each item is assigned a score depending on the quantity consumed. The points are summed up, and the index ranges from 0 to 100, with 0 being the least healthy diet and 100 being the healthiest one. The BRFSS does not have all the items that are in the HEI, which cannot be constructed using this dataset. Nevertheless, the CDC explains that the module is valid and moderately reliable to detect population-level change, while it is not reliable to monitor trends in consumption (Centers for Disease Control and Prevention 2015).

Individual social support is measured using the following question: "How often do you get the emotional support needed?" Responses are (1) always, (2) usually,

(3) sometimes, (4) rarely, and (5) never. A binary measure of social support is created with 0 being rarely or never and 1 the other responses.

Since the BRFSS does not have information on store proximity, I use the number of stores to measure food access. I use data from the County Business Patterns, which compiles annual economic data by industry, to construct measures of food accessibility. The measures include the number of establishments for the following stores using the North American Industry Classification System (NAICS): supermarkets and other grocery stores (not convenience stores), food specialty stores, convenience stores, warehouse stores, full-service restaurants, limited-service eating places, liquor retail stores, and tobacco retail stores. I combine supermarkets with specialty stores and convenience with warehouse stores. A total of six variables count the number of each type of stores.

To measure institutional informal support, I include data on the number of nonprofit food banks and pantries available in each county annually using the National Center for Charitable Statistics (NCCS). The NCCS provides data on the number of registered nonprofit organizations, their revenues, assets, and those that filled out a return of organization exempt from income tax (form 990). I create a variable that indicates the number of nonprofit food banks and pantries in each county.

To account for health behaviors, I include variables indicating smoking status (current smoker, former smoker, or never smoked), the average number of alcoholic beverages consumed per day, the number of days in the past month that the physical health of the respondent was not good, the number of days in the past month that the mental health of the respondent was not good, whether the respondent was in general in poor or fair health, and whether the respondent reported any exercising.

The control variables include age, race/ethnicity (white, black, Hispanic, Asian, or other), gender, marital status (never married, married, divorced, widowed, and separated), number of children, education (less than high school, high school, some college, and college graduate or beyond), and income categories. The analysis uses linear regressions using ordinary least squares to examine food insecurity and diet quality. The regressions use weights to account for the sampling design of the survey and control for state and survey year.

Results

Table 4.1 presents summary statistics for the proportion of food insecure adults and their daily consumption of fruits and vegetables. Approximately 24.7% of adults living in rural households in this sample experienced food insecurity. The adults in this sample consumed fruits and vegetables approximately 3.3 times a day. In comparison, Lutfiyya et al. (2012) use the BRFSS to find that urban residents in this sample consume on average more fruits and vegetables than rural residents. Dean and Sharkey (2011) use a sample of households in a region in Texas and find that the urban respondents in their sample consume more fruits and vegetables than the rural respondents.

Table 4.1 Summary Statistics for the 2009–2012 BRFSS
for Non-Elderly Adults Living in Rural Areas

Variables	Mean
Food insecure (%)	24.7
Daily serving of fruits and vegetables	3.3
Female	61.0
Age	49.2
Race/Ethnicity (%)	
White	83.3
Black	5.8
Hispanic	4.7
Asian	1.1
Other	5.1
Marital Status (%)	
Married	63.3
Divorced	15.5
Widowed	5.9
Separated	3.6
Never married	11.7
Education (%)	
Less than high school	6.9
High school	31.3
Some college	28.9
College graduate or beyond	32.9
Employment Status (%)	
Employed	56.1
Self-employed	11.1
Unemployed	6.7
Homemaker	6.5
Retired	9.3
Unable to work	10.3
Income Categories (%)	
Less than $15,000	11.5
$15,000–$24,999	15.8
$25,000–$34,999	11.1
$35,000–$49,999	15.8
$50,000 or more	45.8
Poor or fair health	18.0
Smoker Status (%)	
Current smoker	20.7

(*Continued*)

Table 4.1 (Continued) Summary Statistics for the 2009–2012 BRFSS for Non-Elderly Adults Living in Rural Areas

Variables	Mean
Former smoker	25.8
Never smoked	53.6
Number of days physical health not good	4.3
Number of days mental health not good	4.1
Has social and emotional support needed (%)	89.3
Number of Establishments	
Supermarkets and specialty stores	22.1
Convenience and warehouse stores	8.4
Full service restaurants	58.9
Limited service restaurants	47.9
Liquor stores	7.6
Tobacco stores	2.1
Number of food banks and pantries	0.9
Number of observations	60,174

Even though the proportion of racial minorities has increased over time in rural areas, the sample remains predominantly white (83%). About 18% of adults in the sample reported being in poor or fair health. The average number of drinks consumed daily was about 1.16. About 46% of the sample reported being current or former smokers. The adults in the sample reported their physical and mental health being not good during about 4.3 and 4.1 days in a month, respectively. About 89% of the respondents reported getting the social and emotional support they needed. The table also reports the average number of establishments by category at the county level. A large proportion of food establishments in these counties are restaurants (full service and limited service). There is on average less than one (0.9) food bank and pantry in these rural counties.

Table 4.2 presents estimates examining the risk of food insecurity using four models. Model 1 shows the associations of the number of stores and food banks on food insecurity controlling for demographic and socioeconomic status. Surprisingly, the number of supermarkets increases the risk of food insecurity while the number of limited-service eating places reduces it. There is no association between the number of convenience stores and full-service restaurants on food insecurity. The number of liquor and tobacco retail stores both increase the risk of food insecurity. On the other hand, the number of food banks reduce food insecurity. Examining individual-level factors, racial minorities except Asians are more likely to experience food insecurity. Being married is a protective factor against food insecurity. Having children, lower levels of education, and lower income are factors that increase the risk of food insecurity.

Model 2 includes the health behavior measures, which do not seem to mediate the association of the type of stores and the number of food banks on food

Table 4.2 Estimates of the Impact of the Number of Stores on Food Insufficiency

	Model 1	*Model 2*	*Model 3*	*Model 4*
Female	0.037**	0.028**	0.167**	0.017*
	(0.007)	(0.007)	(0.030)	(0.007)
Age	0.010**	0.007**	0.003	0.008**
	(0.002)	(0.002)	(0.009)	(0.002)
Age^2	−0.000**	−0.000**	−0.000	−0.000**
	(0.000)	(0.000)	(0.000)	(0.000)
Black	0.035**	−0.023	0.142**	−0.015
	(0.013)	(0.013)	(0.044)	(0.013)
Asian	0.042	0.042	0.105	0.023
	(0.030)	(0.029)	(0.095)	(0.031)
Hispanic	0.086**	0.078**	−0.008	0.095**
	(0.020)	(0.020)	(0.054)	(0.021)
Other race	0.101**	0.088**	0.016	0.092**
	(0.016)	(0.016)	(0.042)	(0.017)
Married	−0.037**	−0.040**	0.002	−0.037**
	(0.012)	(0.012)	(0.043)	(0.012)
Divorced	0.076**	0.055**	0.074	0.041*
	(0.016)	(0.016)	(0.047)	(0.017)
Widowed	0.031	0.021	0.084	0.001
	(0.028)	(0.027)	(0.069)	(0.029)
Separated	0.132**	0.101**	0.036	0.108**
	(0.026)	(0.025)	(0.073)	(0.027)
Number of children	0.015**	0.012**	0.032**	0.010**
	(0.003)	(0.003)	(0.012)	(0.003)
Less than high school	0.068**	0.015	−0.059	0.021
	(0.016)	(0.016)	(0.060)	(0.017)
High school	0.041**	0.023*	−0.085	0.027**
	(0.010)	(0.010)	(0.051)	(0.010)
Some college	0.035**	0.022*	−0.104	0.027**
	(0.010)	(0.010)	(0.054)	(0.010)
Less than $15,000	0.260**	0.219**	0.290**	0.220**
	(0.016)	(0.015)	(0.051)	(0.016)
$15,000–$24,999	0.302**	0.264**	0.369**	0.256**
	(0.012)	(0.012)	(0.042)	(0.012)
$25,000–$34,999	0.172**	0.153**	0.229**	0.150**
	(0.012)	(0.012)	(0.052)	(0.012)
$35,000–$49,999	0.066**	0.057**	0.066	0.060**
	(0.010)	(0.010)	(0.048)	(0.010)
Poor health		0.118**	0.164**	0.115**
		(0.012)	(0.037)	(0.012)

(Continued)

Table 4.2 (Continued) Estimates of the Impact of the Number of Stores on Food Insufficiency

	Model 1	Model 2	Model 3	Model 4
Average drink per day		−0.000	0.011*	−0.001
		(0.001)	(0.005)	(0.001)
Self-employed	−0.039**	−0.039**	−0.215**	−0.029*
	(0.012)	(0.012)	(0.043)	(0.012)
Unemployed	0.102**	0.076**	0.090	0.075**
	(0.014)	(0.014)	(0.050)	(0.014)
Homemaker	0.022	0.018	−0.036	0.022
	(0.015)	(0.015)	(0.078)	(0.015)
Retired	−0.026	−0.048**	−0.012	−0.041*
	(0.018)	(0.017)	(0.080)	(0.018)
Unable to work	0.164**	0.036*	−0.072	0.043*
	(0.015)	(0.017)	(0.049)	(0.018)
Current smoker		0.029**	−0.059	0.035**
		(0.009)	(0.033)	(0.009)
Former smoker		0.009	−0.128**	0.018*
		(0.009)	(0.041)	(0.009)
Number of days poor physical health		0.001*	0.005**	0.001
		(0.001)	(0.002)	(0.001)
Number of days poor mental health		0.007**	0.006**	0.007**
		(0.000)	(0.001)	(0.001)
Social support		−0.104**		
		(0.014)		
Reports exercising		−0.008	−0.070*	−0.015
		(0.008)	(0.031)	(0.009)
Number of supermarkets and grocery stores	0.002*	0.002*	0.008*	0.001
	(0.001)	(0.001)	(0.003)	(0.001)
Number of convenience and warehouse stores	0.002	0.002	0.014*	0.003*
	(0.001)	(0.001)	(0.006)	(0.001)
Number of full service restaurants	−0.000	−0.000	−0.003**	0.000
	(0.000)	(0.000)	(0.001)	(0.000)
Number of limited service eating places	−0.001**	−0.001**	−0.000	−0.001**
	(0.000)	(0.000)	(0.002)	(0.000)
Number of liquor retail stores	0.006**	0.005**	0.022**	0.005**
	(0.001)	(0.001)	(0.006)	(0.001)

(*Continued*)

Table 4.2 (Continued) Estimates of the Impact of the Number of Stores on Food Insufficiency

	Model 1	Model 2	Model 3	Model 4
Number of tobacco retail stores	0.012**	0.010**	−0.004	0.011**
	(0.004)	(0.004)	(0.017)	(0.004)
Number of food banks	−0.012**	−0.012**	−0.090**	0.004
	(0.005)	(0.005)	(0.019)	(0.005)
Observations	12,145	12,145	921	11,224
R-squared	0.230	0.265	0.429	0.247

Note: The models also control for state and survey year. Standard errors in parentheses ** $p < 0.01$, * $p < 0.05$.

insecurity. Those in poorer health and current smokers are more likely to experience food insecurity. Both the number of days in poor physical health and the number of days in poor mental health contribute to a higher risk of food insecurity. The number of alcoholic drinks consumed per day and exercising do not have an association with food insecurity. Those who have social support are substantially less likely to experience food insecurity.

Given that social support substantially reduces the risk of food insecurity, I test whether the number of food stores and food banks have different impacts depending on the level of social support. A model with interaction terms between social support and the number of food outlets was statistically significant (not shown), which suggests that the impact of the number of stores differs by social support status. The estimates are presented for those who report having no social support (Model 3) and those who report having social support (Model 4). Comparing the estimates in Models 3 and 4, the impacts of health behaviors and the number of stores differ. For those with no social support, the number of drinks per day increases the risk of food insecurity while there is no association for those with social support. Similarly, the number of days in poor physical health contributes to food insecurity for those with no social support while there is no association for those with social support. Exercising has protective factors against food insecurity for those with no social support while there is no association for those with social support. Lastly, the number of food banks reduces the risk of food insecurity for those with no social support while there is no association for those with social support.

Table 4.3 presents estimates of examining daily consumption of fruits and vegetables. Similar to Table 4.2, Model 1 presents estimates controlling for demographic and other individual characteristics. Neither grocery stores nor convenience stores affects dietary intake. The number of full-service restaurants increases the daily consumption of fruits and vegetables while fast foods decrease it. The number of food banks does not have a statistically significant association with dietary intake. While health behaviors do not seem to mediate some of these associations, they do change (Model 2) after accounting for health

Table 4.3 Estimates of the Impact of the Number of Stores on Fruits and Vegetable Consumption

	Model 1	*Model 2*
Female	0.579**	0.524**
	(0.017)	(0.017)
Age	−0.031**	−0.026**
	(0.006)	(0.005)
Age²	0.000**	0.000**
	(0.000)	(0.000)
Black	0.067	0.005
	(0.039)	(0.034)
Asian	−0.115	0.191*
	(0.086)	(0.088)
Hispanic	0.324**	0.311**
	(0.041)	(0.037)
Other race	0.153**	0.286**
	(0.038)	(0.042)
Married	0.057	0.069*
	(0.029)	(0.027)
Divorced	−0.081*	−0.080*
	(0.033)	(0.033)
Widowed	−0.136**	−0.051
	(0.046)	(0.054)
Separated	−0.053	−0.125*
	(0.057)	(0.056)
Number of children	0.028**	0.039**
	(0.008)	(0.007)
Less than high school	−0.786**	−0.500**
	(0.037)	(0.032)
High school degree	−0.699**	−0.532**
	(0.022)	(0.023)
Some college	−0.390**	−0.267**
	(0.021)	(0.022)
Less than $15,000	−0.299**	−0.173**
	(0.034)	(0.033)
$15,000–$24,999	−0.252**	−0.054*
	(0.028)	(0.026)
$25,000–$34,999	−0.181**	−0.104**
	(0.028)	(0.027)
$35,000–$49,999	−0.126**	−0.033
	(0.024)	(0.023)
Self-employed	0.334**	0.392**
		(*Continued*)

Table 4.3 (Continued) Estimates of the Impact of the
Number of Stores on Fruits and Vegetable Consumption

	Model 1	Model 2
	(0.027)	(0.027)
Unemployed	0.094**	0.159**
	(0.035)	(0.031)
Homemaker	0.274**	0.272**
	(0.035)	(0.034)
Retired	0.080*	0.069
	(0.032)	(0.036)
Unable to work	−0.082**	0.075*
	(0.031)	(0.035)
Poor health		−0.117**
		(0.027)
Average drink per day		−0.019**
		(0.003)
Current smoker		−0.211**
		(0.021)
Former smoker		0.132**
		(0.020)
Number of days poor physical health		0.009**
		(0.001)
Number of days poor mental health		−0.006**
		(0.001)
Reports exercising		0.644**
		(0.018)
Number of supermarkets and grocery stores	−0.000	0.001**
	(0.001)	(0.000)
Number of convenience and warehouse stores	−0.001	−0.003**
	(0.001)	(0.001)
Number of full service restaurants	0.001**	−0.001**
	(0.000)	(0.000)
Number of limited service eating places	−0.001*	0.001*
	(0.000)	(0.000)
Number of liquor retail stores	−0.001	−0.002
	(0.001)	(0.001)
Number of tobacco retail stores	−0.001	0.007
	(0.005)	(0.004)
Number of food banks	0.007	0.015*
	(0.008)	(0.006)
Observations	60,174	60,174
R-squared	0.087	0.099

Notes: The models also control for state and survey year. Standard errors in parentheses ** $p < 0.01$, * $p < 0.05$.

behaviors. After accounting for health behaviors, the number of supermarkets increases the daily consumption of fruits and vegetables. On the other hand, the number of convenience and warehouse stores decrease it. Also, the association of full-service restaurants becomes negative while that of fast foods becomes positive. Regardless of health behaviors, liquor and tobacco retail stores do not have an association with fruits and vegetable consumption. Furthermore, food banks have a positive association with fruits and vegetable consumption indicating that informal institutional support improves diet quality. The analysis is unable to determine the impact of individual social support because the question was not asked with the fruits and vegetable questionnaire.

Discussion

This chapter sought to understand the interaction between the number and types of food stores, informal social support (both individual and institutional) on food insecurity and diet quality for rural residents. Most of the existing research on the food environment either focus on urban settings or do not examine whether their findings may differ for rural communities (e.g., Rose and Richards 2004; Larson et al. 2009; Bartfeld et al. 2010), even though there is evidence that rural residents have greater risks of food insecurity, face greater transportation costs, have fewer food store outlets, and are in poorer general health (Powell et al. 2007; Larson et al. 2009; Dean and Sharkey 2011). Previous studies on rural communities are limited in their generalizability due to the use of case studies or geographically restricted samples (e.g., Morton et al. 2005; Hendrickson et al. 2006; Dean and Sharkey 2011). Failure to understand whether rural residents' challenges require a different and more tailored approach than urban residents may result in an increase in health disparities between urban and rural communities (e.g., Eberhardt and Pamuk 2004).

Using data from the Behavioral Risk Surveillance Factors System merged with information on the number of stores from the County Business Patterns and food banks and pantry data from the NCCS, I focus on adults living in rural counties. Ordinary least squares models find that the number of liquor stores and tobacco retail stores contributes to food insufficiency. In addition, the number of food banks reduces the risk of food insufficiency. In addition, the impact of the number of stores on food insecurity differs by social support and health behaviors do not mediate these relationships. Similarly, the number of food outlets has an impact on diet quality, and some of these associations can be explained by health behaviors. The number of food banks increases the consumption of fruits and vegetables.

This study shows that the types and number of stores and food outlets have an association with dietary intake but not with food insecurity, which is inconsistent with previous studies (Morton et al. 2005; Smith and Morton 2009). Furthermore, social support and health behaviors appear to play an important role in food insecurity for rural residents in this sample. For example, social support reduces the risk of food insecurity, which is consistent with some previous studies (Walker et al. 2007; Kirkpatrick and Tarasuk 2010; dos Santos Interlenghi and Salles-Costa 2015) and contradicts De Marco and Thorburn (2009) who find no impact of social support. For those with no social support, healthy behaviors and food banks have greater protective factors against food insecurity than those with social support. On the other hand, the negative impacts of liquor retail stores and tobacco retail stores are exacerbated for those without social support.

The findings in this study show that supermarkets increase the consumption of fruits and vegetables while convenience stores decrease it, which is consistent with studies suggesting that store proximity increases the consumption of fruits and vegetables (Rose and Richards 2004; Bartfeld et al. 2010; Dean and Sharkey 2011). In addition, health behaviors explain some of these relationships on dietary intake (Pearson and Biddle 2011). On the other hand, the availability of liquor and tobacco retail stores does not seem to affect the consumption of fruits and vegetables while it increases the risk of food insecurity.

The analysis has several limitations. First, while store density and proximity are some of the most commonly used measures of food access, their main limitation is that they measure potential access rather than realized access. Potential access is where households could shop while they may actually shop somewhere else (realized access) (United States Department of Agriculture 2009). For example, some households may be living close to a supermarket but travel further to go to fast foods or vice versa. However, this type of information is nonexistent in nationally representative surveys. Second, while the BRFSS is one of the largest sources of data for rural populations (after the Census), the BRFSS no longer includes counties with a population of less than 10,000 since 2006 (Bennett 2013). This could lead to potential underrepresentation and underestimation of residents of these communities. The difficulty is that there is no alternative source of data with sample sizes of rural residents that are large enough to analyze. In addition, the BRFSS has extensive information on health, which is not available in many other sources of data. Third, the food insecurity question is only available for 13 states. As a result, it is unclear how generalizable the findings are beyond these 13 states and/or beyond the counties included in this sample (10,000 residents or more). Fourth, participation in formal food assistance programs such as SNAP is not available. It is then not possible to examine any potential interaction between formal and informal support. Fifth, although the County Business Patterns is not subject to sampling error, the U.S. Census Bureau explains that the data are subject to nonsampling errors such as the "inability to identify all cases that should be in the universe; definition and classification difficulties; errors in recording or coding the data obtained," among others. Finally, the BRFSS uses mostly self-reported survey questions. There is evidence that self-reported questions introduce recall and social desirability bias (Dietz et al. 2011; Robbins et al. 2014; Stevens 2016). For example, questions that pertain to negative behaviors (e.g., smoking and drinking) tend to be underestimated while questions related to positive behaviors (e.g., exercising and healthy eating) tend to be overestimated.

This chapter has potential implications for policy. The findings suggest that rather than directly changing the food environment (e.g., increasing the number of grocery stores), improving informal social support (both individual and institutional) could be an alternative option to improve the food security of rural residents. For example, providing informal social support by promoting community engagement, providing assistance to food banks, and encouraging healthier behaviors would improve the dietary intake of rural residents and food security. Some studies suggest that community gardens and farmers' markets could be an alternative that may improve dietary intake and reduce health disparities (Morton et al. 2008; McCormack et al. 2010). These alternatives may also help relieve some of the financial burdens of the SNAP program, which cost approximately $70 billion in 2014, making it one of the largest federal assistance programs. While this chapter was unable to examine SNAP participation, future research should examine the potential interactions between formal and informal support to find potential ways to enhance the SNAP program.

REFERENCES

Allgöwer, A., J. Wardle, and A. Steptoe. 2001. Depressive symptoms, social support, and personal health behaviors in young men and women. *Health Psychology* 20(3):223.

Alpert, J. E. and M. Fava. 1997. Nutrition and depression: The role of folate. *Nutrition Reviews* 55(5):145–149.

Bartfeld, J. S., J.-H. Ryu, and L. Wang. 2010. Local characteristics are linked to food insecurity among households with elementary school children. *Journal of Hunger & Environmental Nutrition* 5(4):471–483.

Bennett, K. J. 2013. Rural population estimates: An analysis of a large secondary data set. *Journal of Rural Health* 29(3):233–238.

Berkman, L. F., T. Glass, I. Brissette, and T. E. Seeman. 2000. From social integration to health: Durkheim in the new millennium. *Social Science & Medicine* 51(6):843–857.

Canter, K. S., M. C. Roberts, and A. M. Davis. 2016. The role of health behaviors and food insecurity in predicting fruit and vegetable intake in low-income children. *Children's Health Care* 46(2):131–150.

Centers for Disease Control and Prevention. 2015. Behavioral Risk Factors Surveillance System. Overview: BRFSS 2014. http://www.cdc.gov/brfss/annual_data/2014/pdf/overview_2014.pdf

Charreire, H., R. Casey, P. Salze, C. Simon, B. Chaix, A. Banos, D. Badariotti, C. Weber, and J.-M. Oppert. 2010. Measuring the food environment using geographical information systems: A methodological review. *Public Health Nutrition* 13(11):1773–1785.

Coleman-Jensen, A., C. Gregory, and A. Singh. 2015. *Household Food Security in the United States in 2014.* USDA Economic Research Report Number 194. Washington, DC.

Dean, W. R. and J. R. Sharkey. 2011. Rural and urban differences in the associations between characteristics of the community food environment and fruit and vegetable intake. *Journal of Nutrition Education and Behavior* 43(6):426–433.

Dean, W. R., J. R. Sharkey, and C. M. Johnson. 2011. Food insecurity is associated with social capital, perceived personal disparity, and partnership status among older and senior adults in a largely rural area of central texas. *Journal of Nutrition in Gerontology and Geriatrics* 30(2):169–186.

De Marco, M. and S. Thorburn. 2009. The relationship between income and food insecurity among Oregon residents: Does social support matter?. *Public Health Nutrition* 12(11):2104–2112.

Dietz, P. M., D. Homa, L. J. England, K. Burley, V. T. Tong, S. R. Dube, and J. T. Bernert. 2011. Estimates of nondisclosure of cigarette smoking among pregnant and nonpregnant women of reproductive age in the United States. *American Journal of Epidemiology* 173(3):355–359.

dos Santos Interlenghi, G. and R. Salles-Costa. 2015. Inverse association between social support and household food insecurity in a metropolitan area of Rio de Janeiro, Brazil. *Public Health Nutrition* 18(16):2925–2933.

Eberhardt, M. S. and E. R. Pamuk. 2004. The importance of place of residence: Examining health in rural and nonrural areas. *American Journal of Public Health* 94(10):1682–1686.

Gantner, L. A., C. M. Olson, E. A. Frongillo, and N. M. Wells. 2011. Prevalence of nontraditional food stores and distance to healthy foods in a rural food environment. *Journal of Hunger & Environmental Nutrition* 6(3):279–293.

Garasky, S., L. W. Morton, and K. A. Greder. 2006. The effects of the local food environment and social support on rural food insecurity. *Journal of Hunger & Environmental Nutrition* 1(1):83–103.

Glanz, K., J. F. Sallis, B. E. Saelens, and L. D. Frank. 2007. Nutrition Environment Measures Survey in stores (NEMS-S): Development and evaluation. *American Journal of Preventive Medicine* 32(4):282–289.

Gundersen, C. and J. P. Ziliak. 2015. Food insecurity and health outcomes. *Health Affairs* 34(11):1830–1839.

Heflin, C. M., K. Siefert, and D. R. Williams. 2005. Food insufficiency and women's mental health: Findings from a 3-year panel of welfare recipients. *Social Science & Medicine* 61(9):1971–1982.

Hendrickson, D., C. Smith, and N. Eikenberry. 2006. Fruit and vegetable access in four low-income food deserts communities in Minnesota. *Agriculture and Human Values* 23(3):371–383.

Irving, S. M., R. S. Njai, and P. Z. Siegel. 2014. Food insecurity and self-reported hypertension among Hispanic, black, and white adults in 12 states, behavioral risk factor surveillance system, 2009. *Preventing Chronic Disease* 11:E161.

King, C. 2016. Food insecurity and housing instability in vulnerable families. *Review of Economics of the Household* 1–19.

Kirkpatrick, S. I. and V. Tarasuk. 2010. Assessing the relevance of neighbourhood characteristics to the household food security of low-income Toronto families. *Public Health Nutrition* 13(7):1139–1148.

Kubik, M. Y., L. A. Lytle, P. J. Hannan, C. L. Perry, and M. Story. 2003. The association of the school food environment with dietary behaviors of young adolescents. *American Journal of Public Health* 93(7):1168–1173.

Larson, N. I., M. T. Story, and M. C. Nelson. 2009. Neighborhood environments: Disparities in access to healthy foods in the U.S. *American Journal of Preventive Medicine* 36(1):74–81.e10.

Lee, J. S. 2013. Food insecurity and healthcare costs: Research strategies using local, state, and national data sources for older adults. *Advances in Nutrition: An International Review Journal* 4(1):42–50.

Lutfiyya, M. N., L. F. Chang, and M. S. Lipsky. 2012. A cross-sectional study of US rural adults' consumption of fruits and vegetables: Do they consume at least five servings daily? *BMC Public Health* 12(1):1.

McCormack, L. Arneson, M. N. Laska, N. I. Larson, and M. Story. 2010. Review of the nutritional implications of farmers' markets and community gardens: A call for evaluation and research efforts. *Journal of the American Dietetic Association* 110(3):399–408.

Monsivais, P. and A. Drewnowski. 2007. The rising cost of low-energy-density foods. *Journal of the American Dietetic Association* 107(12):2071–2076.

Monsivais, P., J. McLain, and A. Drewnowski. 2010. The rising disparity in the price of healthful foods: 2004–2008. *Food Policy* 35(6):514–520.

Moore, L. V., A. V. Diez Roux, and S. Brines. 2008a. Comparing perception-based and geographic information system (GIS)-based characterizations of the local food environment. *Journal of Urban Health* 85(2):206–216.

Moore, L. V., A. V. Diez Roux, J. A. Nettleton, and D. R. Jacobs. 2008b. Associations of the local food environment with diet quality—A comparison of assessments based on surveys and geographic information systems the multi-ethnic study of atherosclerosis. *American Journal of Epidemiology* 167(8):917–924.

Morland, K., S. Wing, and A. D. Roux. 2002. The contextual effect of the local food environment on residents' diets: The atherosclerosis risk in communities study. *American Journal of Public Health* 92(11):1761–1768.

Morton, L. W., E. A. Bitto, M. J. Oakland, and M. Sand. 2005. Solving the problems of Iowa food deserts: Food insecurity and civic structure. *Rural Sociology* 70(1):94–112.

Morton, L. W., E. A. Bitto, M. J. Oakland, and M. Sand. 2008. Accessing food resources: Rural and urban patterns of giving and getting food. *Agriculture and Human Values* 25(1):107–119.

Muirhead, V., C. Quiñonez, R. Figueiredo, and D. Locker. 2009. Oral health disparities and food insecurity in working poor Canadians. *Community Dentistry and Oral Epidemiology* 37(4):294–304.

Pearson, N. and S. J. H. Biddle. 2011. Sedentary behavior and dietary intake in children, adolescents, and adults: A systematic review. *American Journal of Preventive Medicine* 41(2):178–188.

Phipps, E. J., S. Brook Singletary, C. A. Cooblall, H. D. Hares, and L. E. Braitman. 2016. Food insecurity in patients with high hospital utilization. *Population Health Management* 19(6):414–420.

Powell, L. M., S. Slater, D. Mirtcheva, Y. Bao, and F. J. Chaloupka. 2007. Food store availability and neighborhood characteristics in the United States. *Preventive Medicine* 44(3):189–195.

Reynolds, E. H. 2002. Folic acid, ageing, depression, and dementia. *British Medical Journal* 324(7352):1512–1515.

Robbins, C. L. et al. 2014. Core state preconception health indicators-pregnancy risk assessment monitoring system and behavioral risk factor surveillance system, 2009. Morbidity and Mortality Weekly Report. *Surveillance Summaries (Washington, DC: 2002)* 63(3):1–62.

Rose, D. and R. Richards. 2004. Food store access and household fruit and vegetable use among participants in the US Food Stamp Program. *Public Health Nutrition* 7(8):1081–1088.

Rosenbloom, S. 2004. The mobility needs of older Americans. *Taking the High Road: A Transportation Agenda of Strengthening Metropolitan Areas* 227–54.

Sallis, J. F. and K. Glanz. 2009. Physical activity and food environments: Solutions to the obesity epidemic. *Milbank Quarterly* 87(1):123–154.

Seligman, H. K., A. B. Bindman, E. Vittinghoff, A. M. Kanaya, and M. B. Kushel. 2007. Food insecurity is associated with diabetes mellitus: Results from the National Health Examination and Nutrition Examination Survey (NHANES) 1999–2002. *Journal of General Internal Medicine* 22(7):1018–1023.

Seligman, H. K., B. A. Laraia, and M. B. Kushel. 2010. Food insecurity is associated with chronic disease among low-income NHANES participants. *Journal of Nutrition* 140(2):304–310.

Sharkey, J. R. 2009. Measuring potential access to food stores and food-service places in rural areas in the US. *American Journal of Preventive Medicine* 36(4):S151–S155.

Smith, C. and H. Miller. 2011. Accessing the food systems in urban and rural Minnesotan communities. *Journal of Nutrition Education and Behavior* 43(6):492–504.

Smith, C. and L. W. Morton. 2009. Rural food deserts: Low-income perspectives on food access in Minnesota and Iowa. *Journal of Nutrition Education and Behavior* 41(3):176–187.

Stevens, A. C. 2016. Comparison of 2 disability measures, behavioral risk factor surveillance system, 2013. *Preventing Chronic Disease* 13.

Stommes, E. S. and D. M. Brown. 2002. Transportation in rural America: Issues for the 21st century. *Community Transportation* 20(4).

Swanson, J. A., C. M. Olson, E. O. Miller, and F. C. Lawrence. 2008. Rural mothers' use of formal programs and informal social supports to meet family food needs: A mixed methods study. *Journal of Family and Economic Issues* 29(4):674–690.

Tiemeier, H., H. R. van Tuijl, A. Hofman, J. Meijer, A. Kiliaan, and M. M. B. Breteler. 2002. Vitamin B12, folate, and homocysteine in depression: The Rotterdam Study. *American Journal of Psychiatry* 159(12):2099–2101.

United States Department of Agriculture. 2009. *Access to Affordable and Nutritious Food: Measuring and Understanding Food Deserts and Their Consequences.* Economic Research Service, June 2009.

United States Department of Agriculture. 2012a. *Characteristics and Influential Factors of Food Deserts.* Economic Research Report Number 104, August 2012.

United States Department of Agriculture. 2012b. *Access to Affordable and Nutrition Food: Updated Estimates of Distance to Supermarkets Using 2010 Data.* Economic Research Report Number 143, November 2012.

United States Department of Agriculture. 2015. Rural America at a Glance, 2015 Edition. Economic Information Bulletin Number 145, November 2015.

United States Department of Agriculture. 2016. Population & Migration. Accessed on May 17, 2016. http://www.ers.usda.gov/topics/rural-economy-population/population-migration.aspx.

Walker, J. L., D. H. Holben, M. L. Kropf, J. P. Holcomb Jr., and H. Anderson. 2007. Household food insecurity is inversely associated with social capital and health in females from Special Supplemental Nutrition Program for women, infants, and children households in Appalachian Ohio. *Journal of the American Dietetic Association* 107(11):1989–1993.

Whitaker, R. C., S. M. Phillips, and S. M. Orzol. 2006. Food insecurity and the risks of depression and anxiety in mothers and behavior problems in their preschool-aged Children. *Pediatrics* 118(3):e859–e868.

Ziliak, J. P. 2015. Why are so many Americans on food stamps? In *SNAP Matters: How Food Stamps Affect Health and Well-Being*, edited by J. Bartfeld, C. Gundersen, T. M. Smeeding, and J. P. Ziliak. Stanford, CA: Stanford University Press.

5 A case study of a rural food desert

Emily C. Kohls

Food deserts: The pursuit of healthy foods

"Food desert" is a term utilized by the United States Department of Agriculture (USDA) to identify and describe geographical areas in which fresh and healthy foods are not readily available. Food deserts are of concern to public health, as the residents living in these communities may not have the foods available to make healthful choices and reduce their risk for health complications, such as overweight/obesity, diabetes, heart disease, and others. Food deserts can also contribute to food insecurity.

Much of the available literature on food deserts focuses on the characteristics of a geographical area that make up a food desert. Varying definitions exist in the literature, including proximity to the grocery store or supermarket, poverty rates, vehicle ownership, and number of grocery stores in a specified area (i.e., state or county). What is largely unknown about food deserts, particularly those in rural areas, is what the community is doing to overcome the food access issues. What, if any, actions are being taken by individuals, groups, civic leaders, or others to overcome challenges in food access and make healthy foods available to the community?

The focus of this case study is to examine an existing rural food desert county as well as the interventions made by the community and surrounding communities to improve food access. This study will identify previous and existing programs, both formal and informal, and programs in the planning phase. This case study seeks to answer the following research question: What are local rural communities doing to deal with food insecurity and/or limited access to healthy foods?

A rural food desert county in Nebraska was studied to determine the current state of food access within the county. Details about the present grocery stores and recently closed grocery stores were collected, as well as information about formal and informal programs that exist to assist residents with obtaining food. Interviews were conducted with community members, community leaders, nonprofits employees, and others to gather information.

Current research and gaps in the literature

Defining food deserts

Food deserts are fairly well studied in terms of identifying parameters used to define and identify food deserts. The term "food desert" was said to have originated from a Scotland resident of public sector housing in the 1990s (Whelan, Wrigley, Warm and Cannings 2002; Shaw 2006; Walker, Keane and Burke 2010). The term is now used to describe a geographical area experiencing food hardship related to inadequate access to healthy foods. Definitions of food deserts vary in the literature, and while they contain a common theme of inadequate access, the parameters for "adequately accessible" is inconsistent.

The USDA utilizes various parameters to identify food desert areas, such as access to supermarkets and income level. An area is considered low access if 500 or more residents or at least 33% of the census tract population live one mile from a supermarket or large grocery store in urban areas, and more than 10 miles in rural areas. An area is considered low income if the tract's poverty rate is 20% or greater, or median family income is at or below 80% of the statewide or metropolitan area median family income. Other parameters may also be used, such as vehicle availability, public transportation, and number of supermarkets in the area (USDA 2017).

Scholars have questioned if the distance of 10 miles in rural areas is adequate, due to other factors limiting access to grocery stores. "Does the proximity [to grocery stores] have a large impact on food access and food choice, regardless of poverty rates and income levels? For rural areas, the most 'reasonable' distances are less well-established than for urban areas, with some researchers defining 'high accessible' as 'within ten miles of the population'. This variability may be related both to the lesser numbers of rural studies and to the high variability of terrain and weather conditions in rural areas, as well as 'reasonable routes' reported by residents themselves" (Hubley 2011, p. 1225). This uncovers limitations in the study of rural food deserts, as many other factors outside of proximity and poverty level may be in play. Car availability, terrain, weather conditions, and distances much greater than 10 miles can impact on access to healthy foods, even in populations not considered a food desert due to the USDA definition of low income.

Cost and variety of available food items are others factors to consider, rather than solely proximity to the nearest grocery store (Jiao 2012). In areas where access to a grocery store or supermarket is limited, perhaps individuals will be more inclined to choose food items that are more easily accessible. Frequently, this can involve convenience stores that offer more processed foods and less fresh fruits and vegetables. When and if fresh produce is offered, it is often more expensive and of suboptimal quality. "Although nearby small food retailers may be expensive and offer poor choices, residents may make the rational choice to secure food locally rather than devote scarce time and resources to the task of traveling to a major grocery store outside their neighborhood" (LeClair and Aksan 2014, p. 538).

Impacts on health

The 2015-2020 Dietary Guidelines for Americans outline a healthy eating pattern as containing whole, fresh fruits, a variety of vegetables, whole grains, and lean protein sources, and limiting foods containing high amounts of fat, trans fat, sodium, and added sugar. Healthy eating patterns are linked to lower rates of cardiovascular disease, certain types of cancer, overweight, obesity, and Type II diabetes (U.S. Department of Health and Human Services 2017). The challenges in achieving a healthy eating pattern for individuals living in food deserts are often twofold: less access to fresh, healthy, and whole foods, and over-abundant supply of processed foods generally containing higher calories, fat, trans fat, sodium, and added sugar.

Food deserts also contribute to hunger and poor nutrition (Hubley 2011). Rural food deserts have resulted in lower-income and elderly individuals having to travel greater distances to obtain food and thus pay more to be food secure. Furthermore, food deserts and food insecurity may be related, as limited access and barriers to obtaining food can result in food insecurity, particularly in disadvantaged groups (Morton et al. 2005). Food insecurity in communities means that individuals are relying more on other sources to obtain their food, such as food banks and meal services provided by churches. The availability of these sources in rural areas may not be enough to provide adequate food security for their residents.

Interventions in poor access areas and gaps in the literature

Despite the well-documented characteristics of a food desert and the impacts on health, there is a limited amount of research on the topic in the United States (Walker, Keane and Burke 2010). One topic noticeably lacking in the literature is strategies to overcome food access in food deserts, particularly in rural communities. Thus, a gap in the literature has been identified. The existing literature, while sparse, has a common theme: a comprehensive intervention that combines personal relationships, community partnerships, and ideally a community education component, is essential to successful community-based interventions addressing food access.

Two case studies conducted in rural Minnesota and rural Iowa concluded that civic structure combined with personal and/or community partnerships can be successful in addressing poor access to healthy foods. Limited food access is particularly an issue for low-income and disadvantaged individuals, although it impacts all in a community, regardless of income level, according to the authors. Reliance on personal relationships is common. Civic structure in the form of community-based programs and services must be combined with personal relationships to successfully address food access issues, the case study concluded. Using this two-pronged approach, communities can successfully implement programs and services, such as community food pantries, ride sharing, sales or sharing of locally sourced produce and meat, meals served by local organizations, and community gardens. The rural Iowa/Minnesota study stressed the importance of leadership and collaboration among community members for successfully improving healthy food access (Morton et al. 2005; Smith and Morton 2009).

Another case study examined a plan implemented in Los Angeles County with a high prevalence of chronic disease, which involves a grassroots approach targeting community behavior change and the food environment. The strategy includes four levels. The first level addresses individual behavior, with the aim of modifying individual decisions surrounding their food choices. This involved community education and encouraged the residents to engage in improving their food environment. The second level addresses relationships, and focuses on family and networks and how these can support individual behavior and, subsequently, societal behavior. The third level addresses community infrastructure that can support individual and community health. Coalitions and work groups were formed to bring the community and organizations together to develop strategies to address access to healthful foods. The final level addresses societal factors that impact policies surrounding health, economics, education, and social issues. This strategy resulted in the implementation of two policies: one that incentivized existing grocery stores to stay and new grocery stores to be built in the community, and another that halts the opening of new fast food restaurants to allow for officials to address the food environment (Lewis et al. 2011).

This community-based participatory approach in Los Angeles County is significant because it can be applied to the urban or rural setting to address food access challenges. As with the suggestions previously mentioned, a collaborative approach is essential to success: one that engages civic leaders, community partners, and the citizens in the community. The plan resulted in a more engaged community that was eager to work with their policymakers and civic leaders to improve their food environment, as well as policy changes that have the potential significantly improve access to healthy foods and the overall health of the community.

A case study in Leeds, the United Kingdom identified local projects, policies, and strategies to address food access challenges. "Tackling food deserts is clearly a multi-sectoral responsibility and provides the opportunity to apply the principles of health promotion regarding community development, advocacy and partnership working." Initiatives should not be left to individuals, local authorities, or community groups alone. A collaborative approach is encouraged to ensure effective implementation (Reisig and Hobbiss 2000).

The Leeds case study outlined strategies to include many different programs and ideas, such as workshops and courses aimed at educating the public about healthy eating and cooking. Community-based projects were implemented, such as food cooperatives, school breakfast clubs, and food-growing strategies. The intent of these educational programs was to enhance knowledge about the importance of a healthful diet, as well as practical application of ways to prepare healthy foods and incorporate fresh produce into the diet. Supermarket initiative projects were developed to address transportation challenges, such as home deliveries and grocery store buses. Plans were implemented to review the shops and supermarkets in the area to ensure that adequate shops and outlets were present.

Government and political strategies were considered that involved government intervention to keep grocery stores and food outlets in the areas. These plans were limited due to policymakers' hesitation to "interfere with market processes" (Reisig and Hobbiss 2000).

Other researchers further support farmers' markets and community gardens, due to the potential for improved fruit and vegetable intake of participants (Pitts et al. 2014). These activities improve access to healthful foods, and may also reduce the intake of processed foods. Researchers found that those who volunteered in the community gardens reported eating less processed foods and fast foods, spending less money on food, and being more aware of where their food came from and the environmental impact of their food choices (Barnidge et al. 2013). Community gardens and farmers' markets also offer the opportunity for collaboration among community members and civic leaders, a crucial component in improving the food environment and access to healthy foods.

Each of these four case studies on activities to address food access discussed various community-based activities to improve the food environment, but almost all activities contained a common theme of collaboration and not a singular approach. Whether a rural or urban food desert, the researchers concluded that engaging the members of the community with public health officials, civic leaders, and other stakeholders was imperative in addressing food access challenges. An education component is also important in engaging the community and improving health behavior and food choice. These case studies offer a framework for future initiatives implemented in food desert communities. However, the long-term success of improving the food environment and access to healthy foods with this multisectional collaborative approach is unknown, and thus more research in food desert communities is needed.

Case study: A rural Nebraska food desert

To gain a comprehensive understanding of a rural food desert and potential strategies to address food access issues at the community level, a case study was conducted in a rural food desert county in Nebraska. Interviews were conducted with community members, public health officials, and public administrators to assess activities in this food desert community, as well as other areas in the state with poor access to healthy foods. Additional interviewees were identified using the snowball method. The county extension office was contacted, and an employee provided the names of individuals participating in a community-level committee formed with the intention of addressing food access concerns within the county. The structured interview questions were developed based on the themes found in the literature on food deserts. Information was requested on existing and developing programs that may involve community engagement, civic structure, and educational activities. A rural Nebraska county was selected for this study due to the recent classification as a USDA rural food desert. Contact was made with a Nebraska Center for Rural Affairs employee who recommended some counties to consider for this study. One particular county was chosen because it was recently classified a food desert after the closing of a grocery store in November 2014. Furthermore, it was reported that members in the surrounding communities were working on addressing food access, and there was potential to study existing programs underway in the area. The county will not be named to ensure anonymity of the respondents.

Persons below the poverty level from 2009 to 2013 was 11.1%. Median household income from 2009 to 2013 was $37,594 (United States Census Bureau 2015). The entire county is considered to have low income according to the USDA, because the county median family income is less than 80% of the median household income for the state of Nebraska ($51,672). According to Feeding America, 550 people, or 12.3% of the county population, are considered food insecure (feedingamerica.org 2015). Food insecurity is "limited or uncertain availability of nutritionally adequate and safe foods or limited or uncertain ability to acquire foods in socially acceptable ways" (USDA Economic Research Service 2017a).

The USDA Food Environment Atlas, utilizing data from 2007, indicates that there were three grocery stores in the county in 2007 and two grocery stores in 2011 (USDA Economic Research Service 2017b). One of these grocery stores, located in the central portion of the county, closed in November of 2014, the week before Thanksgiving. Currently, the only grocery store in the county is located in the largest town, located at the far southern end of the county. Outside of the county, the nearest grocery store in each county town is located an average of 11.7 miles away, the nearest being 8 miles away and the farthest being 15 miles away.

Case study findings

Nine interviews were conducted: six formal structured interviews and four personal communications with unstructured questions. Interviewees included public administrators with state departments, nonprofits, health departments, and residents living in the county. Figure 5.1 shows a map of current and recently closed grocery stores in the county. Table 5.1 shows the various community programs discussed by the respondents (Table 5.1).

Personal networks to improve access to food

Personal networks are one way that rural communities are dealing with food access issues. When one of two grocery stores in the county closed, a resident of the town put an ad in the paper providing a hotline telephone number through their own locally owned business that residents could call if they wanted to make requests for items to be picked up at the only grocery store in the county. However, not many people have utilized the hotline. "Everybody is watching out for each other. If I'm going to the next town, I'll contact the people I know who have trouble getting out and see if they need anything. There are times that I'll take someone with me or I'll do the shopping for them." Another respondent said that there is likely some personal networks being utilized to address food access, but it is inconsistent and not well known. Some residents may grow their

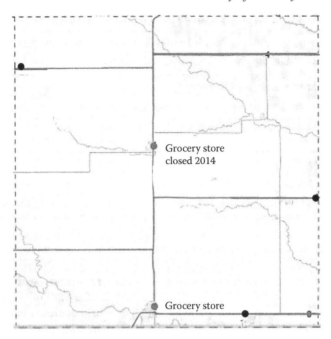

Figure 5.1 With the closing of one centrally located grocery store, the county was left with one store located at the south end of the county. Many county residents must now drive between 8 and 15 miles to the nearest grocery store.

own food and share parts of their harvest with others in the community. One respondent noted that residents in the community will bring their extra harvests, especially produce, to their community churches for others to take. The food sharing was informal and voluntary, and thus likely not a reliable means for the food insecure to obtain food.

Table 5.1 County Programs and Strategies to Address Food Access

Program or Strategy	*Availability in the County*
Personal networks • Sharing of homegrown produce • Informal ride sharing • Grocery shopping for neighbors	• Informal and sparse
Civic engagement and community-based programs • Mobile food pantries • Food banks • Senior Farmers' Market Nutrition Programs • Farmers' markets • Community gardens • Cooperative grocery stores	• Food bank and farmers' market available but only in same town with sole grocery store • Nearest mobile food pantry located over 45 miles away • No community garden • No cooperative grocery store in the area

Programs based on civic engagement and community support

Throughout the interviews, several programs were mentioned that serve areas throughout the state that work to address food access issues in rural communities. Some were programs available throughout the state and some were specific to neighboring counties. There was limited availability of these programs within the county. All of the programs discussed have some level of collaboration between the community receiving the services and a public or nonprofit entity.

Mobile food pantries and food banks

The Lincoln Food Bank and Catholic Social Services created a partnership to conduct a mobile food pantry that serves several rural counties in the state. A truck load of food is driven to 14 small communities on a monthly basis and is parked in a church parking lot. Residents may come to the mobile food pantry to get food items. One respondent indicated that while it is a great program, it does not meet the need of the communities. Another challenge of this program is the lack of anonymity in small communities. This program is not currently offered in the county, and the nearest mobile food pantry is over 100 miles away. Food banks are present in surrounding towns, which may help address food insecurity for the poor. However, they are often present in towns with a grocery store and require travel of greater than 10 miles to obtain the services, so the challenge of proximity to a food source remains.

Senior services

The Nebraska Department of Agriculture operates the Senior Farmers Market Nutrition Program (SFMNP) that provides coupons to low-income senior citizens, obtained through their local senior center, to purchase fresh, locally grown produce at a farmers' market or produce stand. The program publishes a listing of participating farmers' markets that have been certified to accept the coupons. SFMNP serves approximately 5000 senior citizens throughout the state and brings in about $200,000 in federal funds to the local produce market. It aims to market, support, and grow the state produce industry, while improving access to fresh and locally grown produce for low-income seniors. Farmers' markets are not present in every area, so this program does not meet the needs in all food desert areas, including the county studied. Some areas of the state may have senior centers that provide free or reduced-cost meals, but similar to the farmers' markets, they are typically located in larger towns, requiring residents of the surrounding area to drive to obtain their services.

Farmers' markets and community gardens

The Farmers' Market Coalition of Southeast Nebraska was formed by the Public Health Solutions District Health Department of Nebraska, which serves a five-county area, but does not serve the case-study county. The idea for the coalition began after several small communities' consolidated schools and grocery stores closed. The program has been successful in that prior to its inception, there were two to three markets in the area. Now, 4 years into the program, there are nine farmers' markets throughout the five-county area.

The Public Health Solutions District Health Department plays a role in the program by assisting with branding and marketing for the vendors participating in the farmers' markets, as well as providing opportunities for professional development to "equip the farmer's market managers to be more business savvy." The health department also develops informational fliers to distribute throughout the five-county area.

The South Heartland District Health Department serving the food desert county was recently awarded a 1422 federal grant. This grant will be utilized to conduct a survey of the four-county service area to help increase accessibility to healthy foods. Part of the grant will include working with local grocery stores and convenience stores to assess their food offerings as well as to provide more fresh produce and low sodium options. The project is currently in the survey phase, and based on the results of the survey, increasing the number of farmers' markets may be a goal of the program. There is currently one farmers' market located in the county, in the same town with the only county grocery store. There was a second farmers' market in the county but it did not stay open due to lack of participation, according to one respondent.

Community gardens have been successful in other rural towns in the state, according to one Health Department worker interviewed. Two gardens were started by a motivated student from a local college to serve area citizens, particularly those without land or a yard in which to grow their own food. The community is able to sustain the community gardens with the help of leadership from the college. The gardens require a very small fee for participants, and the college even offers gardening education courses to participants. The respondent mentioned that the population of the town with one of the community gardens, which includes a high Hispanic and Latino population living in quarters with limited greenspace, is especially benefiting from having access to the community garden.

Cooperative grocery stores

The Center for Rural Affairs and the Nebraska Cooperative Development Center have partnered with rural communities in the state to open small, community owned and operated grocery stores. The community will unite to decide that they want a local grocery store and, more importantly, will support it. The state partners provide guidance and expertise throughout the process of opening the grocery store.

The partnership has successfully opened grocery stores in rural communities. In Elwood, Nebraska, the local grocery store closed in January of 2012, and the community came together to develop a plan to reopen the store. The community steering committee developed a business plan, marketing plan, and researched the required permits and insurance needs. The committee and the subcommittees met weekly throughout the entire process, which took 14 months. The grocery store is cooperatively owned by 160 shareholders in the community, who support and utilize the grocery store. Nonshareholders in the community can also utilize the grocery store. While the shareholders may see a small return on their investment in the cooperative, the profits and financial return on investment are not the goals of cooperative businesses.

The reason the cooperative was successful was because the committee was extremely motivated and committed to the project. The project was also successful because they had the support of the community in the beginning and maintained that support throughout the cooperative planning process. By moving the process along as quickly as they could, they were able to maintain the community's interest and commitment to the cooperative.

Another success story was about a community-managed, nonprofit grocery store located in Cody, Nebraska, a town with a population of 154 (United State Census Bureau 2015), and 38 miles from the nearest town. Without a grocery store in town, residents must travel nearly 80 miles round trip to purchase groceries. Ranchers who live in even more remote areas might have to drive nearly double that.

The idea to open the grocery store came out of the Cody-Kilgore Unified Schools system. The students pushed for the store, the school supported them, and the community also quickly showed their support for the project. Their community meetings drew great attendance. The students at the school were responsible for developing a business plan, with help from the Nebraska Cooperative Development Center, and the students and community came together to construct the store. Now that the store is open, the school continues to run the grocery store and the students are responsible for every aspect of running the store, including marketing, stocking shelves, managing, and even cashiering. The program is a service-learning opportunity to teach the student about hard work and entrepreneurship. The success of this project was dependent on the support of the community throughout the planning process, and after the store opened.

While some cooperative grocery stores have had great success, there have been some cooperative grocery store projects that did not make it through the planning stages. One respondent stated, "Some failed pretty monumentally because [the community] wasn't committed to the process. If they run into a barrier, they must find a way to overcome it." One particular project in the state ultimately failed due to lack of community support after misinformation about the project began circulating throughout the town. In the next planning meeting, after having great attendance at previous meetings, only a few community members attended. The project had failed. Without the buy-in of the community and shareholders, cooperative grocery stores will not succeed. The respondents working closely with these cooperative grocery stores in Nebraska stressed that community support is paramount to their success. Without it, the projects are likely to fail.

Educational offerings to improve access to foods

While the literature cited community education as a component of strategies of improve food access and food choice, there was limited formal education programs discussed. Some programs in this case study contain a community education component, but it was not present in all programs. Education has become an important component of the programs coming out of the county health departments, particularly the importance of increased fruit and vegetable intake. County extension offices often offer educational services and information, such as materials and guides, on how to grow and preserve food. While these services exist in rural communities, their use or knowledge of their existence appears to be limited.

Lack of collaboration leads to barriers

Since the town's only grocery store, and one of two in the county, closed in November of 2014, new challenges have been presented to individuals in the community. Upon the grocery store closing, about 7–10 citizens developed a committee and began meeting to discuss solutions to their food access issue. A wide variety of options have been discussed, but many roadblocks are present and little progress has been made in finding a long-term solution.

The condition of the building was one contributing factor for why the grocery store closed, and suitable infrastructure has been difficult to find. In an attempt to find a home for a small, basic-needs grocery store in town, the committee has looked into potential buildings to house a small grocery store. Some business owners considered offering space, but due to the requirement of special permits to sell dairy and the needed health inspections, this option was not explored further. An old library owned by the city is currently unoccupied; however, when the committee asked the city council if they could lease the space to open a small grocery store, the city council did not approve their request.

Another challenge related to opening a grocery store is the minimum purchases required by food wholesalers. Many small, locally operated grocery stores struggle to meet the wholesaler minimum for food deliveries. The stores will not receive deliveries from the wholesalers if they cannot meet the minimum dollar amount, even if a delivery truck drives through the town on its route to another store. Some area grocery stores must combine their orders with neighboring towns, and one owner will have to drive to that town to pick up their food order. One grocery store manager in a neighboring community will even go to another grocery store to purchase food items the store has run out of, and will sell the items at cost, simply to have the items available for his customers.

A ridesharing program was discussed in the community, but due to the many challenges, no program has been implemented. The community would have had to buy a vehicle, obtain special service because it was considered a taxi service, and obtain a special permit. If they planned to charge any fee, even $2 per ride, they would have to obtain special insurance. They could try to run the service on volunteers and donations, but that raised concerns about the ability to sustain the service and the community being willing to utilize and support the service.

The community has had difficulty getting more buy-in from the community members and the community civic leaders. Specifically, the city council has not been very receptive to the committee, according to one respondent. The "City council will not help and will not get involved. They worried that if they start helping businesses in need, everyone will come to them for help." One city council member is also a member of the volunteer grocery store committee, and this individual has not been permitted to vote on any matter related to the grocery store, according to one respondent.

The committee reached out to the one convenience store in town and asked if they would consider using a vacant space on their building to open a small grocery store. The convenience store would not consider it, according to one respondent. The store mainly only sells premade sandwiches, in addition to typical convenience foods and beverages found in a convenience store. They do sell some necessity food items; however, it comes at a price. "You can now get a gallon of milk at the c-store, but it will cost you $6.00. You can also get a loaf of bread, but that will cost you $4.50. So, of course no one goes there to buy those things."

The town was awarded a grant to conduct a community survey to develop a comprehensive plan. The survey will ask residents about several issues facing the town, and will include a section about a town grocery store. This survey will be used to help determine if a grocery store might be successful in their community. The survey will be utilized to gauge the community's interest and likelihood to support a cooperative grocery store. Since community involvement and support is a must for a cooperative business to succeed, the results of the survey will be crucial to any future plans for a cooperative grocery store.

Lessons learned from a rural food desert

There are various community resources provided throughout the state of Nebraska that are aimed at improving food access to healthy foods, particularly fresh fruits and vegetables, and addressing food security in rural areas. Some programs have been implemented and sustained over a period of time, and have increased their offerings of food in their communities. Since some of the programs discussed in this study are fairly new, having been implemented in the past 2–5 years, the long-term success and sustainability of these programs is not yet known.

The concern is that these successful programs are not always accessible or replicated in areas of need. The county studied appears to be a prime example of an area of great need related to food access, and not enough community or state-run programs to address the need. While there are some informal personal networks forming, there appears to be a lack of civic engagement and community-driven programs. In fact, there appears to be a lack of support, and perhaps even apathy, concerning the need for programs to address food access issues in the community.

The county is low income, and the majority of residents in the county must drive at least 8 miles, but usually more, to access the nearest grocery store. There are not many community programs available to all residents in the county. Without ready access to not only healthy food options, but also the basic food necessities, how will these residents cope? How will low-income and elderly residents cope? What might the long-term effects be if residents are required to shop at their local convenience store or perhaps go without? These important questions remain unanswered.

Replication of existing programs to areas of need

The lack of programming in areas of need reflects a need for additional funding to support the replication of successful programs. It should also be noted that some of the programs outlined are fairly new, and the program managers may not have had ample opportunity to collaborate with neighboring communities to replicate their programs. A plan for collaboration is needed to ensure that these programs can be replicated in rural areas throughout the state. A state agency may need to step in to identify the successful programs, and begin developing a plan to spread the programs to other food desert communities.

A common theme found in existing programs is collaboration between city leaders and the community, with input and assistance from the professionals from organizations around the state. Collaboration appears to be lacking in the county, particularly among community members in towns with a grocery store and their city council members. The literature and the findings strongly support the need for strong city leadership and civic engagement to develop successful community interventions.

Policy implications and the role of government

The results of this study indicate that while some communities are able to successfully develop community-based programs to meet the needs of their residents, not all communities are able to do so on their own. This provides a foundation for the argument that state and federal agencies must do more to identify areas of need related to food access and food security and assist in program implementation in these areas, including funding in the long term for these programs. It may be ideal to develop community-based programs at the grassroots level to gain support and buy-in from the community that will receive the services, but the concern remains for communities that are not receiving the adequate services they need.

The literature review and the findings of this study strongly support the argument that educational outreach and civic engagement must serve as the foundation for successful community interventions and programs. Some programs discussed in this study utilize an education component, including education and training for the community, for farmers' market managers, or for a group of citizens who will soon own their own cooperative business. Civic engagement and strong city leadership help to ensure successful collaboration and mutual support among the key players and stakeholders. This has already led to several programs being successful in rural areas throughout the state, and is strongly supported by the key players and stakeholders involved in these programs.

Since strong leadership from city officials is not always guaranteed in these communities, there should be a strategy in mind to educate and engage city leaders on the importance of community-based grassroots efforts. City leadership must take an active role in supporting these efforts, particularly those that benefit the livelihood of their communities. Lack of support and apathy on the part of city leadership can be detrimental to the efforts of the community, and prevent successful programs from developing in their communities. City leadership should take an active role in the planning for these programs and engage their citizens to get involved in the process.

It may be necessary to consider policies that benefit and support small grocery store owners in rural areas. Small grocery stores are facing additional challenges, such as aging infrastructure, difficulty with transportation, difficulty in meeting food order minimums, and competition with large, nationally owned retail outlets. Policy intervention may be needed to support these small businesses, which are essential to the health and livelihood of the community. Policies should also be considered to improve offerings of alternative food sources in rural food deserts, such as farmers' markets, community gardens, and educational sessions, so that residents may learn how to grow and preserve their own foods. With the success of the cooperative business program in the state, additional funds would help to expand the program and help more rural communities in need of small businesses in their communities.

Conclusion

The literature points to the need for community engagement, civic structure, and educational activities to improve food access in food desert areas. This case study supports the findings in the literature, as the existing programs in Nebraska, particularly cooperative grocery stores and Farmers' Market coalition, incorporate these components into their programs in the planning, implementation, and sustaining phases. Additional research is needed to understand the current state of community-based programs in rural areas throughout the country, and may help to promote a more wide spread approach to food access in rural food deserts. This will also provide a better understanding of how many rural food desert communities are being underserved. More research is needed to better understand the challenges faced by rural communities throughout the United States and to develop interventions to assist rural areas in overcoming them.

REFERENCES

Barnidge, E. K., P. R. Hipp, A. Estlund, K. Duggan, K. J. Barnhart, and R. C. Brownson. 2013. Association between community garden participation and fruit and vegetable consumption in rural Missouri. *Journal of Behavioral Nutrition and Physical Activity* 10:128. http://www.ijbnpa.org/content/10/1/128

Feeding America. 2015. Retrieved from http://www.feedingamerica.org/.

Hubley, T. A. 2011. Assessing the proximity of healthy food options and food deserts in a rural area in Maine. *Applied Geography* 31:1224–1231. doi: 10.1016/j.apgeog.2010.09.004.

Jiao, J., A. V. Moudon, J. Ulmer, P. M. Hurvitz, and A. Drewnowski. 2012. How to identify food deserts: Measuring physical and economic access to supermarkets in King County, Washington. *American Journal of Public Health* 102(10):e32–e39. doi: 10.2105/AJPH.2012.300675.

Jilcott Pitts, S. B., A. Gustafson, Q. Wu, M. L. Mayo, R. K. Ward, J. T. McGuirt, A. P. Rafferty, M. F. Lancaster, K. R. Evenson, T. C. Keyserling, and A. S. Ammerman. 2014. Farmers' market use is associated with fruit and vegetable consumption in diverse southern rural communities. *Nutrition Journal* 13:1. doi: 10.1186/1475/2891-13-1.

LeClair, M. S. and A. Aksan. 2014. Redefining the food desert: Combining GIS with direct observation to measure food access. *Agriculture and Human Values* 31:537–547. doi: 10.1007/s10460-014-9501-y.

Lewis, L. B., L. Galloway-Gilliam, G. Flynn, J. Nomachi, L. C. Keener, and D. C. Sloane. 2011. Transforming the urban food desert from the grassroots up: A model for community change. *Family Community Health* 34(1S):92–101.

Morton, L. W., E. A. Bitto, M. J. Oakland, and M. Sand. 2005. Solving the problems of Iowa food deserts: Food insecurity and civic structure. *Rural Sociology* 70(1):91–112.

Reisig, V. M. T. and A. Hobbiss. 2000. Food deserts and how to tackle them: A study of one city's approach. *Health Education Journal* 59:137–149.

Shaw, H. J. 2006. Food deserts: Towards the development of a classification. *Geografiska Annaler: Series B, Human Geography* 88B(2):231–247.

Smith, C. and L. W. Morton. 2009. Rural food deserts: Low-income perspectives on food access in Minnesota and Iowa. *Journal of Nutrition Education and Behavior* 41(3):176–187. doi: 10.1016/j.jneb.2008.06.008.

United States Census Bureau, State and County Quick Facts. 2015. Retrieved from https://www.census.gov/quickfacts/

United States Department of Agriculture (USDA) Economic Research Service, Food Access Research Atlas. 2017. Retrieved from https://www.ers.usda.gov/data-products/food-access-research-atlas/documentation/#indicators

United States Department of Agriculture Economic Research Service. 2017a. Retrieved from https://www.ers.usda.gov/topics/food-nutrition-assistance/food-security-in-the-us/measurement/

United States Department of Agriculture Economic Research Service, Food Environment Atlas. 2017b. Retrieved from https://www.ers.usda.gov/data-products/food-environment-atlas/go-to-the-atlas/

U.S. Department of Health and Human Services. 2017. 2015-2020 Dietary Guidelines for Americans. Retrieved from https://health.gov/dietaryguidelines/2015/guidelines/introduction/nutrition-and-health-are-closely-related/

Walker, R. E., C. R. Keane, and J. G. Burke. 2010. Disparities and access to healthy food in the United States: A review of food deserts literature. *Health and Place* 16:876–884. doi: 10.1016.j.healthplace.2010.04.013.

Whelan, A., N. Wrigley, D. Warm, and E. Cannings. 2002. Life in a "food desert." *Urban Studies* 39(11):2083–2100. doi: 10.1080/0042098022000011371.

Part III

Exploring the regulation of food

6   When is food (not) functional?

Courtney I. P. Thomas

We all should have known that it was too good to be true when the announcement began popping up on our social media pages, shared by like-minded friends who were equally determined to embrace the possibility of the unlikely: Eating chocolate can help you LOSE weight! We have all seen similar claims in the past that have transformed our culinary vices into health virtues. Yahoo News tells us, "Don't feel guilt the next time you order a bottle of Shiraz or a Pinot Noir for your dinner date. It may actually prove to be good for your health" before extolling seven health benefits of red wine from the hardening of tooth enamel to the reduction of saturated fat accumulation in the arteries to reducing the appearance of fine lines and wrinkles (Yahoo! News 2015). The Huffington Post gives us 11 reasons to drink coffee every day: coffee provides more antioxidants than fruits and vegetables, may help people with Parkinson's disease control their movements, may reduce the risk of liver cirrhosis, can reduce the risk of developing Type 2 diabetes, and may even make you more intelligent (Jacques 2013). Even Lucky Charms™ with 25 g of carbohydrates per cup claims to be not only "magically delicious"™ but also nutritious with "more whole grains than any other ingredient." How did we get to a place where marketers could extol the nutritional benefits of Lucky Charms?

In 1999, General Mills, the company that makes Lucky Charms, submitted a notification of a prospective health claim about the relationship of whole grain foods and heart disease and certain cancers to the United States Food and Drug Administration (FDA). The FDA determined that for purposes of this claim "whole grain foods" would be defined as foods that contain 51% or more whole grain ingredients by weight. It ruled that manufacturers could use the following claim on the label and in labeling of any eligible product: "diets rich in whole-grain foods and other plant foods and low in total fat, saturated fat, and cholesterol, may help reduce the risk of heart disease and certain cancers" (FDA 1999). With its whole grains, added vitamins and minerals, and calcium, Lucky Charms are considered a functional food, so called because they give an additional function, often one related to health promotion or disease prevention, by adding new ingredients or more of existing ingredients (General Mills 2016). Marion Nestle, who classifies functional foods under the banner of techno-foods, says that functional foods put in the good instead of taking out the bad, but this is not entirely true. To the contrary, many functional foods are simply conventional foods whose ingredients or properties provide a health benefit beyond nutrition, and in 2015 it looked as though chocolate was joining their ranks with a health benefit—weight loss—that was a marketing dream. The problem? The claim was bogus.

In this case, the scientist behind the research, John Bohannon, was part of a project designed to expose the "junk-science of the dieting industry" (Bohannon 2015). He called the research "a fairly typical study for the field of diet research. Which is to say: It was terrible science. The results are meaningless, and the health claims that the media blasted out to millions of people around the world are utterly unfounded" (Bohannon 2015). In this case, the chasm between the health claims associated with chocolate and the scientific research were purposefully glaringly obvious. Bohannon and his colleagues published their research in a for-pay scientific journal before sending out their press release to the mainstream media. Anyone could have looked at the original story and reported, not about the health benefits of chocolate, but about the fundamental flaws in the research, but, even with the benefit of transparency, they did not. Instead, headlines informed millions of readers that "Those who eat chocolate stay slim!"

It would be easy to condemn this study as an outlier, a farce intentionally designed to discredit legitimate food science research and cast consumer doubt on the functional foods industry. However, between 1978 and 1994, Quaker Oats™ submitted 37 studies to the U.S. FDA in support of its health claim petition about the cholesterol-lowering benefits of oat cereals. The FDA said that just 20 of these studies produced statistically significant results. One of the remaining 17 was disqualified for poor methods while the remaining 16 were found to have yielded equivocal effects at best (Nestle 2007, pp. 322–333). Nevertheless, the FDA agreed that "the preponderance of evidence supported a cholesterol-lowering effect—although a small one—from eating oat fiber as part of an otherwise low-fat diet" and approved a health claim to that effect (Nestle 2007, p. 333). What does this say about functional foods—the science and the politics? Are functional foods about health or marketing or both? Also, can the claims they profess be trusted or are they, as Bohannon suggests, part of a study design process that is a recipe for false positives? (Bohannon 2015).

Functional foods are a growing niche of the global food market, but their proliferation has sparked controversy among nutritionists, policymakers, consumers, and producers. Functional foods tempt consumers with a variety of health and welfare claims from the prevention of heart disease to better gastrointestinal health to cancer prevention. The producers who design and market them seek to capture consumer dollars and if the claims made by functional food proponents are to be believed, these products create a new bridge, lucrative both to the corporations that produce them and beneficial to the people who consume them, between food and health. However, to what extent are the health claims advanced by these producers and attached to these foods legitimate? Who conducts the research into the authenticity of these claims and how are those researchers held accountable? Finally, how do policymakers confront the regulatory challenges posed by foods that are linked to a wide variety of health claims?

The first generation of functional foods (1990–2010) featured foods that were enhanced with ingredients linked to specific health claims. At that time, "companies tried to shoehorn ingredients such as plant sterols, omega-3s, conjugated linoleic acid (CLA), coenzyme Q10, glucosamine, GABA—to name just a few—into foods in order to market medicalised benefits, such as lowering cholesterol or supporting joint health" (Mellentin 2015). These ingredients may (or may not) have had health benefits but their obscurity limited their marking potential, and many of these first-generation functional foods failed to capture consumer interest. Most are no longer on the market. Omega-3 yogurt, high fiber chicken, and fish oil Tropicana orange juice are among the 95% of first-generation functional foods to fail.

However, a second generation of functional foods learned from these early failures to transform the food industry and food labeling. Today, food companies "avoid positioning foods as a competitor with food supplements or with drugs" and "instead the emphasis is on what consumers really want—which is ingredients and foods that are *naturally functional*' and make a logical fit with foods" (Mellentin 2015). The key is marketing foods such as almonds, coconut water, whole grains, blueberries, and quinoa, foods that have some kind of intrinsic health benefit while simultaneously appearing "natural" to consumers. In this new market, the foods have to taste good and make sense in the mind of the consumer as well as proclaim some kind of additional health benefit. Consumers are familiar with the idea that yogurts can contain live cultures that can have digestive benefits. Probiotic yogurts make sense, therefore, whereas probiotic pizza did not. While the first generation of functional foods largely failed, this second generation has found enormous success in the food marketplace. This success brings with it serious regulatory challenges.

This chapter analyzes functional foods as they are marketed and regulated in the United States. It examines the regulatory questions that have attended the growth of this food market niche as they have played out in both the executive and judiciary branches of the federal government. In the case of functional foods, both regulatory administrators and federal jurists have been challenged to establish frameworks that protect consumers from misinformation without infringing on the first amendment rights of food producers. The regulatory outcome is one that differentiates between qualified and unqualified health claims and emphasizes the importance of food labeling as a mechanism of consumer education. To demonstrate alternative approaches in food regulation, this chapter compares the U.S. approach to that of the European Union's food safety authorities and reveals dramatic differences between the political and regulatory cultures of the United States and the European Union that are applicable to food regulation and beyond. Finally, it contextualizes the regulation of functional foods within the broader U.S. food safety regulatory regime, a regime that continues to be, in many ways, fundamentally dysfunctional and examines the potential impact of the Food Safety Modernization Act on the functional foods niche.

It's a jungle out there

Since the late 1800s, the American food industry had been plagued by corporate malevolence and market failures that have threatened the health and safety of consumers and prompted regulatory responses from the federal government. Adulteration, or the addition of extraneous materials to foods, was rampant throughout the industry as bread was cut with chalk and sawdust; pepper with burnt metal, mustard, cayenne, buckwheat hulls, and more; and chocolate was heavily adulterated with wheat flour, potatoes, egg yolks, almonds, soap, and red oxide of mercury. Consequently, the 1906 Pure Food and Drug Act declared that a food would be considered adulterated if it "was missing a key ingredient (such as flour in bread), or if its inferior quality was masked by coloring, powdering, coating, mixing, or staining" (Hilts 2003, p. 54). Adulteration would be the foundation of the U.S. food safety regulatory regime for more than a century, but how would the FDA regulate functional foods, foods that are valued for their health enhancing additives?

Although terms such as "functional foods," "nutraceuticals," and "technofoods" are widely used in the marketplace and popular culture, they are not legally defined in law. Therefore, although the FDA regulates functional foods under an authority that stems from the 1906 Pure Food and Drug Act and the 1938 Food, Drug, & Cosmetic Act (FDCA), their approach has been to regulate, not the safety of functional foods, but the claims that the manufacturers make regarding the health benefits of these products. According to FDA rules, health claims may not be made if the product "exceeds disqualifying levels for total fat, saturated fat, cholesterol, or sodium or if, prior to fortification, the food does not contain at least 10% of the Reference Daily Intake of Vitamin A, Vitamin C, iron, calcium, protein, or fiber" (Silverglade and Heller 2010, p. 58). For qualifying foods, the FDA classifies health claims as either qualified or unqualified.

Unqualified health claims are those for which enough evidence exists to support the relationship between a food product and the risk of disease that the claim is authorized by the FDA for unqualified use. For example, the FDA allows the following unqualified health claims in food marketing: fiber-containing fruits, vegetables, and grains reduce the risk of coronary heart disease; fruits and vegetables reduce the risk of cancer; dietary saturated fat and cholesterol increase the risk of coronary heart disease; calcium reduces the risk of osteoporosis; salt increases the risk of hypertension; folic acid reduces the risk of neural tube birth defects. Qualified health claims are those for which there is emerging evidence of a health benefit linked to a food or additive, but that evidence is not sufficient or established enough to meet the FDA standards for an unqualified claim. In these cases, the claim must use qualifying language. In *Pearson v. Shalala* (1999), the federal court for the District of Columbia ruled that the FDA was "obligated by the First Amendment to favor disclosure with accurate, succinct, and reasonable disclaimers over suppression and to rely on claim qualifications rather than outright suppression," in that case of dietary supplements (Emord & Associates. PC

2016b). In 2002, the FDA applied this framework to the food industry. Examples of qualified health claims include the following:

> One study suggests that consumption of tomato sauce two times per week may reduce the risk of ovarian cancer; while this same study shows that consumption of tomatoes or tomato juice had no effect on ovarian cancer risk. FDA concludes that it is highly uncertain that tomato sauce reduces the risk of ovarian cancer;
>
> Supportive but not conclusive research shows that consumption of EPA and DHA omega-3 fatty acids may reduce the risk of coronary heart disease. One serving of [Name of the food] provides [ ] gram of EPA and DHA omega-3 fatty acids. [See nutrition information for total fat, saturated fat, and cholesterol content.];
>
> Very limited and preliminary scientific evidence suggests that eating about 1 tablespoon (16 grams) of corn oil daily may reduce the risk of heart disease due to the unsaturated fat content in corn oil. FDA concludes that there is little scientific evidence supporting this claim. To achieve this possible benefit, corn oil is to replace a similar amount of saturated fat and not increase the total number of calories you eat in a day. One serving of this product contains [x] grams of corn oil (U.S. Food and Drug Administration 2017).

However, unlike its European counterpart, the FDA does not actually research health claims made by food manufacturers. Instead, it reviews the research that is submitted to it, research that is usually conducted or funded by the food industry itself, an industry that has a vested interest in marketing functional foods with health claims to consumers in an increasingly health conscious society. From the perspective of public health or even market economics, however, what is the consequence of the FDA's reliance on the food industry to supply the research upon which these claims are based? What constitutes scientific consensus? Does the FDA have access to the full population of studies conducted on a food-health linkage, or only those submitted by the food manufacturers, a sample likely to be skewed in favor of the industry? Also, in a legal environment in which *Pearson v. Shalala* (1999) governs the FDA's regulation of functional food claims, is any amount of scientific evidence, however, limited or unsubstantiated, sufficient so long as the claim is accompanied by a disclaimer to that effect? Could the chocolate industry legally claim that "One study suggests that the consumption of bittersweet chocolate may accelerate weight loss. Based on this study, FDA concludes that it is highly uncertain that chocolate accelerates weight loss."? Qualified health statements for supplements such as selenium would suggest that, in fact, this would be a legal, if not legitimate, claim according to FDA standards.

A zero-sum game

From the perspective of the food industry, functional foods represent an important market niche in what is essentially a zero-sum game. Most consumers do not spend significantly more on food from year to year. The key to increasing share-holder value and profits, therefore, is to capture consumer dollars, to entice consumers to spend their resources on one product instead of another. Market niches are often associated with food fads, some more resilient than others. In 2016, there is an abundance of organic and gluten-free foods on supermarket shelves, but there are also warehouses of Adkins diet products rotting, relics of a fad that has been replaced, of consumers who have moved on, of food dollars lost to a new niche. Functional foods seem to be a good bet from an industry perspective for while U.S. food sales have seen very slow and slight increases overall, functional food sales have increased enormously and rapidly by comparison.

In many cases, especially cases where issues of intellectual property law apply, companies must be the first to get FDA approval for their innovative products. However, in functional food cases, this is not always true. Many companies may benefit from the approval of a new health claim. That said, companies that dominate a market segment can secure a comparative and competitive advantage in the marketplace by pushing for FDA approval of specific claims. For example, Quaker Oats, a PepsiCo holding, petitioned for a claim that oat fiber reduced the risk of coronary heart disease. While the FDA required the additional qualifying phrase "as part of a diet low in saturated fat and cholesterol," this was a victory, certainly for Quaker, but also for General Mills, Kellogg's, and other food producers. The question remains, however, is the claim true or is oat bran no better than any other high-fiber cereal when it comes to lowering cholesterol? More importantly, from a legal perspective, does it matter? It seems that the answer is no.

The industry is careful to phrase its legal defense of functional foods in terms of freedom of speech, health freedom, and health sovereignty. Challenges to FDA crackdowns on functional food marketing and health claims are decried as censorship. If a food manufacturer's petition for FDA approval of a health claim is denied, that manufacturer can sue for approval. Several law firms, including D.C. based Emord & Associates, advertise their success in suing the FDA on First Amendment grounds in health claims cases and report that commercial speech standards are shifting as courts favor more freedom in the marketplace (Emord & Associates, PC 2016a). This shift undoubtedly benefits the food industry and, many would argue, consumers as well. Others, however, question whether more information is necessarily better and choose to frame the functional foods regulatory debate in terms of truth in advertising rather than freedom of speech. From their perspective, functional foods represent a risk to consumers that is not justified by any significant benefit.

The critics

In 2010, the Center for Science in the Public Interest, a D.C. based nonprofit health advocacy organization, sent the FDA a report entitled "Food Labeling Chaos: The Case for Reform." In it, the CSPI identified several problems relating to conventional foods, functional foods, and health claims. One problem, argued the CPSI, is that "companies will often make 'structure/function' claims, claims that a nutrient in a conventional food can benefit the normal structure or function of a bodily system, without expressly mentioning the role that such nutrient plays in the prevention of any disease" (Silverglade and Heller 2010, p. 57). Therefore, while a company would need FDA approval to state that a food "may reduce the risk of heart disease," it does not need the FDA green light to say that that the same food "helps maintain a healthy heart." However, do consumers understand the difference between such structure/function claims and health claims?

Research indicates that they do not. A study by the food industry-funded International Food Information Council (IFIC) concluded that "Consumers do not perceive a difference among unqualified textual health claims [e.g., those based on 'significant scientific agreement'], structure-function claims, and dietary guidance statements with respect to scientific evidence" (International Food Information Council 2005, p. 59). An AARP study revealed that "more than a third of respondents could not distinguish between health claims and structure/function claims" (Eskin 2001, p. 59). In 1999, the FDA itself confirmed that consumers in numerous focus group studies "could not tell the difference between structure/function claims and health claims" (General Accounting Office 2000). So why would the FDA not apply the same regulatory standards to structure/function claims as they make health claims? High standards would not only advance consumer knowledge and public health but also consumer confidence in food labeling. As President of the American Council on Scientific Health Elizabeth Whelan, ScD, MPH observed, "People are confused enough. Why do we want to give food companies more leeway in what they claim?" (Mitka 2003).

However, structure/function claims are only part of the problem, according to CSPI. The report further argued that the Grocery Manufacturers of America persuaded the FDA under the George W. Bush administration to apply an unnecessarily broad reading of the *Pearson* case to allow qualified health claims for functional foods. Some of these claims are downright bizarre such as the one that states "Two studies do not show that drinking green tea reduces the risk of breast cancer in women, but one weaker, more limited study suggests that drinking green tea may reduce this risk. Based on these studies, FDA concludes that it is highly unlikely that green tea reduces the risk of breast cancer" (Silverglade and Heller 2010, p. 70). This language was, in fact, so convoluted that the U.S. District Court for the Northern District of North Carolina ruled that it was so strongly worded that it "effectively negated" the claim it was designed to qualify and thus violated the First Amendment (Watson 2012). The ruling stated that "There are less burdensome ways in which the FDA could indicate in a short, succinct, and accurate disclaimer that it has not approved the claim without nullifying the claim all together" (Watson 2012).

But are there? The American Medical Association (AMA) is not sure. Michael D. Maves, MD, of the AMA wrote, "In an era when consumers are constantly being bombarded with questionable health information (e.g. via television, the Internet, and other avenues), allowing equivocal qualified health claims on conventional foods will only add to consumers' confusion, and not help them to sort out the conflicting claims of food marketers" (Mitka 2003). Thus, the AMA has "opposed qualified health claims in the labeling of conventional foods for three reasons. First, the AMA believes that the FDA does not have the regulatory authority to allow qualified health claims on labels. Second, the organization says the FDA's use of 'weight of the scientific evidence' to label each claim will lower standards. And finally, the AMA opposed the initiative because it believes that qualified health claims will not help consumers and could, in fact, confuse people" (Mitka 2003).

Moreover, CSPI observes that food manufacturers tend to push the regulatory envelope even beyond the low bar for qualified health claims with little to no retribution by the FDA. For example, while the aforementioned qualified green tea claim was approved by the FDA, a Kashi™ Heart to Heart Oatmeal label "hyped the presence of green tea to support healthy arteries," a claim not at all addressed or approved by the FDA (Silverglade and Heller 2010, p. 72). In another case, Olitalia™ olive oil included only the health claim on the label, omitting the qualifying statement altogether. The FDA's budget for food safety is extremely limited, and according to the bipartisan National Association of State Departments of Agriculture (NASDA) "falls far short of the next investment needed in our new preventative approach to food safety and public health" (Flynn 2016). Even if its enforcement powers exist *de jure*, to what extent do they exist *de facto* in a marketplace of thousands of food items in which the FDA faces the herculean challenges associated with implementing the Food Safety Modernization Act while being understaffed and underfunded? In this, the FDA seems to be acknowledging both its limitations and intentions. Although it sends letters to food manufacturers that exaggerate claims, fail to use qualifying language, include health claims on foods, such as eggs, that are ineligible for such claims, or fail to meet the "significant scientific agreement standard" for a claim made on their labels, many of these letters state that the FDA will not take enforcement action against the company making the claims. The CSPI asserts that this strategy by the FDA "signals an 'anything goes' regulatory environment that contributes to the dissemination of a variety of nutrition misinformation" (Silverglade and Heller 2010, pp. 76–77). This problem is exacerbated by the fact, according to CSPI, that the "Federal Trade Commission, which regulates food advertising, has no premarket procedure for reviewing advertising claims. Thus, deceptive claims can only be stopped after the fact, often through a time-consuming process that sometimes involves ligation that can take years to complete" (Silverglade and Heller 2010, p. 77).

While the FDA uses its enforcement discretion to ignore many flagrant violations of its qualified health claims regulations, this is not always the case. For example, when Nestle produced Juicy Juice™ advertised a "Brain Development Fruit Juice Beverage" that claimed that it "helped support brain development in children under two years old," the FDA intervened. It argued that the claim was not a qualified or unqualified health claim, but a drug claim, and required evidence of both the efficacy and safety of the product or the removal of the statement from the label. Clearly, therefore, there is a line that food manufacturers cannot cross, but FDA inaction on qualified health claims alongside action on drug claims indicates where it has decided that line will be, in practice if not in policy. This gives food producers a great deal of latitude in marketing functional foods.

The other side of the pond

Functional foods are a global market niche, not merely an American fad. However, regulatory structures vary around the world and in Europe, food safety regulators have taken a very different approach when it comes to functional foods and health claims. In December 2006, the European Union adopted Regulation 1924 on the use of nutrition and health claims for foods. This harmonized EU-wide rules and mandated that claims made on food labels be clear and substantiated by scientific data (European Food Safety Authority 2016).

The regulation worked "to ensure a high level of protection for consumers and to facilitate their choice" and to "create equal conditions of competition for the food industry" (EC 2006). It mandated that "scientific substantiation...be the main aspect to be taken into account for the use of nutrition and health claims and the food business operators using claims should justify them" (EC 2006). It warned that "a nutrition or health claim should not be made if it is inconsistent with generally accepted nutrition and health principles or if it encourages or condones excessive consumption of any food or disparages good dietary practice" (EC 2006). In this, European authorities were quick to seek to protect consumers against self-medicating with functional foods to the detriment of their nutritional health. To facilitate the implementation of this regulation, the EFSA pledged to develop a list of permitted nutrition claims and their specific conditions of use and required that the list be regularly updated in light of scientific and technological developments. Moreover, EFSA required that "health claims should only be authorized for use in the Community after a scientific assessment of the *highest possible standard*. In order to ensure harmonized scientific assessment of these claims, the *European Food Safety Authority should carry out such assessments*" [emphasis mine] (EC 2006).

These stipulations demonstrate that, as with many regulatory issues, EFTA is committed to the precautionary principle. That is, what they do not know to be safe they assume to be dangerous and regulate proactively. Conversely, U.S. agencies like the FDA tend to rely on risk assessment. That is, what they do not know to be dangerous they assume to be safe and regulate reactively. For this reason, a centralized, harmonized approach to health claims associated with functional foods is consistent with widespread European regulatory commitments and the culture that dictates them. Moreover, the European approach displays far more cooperation with national and international agencies than does that of the United States.

One such agency is the International Life Sciences Institute Europe (ILSI Europe), an organization which "fosters collaboration among the best scientists to provide evidence-based scientific consensus on the areas of nutrition, food safety, toxicology, risk assessment and the environment. By facilitating their collaboration, ILSI Europe helps scientists from many sectors of society—public and private—to best address complex science and health issues by sharing their unique knowledge and perspectives" (ILSI Europe 2016a). Its Functional Foods Task Force acknowledges that "specific components of the diet can bring benefits beyond those of basic nutrition" but cautions that "these beneficial effects need to be supported by scientific evidence before they can be communicated to consumers and others via health or nutrition claims and other relevant channels" (ILSI Europe 2016c). When the EFSA first evaluated health claim dossiers, the ILSI task force "reviewed and evaluated the quality of published results of human intervention studies" and in 2011 "published guidelines for designing, conducting, and reporting human intervention studies for the substantiation of health claims in the *British Journal of Nutrition*" (ILSI Europe 2016b).

EFSA regulations also reference the Guidelines for Nutrition and Health Claims established by the Codex Alimentarius Commission in 1997. These guidelines state that "health claims should be consistent with national health policy, including nutrition policy, and support such policies where applicable" (Codex Alimentarius Commission 1997). Moreover, "health claims should be supported by a sound and sufficient body of scientific evidence to substantiate the claim, provide truthful and nonmisleading information to aid consumers in choosing healthful diets and be supported by specific consumer education" (Codex Alimentarius Commission 1997). Finally, "the impact of health claims on consumers' eating behaviors and dietary patterns should be monitored, in general, by competent authorities" (Codex Alimentarius Commission 1997). Thus, "health claims should have a clear regulatory framework for qualifying and/or disqualifying conditions for eligibility to use the specific claim, including the ability of competent national authorities to prohibit claims made for foods that contain nutrients or constituents in amounts that increase the risk of disease or an adverse health-related condition. The health claim should not be made if it encourages or condones the excessive consumption of any food or disparages good dietary practice" (Codex Alimentarius Commission 1997). From these guidelines, the EFSA has developed strict limitations on food-based health claims and has enforced those limitations consistently.

What is interesting, however, is that these very high standards do not prevent European consumers from eating functional foods. To the contrary, in 2014, 56% of Europeans reported using food and drink to improve their health with 19% specifically eating functional foods at least a few times a week (Moloughney 2014). Even without heavy marketing, some functional foods are taking European markets by storm. Coconut water, for example, has become a huge seller in European markets with retail sells growing by more than 100% in recent years despite the fact that food manufacturers are not legally permitted to make a health claim on coconut water within the European Union (Beverage World 2012; IPD 2016). Nevertheless, the regulatory framework established by EFSA for health claims has created a very strict, some would argue hostile, environment for functional foods. For example, EFSA has consistently rejected probiotic health claim submissions because the science does not adequately support the marketing claims made by food producers. In 2008, Dannon was forced to pay $35 million in damages to consumers because of misleading health claims on Activia™ and DanActive™ yogurts and had to withdraw its claim that Activia improves digestion.

The fact that high science-based standards for health claims and thriving markets for functional foods coexist across Europe is evidence that the two are not mutually exclusive. Regulatory agencies need not sacrifice consumer confidence in food labels or undermine public health through lax standards for health claims in order to allow the functional foods industry to thrive. Many nutritionists and healthcare professionals in the United States would argue that this justifies a change to the FDA's approach despite claims from some corners that existing U.S. standards threaten to cripple the functional foods market (AHN-USA 2015).

The future of function

In today's market, most functional foods are not fortified or enhanced, or (one might say) adulterated with additives designed to produce a desired health benefit. To the contrary, food producers have found that functional foods hold more market appeal when they appear as natural as possible. The market proliferation of "superfoods" is the latest fad in this vein. Superfoods are foods that are considered to be very good for your health and are often thought to be preventative or medicinal relative to specific medical conditions. While the use of the term in marketing is prohibited by the European Union unless accompanied by specific medical claims backed by sufficient scientific consensus, the superfood designation is unregulated in the United States and the market is thriving (Clark 2015). From 1998 to 2013, blueberry production in the United States grew from 17 million pounds to 90 million pounds and is expected to hit 150 million pounds by 2018 (Clark 2015). Quinoa crop prices tripled between 2006 and 2013, but teff, freekeh, kamut, fonio, and lupin are heralded as the new up-and-coming super grains (Spiegel 2014). Similarly, mentions of kale on restaurant menus increased 223% from 2012 to 2014 while the popularization of kale chips, kale smoothies, and kale pesto alongside raw kale itself has more than doubled the size of the industry (Rovell and Meredith 2014). However, what do consumers believe about superfoods and how much of it is true? Also, to what extent can that information be regulated by U.S. agencies?

The answers are what they hear in the media and read online; the jury is out, and potentially nothing. Nutritionist Marion Nestle argues that "The term 'superfood' as we know it today is silly because it is basically code for 'grown 15,000 miles away in a remote mountain range and sold at a premium.' As far as I am concerned, all whole, minimally processed, plant-based foods are superfoods. Are goji berries healthy? Sure. But so is an orange" (Clark 2015). In this political and economic climate, regulators face a lose–lose situation when it comes to functional foods. They have little to no control over how these foods are portrayed in the media, they have an extremely limited budget for nutrition education for consumers, they are constrained by judicial interpretations of the First Amendment relative to limitations on health claims on food labels, and they lack the resources necessary to enforce existing regulations, let alone to develop new ones as new niches emerge. By the time the federal government legally defined and established regulations for "organic" food, the market had moved on to "natural" and "super" foods. The FDA cannot keep up, and as food safety demands associated with the Food Safety Modernization Act overwhelm their resources, functional food and health claim regulations and enforcement are likely to go undeveloped and unenforced.

REFERENCES

AHN-USA. 2015. *FDA Doubles Down on Censoring Food Labels.* April 21. Accessed May 25, 2016. http://www.anh-usa.org/fda-doubles-down-on-censoring-food-labels/

Beverage World. 2012. *The Outlook for Coconut Water in Europe is Sweet.* May 7. Accessed May 25, 2016. http://www.beverageworld.com/articles/full/15031/the-outlook-for-coconut-water-in-europe-is-sweet

Bohannon, J. 2015. *I Fooled Millions into Thinking Chocolate Helps Weight Loss. Here's How.* io9. May 27. Accessed May 24. 2016. http://io9.gizmodo.com/i-fooled-millions-into-thinking-chocolate-helps-weight-1707251800

Clark, L. 2015. Are "superfoods" over: A closer look at a wildly popular. Totally unregulated food label. *Civil Eats.* July 23. Accessed May 25, 2016. http://civileats.com/2015/07/23/are-superfoods-over/

Codex Alimentarius Commission. 1997. *Guidelines for Use of Nutrition and Health Claims.* Accessed May 25, 2016. http://www.fao.org/fao-who-codexalimentarius/sh-proxy/en/?lnk=1&url=https%253A%252F%252Fworkspace.fao.org%252Fsites%252Fcodex%252FStandards%252FCAC%2BGL%2B23-1997%252FCXG_023e.pdf

EC. 2006. *Regulation (EC) No 1924/2006 of the European Parliament and of the Council of 20 December 2006.* Accessed May 25, 2016. http://eur-lex.europa.eu/legal-content/EN/TXT/PDF/?uri=CELEX:32006R1924&from=en

Emord & Associates, PC. 2016a. *Commercialization of Qualified Health Claims.* Accessed May 24, 2016. http://emord.com/blawg/commercialization-of-qualified-health-claims/

Emord & Associates, PC. 2016b. *Health Claims.* Accessed May 24, 2016. http://www.emord.com/FDA_health_claims.html

Eskin, S. B. 2001. AARP Public Policy Institute. Dietary supplements and older consumers. December. In *Food Labeling Chaos: The Case for Reform*, edited by B. Silverglade and I. R. Heller Washington. D.C.: Center for Science in the Public Interest, 2010. Available online: https://www.cspinet.org/new/pdf/food_labeling_chaos_report.pdf

European Food Safety Authority. 2016. *Nutrition and Health Claims.* Accessed May 24, 2016. https://www.efsa.europa.eu/en/topics/topic/nutrition.

FDA. 1999. *Health Claim Notification for Whole Grain Foods.* July. Accessed May 24, 2016. http://www.fda.gov/Food/IngredientsPackagingLabeling/LabelingNutrition/ucm073639.htm

Flynn, Dan. 2016. Obama's 2017 budget not enough for a food safety legacy. *Food Safety News.* February 10. Accessed May 24, 2016. http://www.foodsafetynews.com/2016/02/obamas-2017-budget-not-enough-for-a-food-safety-legacy/#.V0Sq3miDGko

General Accounting Office. 2000. Food safety. Improvements needed in overseeing the safety of dietary supplements and "Functional Foods." (23 GAO/RCED-00-156. July). In *Food Labeling Chaos: The Case for Reform*, edited by B. Silverglade and I. R. Heller Washington. D.C.: Center for Science in the Public Interest, 2010. Available online: https://www.cspinet.org/new/pdf/food_labeling_chaos_report.pdf

Hilts, P. J. 2003. *Protecting America's Health: the FDA. Business and One Hundred Years of Regulation.* New York, NY: Alfred A. Knoph

ILSI Europe. 2016a. *About Us.* Accessed May 24, 2016. http://www.ilsi.org/Europe/Pages/HomePage.aspx#

ILSI Europe. 2016b. *Functional Foods.* Accessed May 24, 2016. http://www.ilsi.org/Europe/Pages/HomePage.aspx#

ILSI Europe. 2016c. *Functional Foods Task Force.* Accessed May 24, 2016. http://ilsi.eu/europe/wp-content/uploads/sites/3/2016/05/Functional-Foods_TFonepager-1.pdf

International Food Information Council. 2005. *Qualified Health Claims Consumer Research Project.* March. Available http://www.ific.org/research/qualhealthclaimsres. cfm. In *Food Labeling Chaos: The Case for Reform*, edited by B. Silverglade and I. R. Heller Washington. D.C.: Center for Science in the Public Interest, 2010. Available online: https://www.cspinet.org/new/pdf/food_labeling_chaos_report.pdf).

IPD. 2016. *CBI Product Factsheet: Coconut Water in Germany.* Accessed May 27, 2016. https://www.cbi.eu/sites/default/files/study/product-factsheet-coconut-water-germany-processed-fruit-vegetables-edible-nuts-2014.pdf

Jacques, R. 2013. 11 reasons you should drink coffee every day. *Huffpost Taste.* October 17. Accessed May 24, 2016. http://www.huffingtonpost.com/2013/10/17/coffee-health-benefits_n_4102133.html

General Mills. 2016. *Lucky Charms.* Accessed May 24, 2016. http://www.generalmills.com/en/Brands/Cereals/lucky-charms

Mellentin, J. 2015. Functional Foods 2.0: Beyond the nutritional shoehorn. *Nutra Ingredietns.com.* April 29. Accessed May 24, 2016. http://www.nutraingredients.com/Markets-and-Trends/The-evolution-of-functional-foods

Mitka, M. 2003. Food fight over product label claims. *Medical News and Perspectives* 7:871–875. Accessed May 24, 2016. doi: 10.1001/jama.290.7.87.

Moloughney, S. 2014. Functional food and drink trends in Europe. *Nutraceuticals World.* May 27. Accessed May 25, 2016. http://www.nutraceuticalsworld.com/contents/view_online-exclusives/2014-05-27/functional-food-drink-trends-in-europe

Nestle, M. 2007. *Food Politics: How the Food Industry Influences Nutrition and Health. Revised and Expanded Edition.* Berkeley, CA: University of California Press.

Rovell, D. and F. Meredith. 2014. The economy of kale: Leafy green is taking over. *ABC News.* August 4. Accessed May 25, 2016. http://abcnews.go.com/Business/economy-kale-leafy-green-taking/story?id=24840049

Silverglade, B. and Heller I. R. 2010. *Food Labeling Chaos: The Case for Reform.* Washington. D.C.: Center for Science in the Public Interest. Available online: https://www.cspinet.org/new/pdf/food_labeling_chaos_report.pdf

Spiegel, A. 2014. Super grains: What's the new Quinoa? *Huff Post: Food for Thought.* January 27. Accessed May 25, 2016. http://www.huffingtonpost.com/2014/01/27/super-grain_n_4659293.html

U.S. Food and Drug Administration. 2017. *Summary of Qualified Health Claims Subject to Enforcement Discretion.* Accessed January 26, 2017. http://www.fda.gov/Food/IngredientsPackagingLabeling/LabelingNutrition/ucm073992.htm#birth

Watson, E. 2012. Green tea qualified health claim ruling. *Nutra Ingredients-USA.com.* March 15. Accessed May 24, 2016. http://www.nutraingredients-usa.com/Regulation/ Green-tea-qualified-health-claim-ruling-Once-again-FDA-is-taken-to-task

Yahoo! News. 2015. *7 Amazing Health Benefits of Drinking Red Wine.* September 30. Accessed May 24, 2016. https://www.yahoo.com/news/7-amazing-health-benefits-drinking-red-wine-144532108.html?ref=gs

7 Chlorpyrifos contamination across the food system

Shifting science, regulatory challenges, and implications for public health

Bhavna Shamasunder

Introduction

Chlorpyrifos is one of the most widely used pesticides in the world since it was developed in the 1960s, yet it is little known by the public despite the growing certainty of its harm to human health and the environment. This chapter traces chlorpyrifos' legacy on the eve of its ban by the Environmental Protection Agency (EPA), more than three decades since it became the majority replacement pesticide following the ban of DDT. Chemical exposures, such as widespread exposures to chlorpyrifos as it moves through the food system, are of public health significance. Intersectional research connecting food studies and environmental health sciences about chemical exposures is limited, resulting in gaps that deter effectively addressing the long-term and systemic public health threats of chemicals as an integrated part of our food system. Chlorpyrifos is part of a class of insecticides termed organophosphates that can trigger neurotoxic effects in humans when touched, inhaled, or eaten. It came to be one of the dominant replacements for DDT after its ban in 1972 because it seemed to be an improvement in the chemistry that caused DDT to persist in the environment and accumulate in wildlife. However, over the past three decades, farmworkers' advocates, environmentalists, and environmental health scientists have documented harm in exposed groups and exerted ongoing pressure on regulatory agencies to curb the chemical's use.

Advocacy groups pressured the EPA to revoke chlorpyrifos tolerances as early as the 1980s given the scientific evidence of harm. They succeeded in 2000 in ending over-the-counter sales of the chemical because of the overwhelming evidence of damage to children, but agricultural uses persisted. In 2007, the Natural Resources Defense Council (NRDC) and Pesticide Action Network North America (PANNA) filed a petition with the EPA to ban the chemical. The EPA dragged out response to the petition for 9 years. In December 2014, the EPA acknowledged peer-reviewed science linking chlorpyrifos exposure with brain damage in children, including reduced IQ, delayed development, and loss of working memory. By December 2015, the U.S. Ninth Circuit Court of Appeals declared EPA's in action on chlorpyrifos to be "egregious" and constituted a "cycle of incomplete responses, missed deadlines, and unreasonable delay" (U.S. Court of Appeals for the Ninth Circuit 2015). The EPA, forced by the hand of the court, is currently weighing the scientific evidence to discontinue all chlorpyrifos uses in agriculture by revoking food tolerances (US EPA 2016) since the primary form of population exposure is through pesticide residues in food. This article examines the conflict over chlorpyrifos and argues for a food system and precautionary public health-based approach to regulatory decision-making over pesticides. Ongoing contestations by scientists over the meaning and interpretation of chemical exposures despite mounting evidence of wide-spread population exposures to multiple chemicals require new frameworks for approaching pesticide regulation (Shamasunder and Morello-Frosch 2015).* The case of chlorpyrifos also raises important questions about replacement chemicals which themselves can prove to be problematic.

Bridging food studies and environmental health

The food studies literature straddles an interdisciplinary swath of social scientific analyses of food systems. Pesticides are often examined at the point of consumption, such as tensions between organic versus conventionally produced food with a predominant focus on consumer perceptions or the cooptation of organic labeling by agribusiness (i.e., Guthman 1998; Yiridoe et al. 2005). Scholars have noted the overlaps of food activism with social movements, coining the term "food justice" (Gottlieb and Joshi 2013), to examine inequities in the food system, for example situating lack of access to quality produce in low-income communities and communities of color as an environmental justice issue.

Research on pesticide regulatory regimes has focused on harm to workers and fenceline communities from pesticide exposures and describes the entrenched regulatory neglect by pesticide agencies in vulnerable communities that dismiss routine poisonings as "accidental" (Harrison 2006). However, there has been little examination of how worker exposures on the frontline of pesticide exposures then pervades the entire food system, continuing along the food chain, and resulting in significant costs to public health. The U.S. agricultural system is extensively industrialized, driven by large-scale corporate agricultural interests, and deeply dependent on pesticide use. Agricultural history is rooted in the massive exploitation of natural resources and the subordination of immigrant workers who suffer from tenuous economic and political circumstances (McWilliams 1939; Walker 2004). The system is absolutely dependent on temporary and marginalized farm labor. Even efforts that work toward alternatives to the industrialized system, such as community supported agriculture or organic farming, are dependent on a steady supply of mostly immigrant and undocumented farmworkers (Guthman 2004). This heavy reliance on vulnerable workers in all agricultural sectors makes the system at its core unwilling to address poor working conditions.

---

* For depth on scientific contestations over biomonitoring and for methods for collecting the scientists' interviews referenced in this paper, see Shamasunder and Morello-Frosch (2015).

The literature on pesticides and agrifood activism points to an increasingly neoliberal and market-driven agenda by both the federal government and environmental and food-centered social movements, where consumer choice and the ability to purchase organic foods are prioritized over worker concerns (Guthman 2004). Studies of pesticide drift find that market-based efforts actually exacerbate drift and worker exposures. Workers are expected to be protected through safety equipment and suggested reentry periods to limit pesticide poisoning. Ultimately, market efforts do not address ongoing pesticide exposures. Additionally, there is regulatory resistance to restrict drift-prone pesticides since these chemicals are often less persistent in the environment despite their often greater acute toxicity to workers (Harrison 2008). For example, the pesticide methyl bromide was banned because it was found to deplete the ozone layer, but growers sought to replace it with methyl iodide, which does not deplete ozone but is far more toxic to workers. Despite these tendencies in the realm of pesticide protections toward consumer and market-driven reforms, the current scientific evidence demonstrates that worker exposures can lead down the line to consumer exposures.

Environmental justice, workers' rights, environmental, and environmental health movements have often strategically parted ways in the fight to curb pesticide use due to differing movement priorities and structural challenges posed by different regulatory mechanisms for workers and consumers. One overarching commonality has been the lack of sustained attention by environmental movements to farmworkers' multiple vulnerabilities despite their acute and chronic exposures to the pesticides (Pulido 1996). When DDT was banned, it was quickly replaced by organophosphate pesticides. As evidence mounted that workers suffered severe neurotoxic effects from chlorpyrifos exposure, California became the first state in the country to adopt cholinesterase monitoring in 1974. Cholinesterase testing sought to manage against the worst health effects from organophosphate poisoning in workers. Nonetheless, the California program is now widely considered to be a failure since it is lax, there is no central reporting, and industries only participate on a voluntary basis.

Studies of pesticide exposure in the environmental health sciences literature are vast, spanning toxicology to epidemiology, and data published on often chemical-specific linear and measurable impacts. Much recent chlorpyrifos research has been conducted through biomonitoring studies that measure metabolite (chemical breakdown) levels primarily in urine and sometimes blood. Biomonitoring is the technology that allows for measurements of chemicals in human blood, breast milk, and other tissues. Chlorpyrifos studies using biomonitoring are undergirded by national chemical biomonitoring surveillance conducted by the Centers for Disease Control (CDC) through the National Biomonitoring Program, which tests a subset of the U.S. population for over 200 chemicals, one of which is chlorpyrifos. The CDC detects chlorpyrifos in over 90% of the U.S. population (Centers for Disease Control and Prevention 2009), showing widespread exposure. These exposures are primarily through food, though some communities such as agricultural fenceline communities face higher exposures given proximity to spraying (Schafer 2004; Eskenazi et al. 2007).

The collective body of data, when connecting disparately produced studies, reveals chlorpyrifos along the food chain in bodies from production to consumption, in workers, communities living on the fenceline of intensive agricultural production, and consumers. "Following the molecule" can be a generative method for understanding the complex patterns of industrial chemicals as they move across sites where they have come to inhabit people, communities, and landscapes (Casper 2003). More recent scientific studies show chlorpyrifos to be an endocrine disruptor, leading to adverse health outcomes at very low-level exposures. In utero exposures and exposures to children are of most concern because they are still invulnerable periods of development (Viswanath et al. 2010). The chemical can also persist in ground water, which worsens exposure when combined with food intake. Agricultural, chemical, and crop protection trade groups argue that exposure alone does not constitute harm and have questioned some of the scientific data in order to stop the EPA from considering a chlorpyrifos ban. The EPA faces strong industry pressure to retain the chemical's use.

Background and health effects

Developed during World War II by the Dow Chemical Company (Doyle 2004), chlorpyrifos is no longer patent protected and is the active ingredient in dozens of pesticide formulations made by global companies such as Bayer and BASF. In the United States, chlorpyrifos is used in numerous crops at a million pounds per year on over two million acres of cropland. It is also used in crop applications globally. Chlorpyrifos is used on corn as well as soybeans, fruit, nuts, brussel sprouts, cranberries, broccoli, and cauliflower, as well as others. It also has non-agricultural uses such as on golf courses, turf, greenhouses, and nonstructural wood treatments. DDT, its predecessor, was banned because it was found to persist in the environment and bioaccumulate across the food chain. The primary concern over DDT was for wildlife and ecosystems. Worker exposures was not a guiding concern for environmentalists of the 1960s and 1970s who sought a ban on DDT (Pulido and Peña 1998). Chlorpyrifos seemed an effective improvement in pesticide chemistry since it does not persist in the environment, does not bioaccumulate across the food chain, and is metabolized by the human body. For decades, chlorpyrifos was the most extensively used home and garden pesticide, sold over the counter under the names Dursban and Lorsban, and the active ingredient in hundreds of consumer products such as flea sprays and roach killers. In 2000, the EPA phased out consumer sales of chlorpyrifos following what was then the most extensive scientific assessment of a pesticide in EPA history (Brown and Warrick 2000), with the scientific data linking it to dangerous neurological and developmental toxicity in children. Chlorpyrifos remains in widespread agricultural uses, propelling the scientific research published over the past 15 years on continued impacts to farmworkers, fenceline communities, and consumers.

Chlorpyrifos works by inhibiting the action of the enzyme acetylcholinesterase that controls the messages that travel between nerve cells. It is a neurotoxin and exposure results in overstimulation of the nervous system (Kwong 2002) and nervous system malfunction. In the 1960s, Dow Chemical secretly tested 16 prisoners at the Clinton Correctional Facility in Dannemora, New York. At higher exposure levels, Dow noted sharp drops in plasma cholinesterase levels (Doyle 2004). However, they deemed the chemical safe for workers with use of protective equipment and routine testing of cholinesterase levels. Higher levels of chlorpyrifos exposure result in acutely neurotoxic effects (Richardson 1995) that can include salivation, irregular heartbeat, convulsions, and death. Low-dose exposures documented in farmworkers include impaired memory and concentration, disorientation, severe depression, irritability, confusion, headaches, nightmares, sleepwalking, drowsiness, insomnia, and flu-like conditions (Barr and Angerer 2006). Physicians can mistake chlorpyrifos exposure for the common flu, leading to misdiagnoses and underreporting of farmworker pesticide poisoning cases (Nash 2004). Chlorpyrifos exposure has been associated with developmental delays, and prenatal exposures are being linked with attention deficit and hyperactivity disorder problems (Rauh et al. 2006). There is also growing animal evidence pointing to chlorpyrifos' role as an endocrine disruptor, a class of toxins that disrupt hormone systems associated with reproduction and development at very low exposure levels (Haviland, Butz, and Porter 2010) making these exposures significant for children. Levels that can cause endocrine disruption are below those that trigger cholinesterase inhibition and also below levels at which the pesticide is regulated.

Chlorpyrifos regulation: A contentious history

Two federal statutes, the Federal Insecticide, Fungicide, and Rodenticide Act (FIFRA) and the Food Quality Protection Act (FQPA), regulate chlorpyrifos. Both of these fall under the purview of the EPA. FIFRA provides the basis for the regulation, sale, distribution, and use of pesticides. In 1996, the FQPA amended FIFRA and set more stringent safety standards for new and old pesticides, creating more uniform requirements for processed and unprocessed foods. The FQPA required the EPA to set standards for the levels allowable as food residues, to consider risks to infants and children when setting these standards (termed tolerances), to consider "aggregate risk" from an exposure to one pesticide from multiple sources, and to address "cumulative risk" for pesticides that share a common mechanism of toxicity, which includes the class of organophosphate pesticides like chlorpyrifos. Some heralded the FQPA as groundbreaking when it first passed since it is the first federal environmental statute to consider the unique exposures and vulnerabilities of fetuses, infants, and children rather than only adult exposures. The FQPA drove the chlorpyrifos ban in consumer products (Landrigan and Goldman 2011).

Chlorpyrifos' scientific assessment in 2000 had been called the most extensive and contentious for a pesticide in history (Brown and Warrick 2000), though the current 2016 assessment rivals the contention of 16 years ago, with more than 80,000 people submitting public comments over the EPA's proposed ban of all chlorpyrifos' uses on all crops by revoking food tolerances. In April 2000, 12 prominent scientists including Philip Landrigan, a pediatrician, and a former

EPA executive, penned a letter to the then EPA Administrator Carol Browner calling on the EPA to "tightly restrict" agricultural uses of chlorpyrifos and "ban outright" its uses in schools and homes. In October 1999, the EPA proposed lowering the acceptable exposure level for the chemical to one-third of its then allowable level and finally restricted it to one-tenth of its then allowable level. Typically, the EPA sets safety exposure levels for pesticides such as chlorpyrifos at one 100th of the maximum concentration at which there are no detectable effects on an adult animal. Under the FQPA, the 100-fold safety margin increases 10-fold if evidence is found that there are any impacts on infants and children. Studies leading up to the decision showed that children absorb more pesticides from their environment than adults; chlorpyrifos persisted in furniture, rugs, and other household items, and children were less able to excrete and detoxify themselves through natural bodily processes than adults (Landrigan and Goldman 2011). These physical and behavioral patterns of children, combined with evidence that chlorpyrifos could likely be a developmental and behavioral neurotoxin, pressured the EPA to take action. The new standard essentially eliminated home uses and lowered the amount of residue allowed on food.

In 2000, thousands of public comments were submitted emphasizing the country's economic dependence on chlorpyrifos, protesting limits on the chemical's sale, chiding the EPA for harming food systems or encouraging the EPA to protect consumers, to name a few. The State of California's Department of Food and Agriculture, linked to the nation's largest agri-industry, argued that the decision would affect consumers who depend on an affordable, reliable food supply. Numerous advocacy organizations challenged the EPA's lack of attention to pervasive population exposures from agriculture. Also, the Attorney General of the State of New York submitted extensive public comment critiquing chlorpyrifos' continued use in agriculture and the residual presence on food. The New York AG argued that the Final Risk Assessment (FRA) failed to address the metabolite TCP (the breakdown product of chlorpyrifos measured in the body) found in 92% of adults and 100% of children tested, as well as the neurological and developmental impacts at low levels, and did not consider environmental justice by neglecting farmworker exposure and communities affected by drift.*

When asked about the agreement in 2000, a Federal EPA scientist was surprised by the criticism that EPA garnered from advocates who criticized the agency as being captured by industry. She stated,

> In risk management, it's really our practice to sit down with companies and get them to voluntarily withdraw chemicals when there's a problem. The reason we do that is because it happens pretty quickly and in fact, we got chlorpyrifos out of people's houses in record time with the help of industry. If they don't agree, our recourse is to go to court. We're doing that on carbofuran right now, and four years later it's still being used, so from a management perspective

---

* The Honorable Eliot Spitzer, Attorney General, State of New York, Albany, NY, letter to Arthur M. Blank, President/CEO, Home Depot, Inc., June 8, 2000.

of getting the hazard away from people, that's how you do it. And I don't think that people realize that. It hurts me to hear that it's an industry friendly deal because we think that we got it away from houses as quickly as possible. I don't think there was any way we could've done that any faster than we did. I mean we actually cancelled the products, changed the numbers so the products couldn't be used. (EPA Government Scientist, Personal Communication)

Whether or not the 2000 tolerance reduction was the swiftest action the EPA could have taken at the time, in the following 15 years, the agency was accused of dragging its feet in the face of new science that showed allowable uses in agriculture to constitute harm to public health.

A growing scientific consensus on chlorpyrifos

In the decade after the 2000 ban, the scientific research on chlorpyrifos burgeoned. Studies from UC Berkeley to Columbia University showed the impacts of prenatal exposures on the neurological development of children. Scientists monitored pregnant women's exposures via umbilical cord blood and found dramatic IQ deficits in exposed children living in low-income public housing and developmental deficits in exposed farmworker children. Dr. Phil Landrigan, who was instrumental in the 2000 consumer ban, called these new findings "shocking" in a *New York Times* health blog and stated, "when we took lead out of gasoline, we reduced lead poisoning by 90 percent, and we raised the I.Q. of a whole generation of children four or five points. I think these findings about pesticides should generate similar controversy" (Parker-Pope 2011).

The following section follows some of the key debates and studies that track the chlorpyrifos molecule in the bodies of workers, fenceline communities, and consumers.

Workers

I think there's a divide between occupational exposure and exposure of consumers. I think it's wrongly termed as "involuntary exposure" of the consumer versus "occupational exposure" in workers. Workers seem to accept a certain level of risk...I don't prescribe to that theory...Medical monitoring has been occurring in workers and workers are exposed to a certain level but that hasn't resulted in so much regulatory change. But those same chemicals measured in consumers or people who aren't working in those chemicals might result in change. (Scientist, California Department of Public Health, Personal Communication)

Worker exposures have been a secondary consideration in any pesticide ban, the primary focal point being consumers or the ecosystem. The story of chlorpyrifos a legacy of the story of DDT. DDT was a widely applied agricultural insecticide and used to control malaria beginning in World War II. DDT biomonitoring began in countries such as Sweden in 1967, one of the first countries to conduct long-term population level chemical biomonitoring (Norén and Meironyté 2000). Studies found that DDT is persistent and bioaccumulative, concentrates in fat and tissues, moves up through the food chain, and the body does not easily rid itself of the chemical. It is found in humans and animals in far-flung regions of the world, even in nonindustrialized areas in the circumpolar North through transboundary transport. Bans on DDT were enacted by countries around the world, and international agreements such as the Stockholm Convention continue to use biomonitoring to document declines in DDT in breast milk worldwide. Chlorpyrifos, which is metabolized and excreted by the body, became a favored replacement chemical.

Organophosphate monitoring in workers serves as a method for keeping workers from the worst effects—essentially monitoring for effect. Cholinesterase monitoring measures workers' physiological reaction to exposure, removing them from the field when they begin to show a physiological response. It is one of the only forms of protection for workers exposed to organophosphate pesticides (DeCaprio 1997). It is used in only a few states where chlorpyrifos is applied. All workers who work with Class I and Class II organophosphate or carbamate pesticides with more than 6 days of exposure in a month are to be tested. Reentry periods have been established to define how long a worker must wait to resume work to give their plasma cholinesterase levels an opportunity to rebound (Lessenger 2005). In Washington state, a cholinesterase monitoring program was established when a pesticide poisoned farmworker Juan Rios sued the Department of Labor & Industries, which administers the Washington Industrial Safety and Health Act. In 2002, the Washington State Supreme Court found that the Department had violated the Act of 1973 when it denied the farmworker's request for a mandatory cholinesterase monitoring program. In doing so, they had failed to comply with their own mandate to protect workers. The program now has a network of state workers and physicians who provide services to farmworkers.

Worker exposures can be contextualized in the long struggle to recognize environmental illness. Environmental illness was rendered invisible for decades because regulators saw human bodies as separate from their environments. When workers came down with illness, they were accused of uncleanliness, lack of hygiene, and failure to follow proper farm protocols. Cholinesterase testing, emerging in the late 1950s and early 1960s, was a move toward acknowledging the body as intimately connected to the environment. It provided a litmus test for exposure and gave occupational health regulators stronger toxicological knowledge of pesticide-related illness. However, prediction proved unwieldy since baseline cholinesterase levels vary widely among individuals and levels in the blood are sometimes a poor approximation for levels in the brain (Nash 2004). Additionally, rather arbitrary regulations emerged to determine "reentry levels" so neurotoxic pesticides could continue to be used while "protecting" worker health. Complex monitoring systems were put in place in lieu of regulations to limit pesticide use. Despite these limitations, cholinesterase testing can corroborate workers' experiences and protect farmworkers from the worst effects of pesticide exposure, though these programs are limited since they are voluntary and exist in very few states. There is no federal farmworker program to regulate pesticide overexposure. There is also poor employer compliance with physician recommendations (Fillmore and Lessenger 1993). Even in Washington State where the program is the strongest, its voluntary structure leaves many workers exposed and untreated. Most farmworkers lack legal status, so they fear the visibility of seeking out testing. This leads to a very low return rate of farmworkers for testing even if they might have registered for the program. Poor industry response and regulatory inaction are the norm despite any testing programs that may exist. Finally, the state rather than the grower shoulders the economic burden of administering the program, making it vulnerable to budget cuts.

Monitoring is equivalent neither to public health surveillance nor to systematic protections. Farmworkers themselves, as evidenced by the Juan Rios lawsuit, are seemingly dissuaded from pursuing pesticide bans. Farmworkers at the local level have not sought out solidarity with consumers or other forms of national pesticide regulation. Rather, since the DDT ban, workers have more narrowly focused on not getting sick. This was the case until the joint lawsuit to ban chlorpyrifos filed by a group of farmworker rights and environmental groups in 2007. Large environmental organizations such as Earthjustice and the NRDC, driven by long-lived contamination in drinking water and public health impacts, merged some of their historical disconnects to find common cause with farmworker movements and petitioned the EPA to discontinue chlorpyrifos uses. Agrifood activism and the organic food movement, probably the most visible front of antipesticide organizing, have spoken broadly about food justice without successfully merging rhetoric with practice. Food scholars note that their efforts have done little to address the concerns of the poorest and most vulnerable in the food system (Allen 2008).

Fenceline Communities

> Look at what the general population is exposed to just from eating food and look at what farmworker children are getting exposed to and realize that these kids are getting hit directly through the air, from hugging their parents when they get home, and through playing in their house and in their yards, which are contaminated. (Advocacy Scientist; Personal Communication)

Agricultural pesticide drift is the offsite, airborne movement of pesticides away from their target location. Drift lands in towns adjacent and downwind from areas where pesticides are applied. Chlorpyrifos poses significant drift problems. In California in 2008, there were 334 documented reports of illness and injury associated with drift, of which 229 were considered by the California Department of Pesticide Regulation to be definitely or probably due to exposure to pesticide drift (California Department of Pesticide Regulation 2011). Pesticide drift is poorly regulated. Though the pesticide regulatory apparatus is elaborate and large, it is highly devolved and fragmented, often captured by industry, and has been weakened by market-oriented approaches to environmental problem-solving. As a result, there are extensive data collected by multiple offices, but there is little actually done to reduce harm (Harrison 2006).

In the face of continuing drift exposures and limited regulatory response, farmworker rights groups aligned with scientists to examine fenceline community exposures, showing that they face much higher exposure levels to chlorpyrifos than the national average. Farming communities, from young children to the elderly, have chlorpyrifos "body burdens" above the national average. The most comprehensive study of chlorpyrifos in an agricultural study is the CHAMACOS* study in Salinas Valley, California, home to a 2 billion dollar per year agricultural industry that employs over 35,000 people. This ongoing study began in 2000 and follows 601 pregnant women in the Salinas Valley, tracking both the mothers and their infants into adolescence. Data from this study have proven invaluable in the current effort to seek a full chlorpyrifos ban. Pregnant women in this community show higher levels of organophosphates in their urine than women in the national sample and these higher levels are associated with shorter gestation periods, diminished reflexes in their babies, and lower cognitive function in older children (Bradman et al. 2005; Eskenazi et al. 2007). Other fenceline communities have collected their own data, conducted biomonitoring with residents, and waged efforts for local zoning to institute buffer zone protections to keep chlorpyrifos spraying at a safe distance. The success of such local efforts has been mixed and is ongoing (Pesticide Action Network, North America 2016).

Despite growing scientific evidence from farmworkers and fenceline communities, much pesticide advocacy centers on the organic food movement and consumer access to pesticide-free produce. This movement has focused on making foods safer at the point of sale, increasing organic options, and limiting direct-to-consumer pesticide sales. Organic foods have become a consumer-driven substitute for larger scale chemical regulatory failures. In a federal government climate that prefers voluntary regulations, market-driven efforts have been easier to enact than government regulations (Cashore, Auld, and Newsom 2004; Szasz 2007).

Consumers

Consumers continue to be exposed to potentially harmful levels of chlorpyrifos despite the over-the-counter sales ban. For residents who were exposed to chlorpyrifos when it was used to combat pests in the home, the exposure impacted health over time, adversely affecting children's health in the long term. In 1998, the Columbia Center for Children's Environmental Health research group began tracking a cohort of inner city, urban New York children from in utero through school age. In 1998, chlorpyrifos was one of the most heavily applied indoor pesticides in urban areas. Columbia University researchers found that insecticide

---

* Center for the Health Assessment of Mothers and Children of Salinas (CHAMACOS) is a multi-generational study and intervention project in a partnership among researchers at the University of California, Berkeley, Natividad Medical Center, Clinica de Salud de Valle de Salinas, http://cerch.berkeley.edu/research-programs/chamacos-study

levels in the blood of their study participants rapidly decreased between 1998 and 2001 after the 2000 ban (Whyatt et al. 2003; Carlton et al. 2004), demonstrating the immediate effectiveness of regulatory interventions on reducing chemical exposures. Later studies showed that children who had been exposed to higher levels of pesticides before the ban showed measurable neurodevelopmental problems, such as weakened motor skills, developmental delays, developmental disorders, and increased risk of attention deficit hyperactivity disorder (ADHD) (Lovasi et al. 2011).

Since the over-the-counter sales ban, pesticide residues in food comprise one of the key sources of pesticide exposure to young children (Landrigan and Goldman 2011). Dietary studies show that chlorpyrifos levels dramatically decrease when organic diets replace conventional diets in young children (Lu et al. 2006). Even low-level exposures are worrisome for children since growing evidence shows that chlorpyrifos acts as an endocrine disruptor and can harm hormone systems (Diamanti-Kandarakis et al. 2009; Viswanath et al. 2010).

Combined, the data on bans and dietary interventions show that interventions, whether regulatory or voluntary, reduce exposures with long-term benefits to public health, particularly for children, with government regulation extending protections to the poor and most vulnerable.

Conclusion

The fragmented regulatory history and scientific trajectory of chlorpyrifos tells the story of a chemical used since 1965 on crops with significant implications for public health across our food system. Its impact on public health spans workers, communities, and consumers and gives insight into how scientific understanding of toxicity evolves over time, but is unmatched by regulating agency decision-making. The fate of chlorpyrifos is yet to be determined, but the Ninth Circuit Court that handed down the ruling compelling the EPA to make a decision noted, "We recognize the scientific complexity inherent in evaluating the safety of pesticides and the competing interests that the agency must juggle. However, EPA's ambiguous plan to possibly issue a proposed rule nearly nine years after receiving the administrative petition is too little, too late…We order EPA to issue a full and final response to the petition no later than October 31, 2015." The EPA asked for an extension through June 2017, and the court provided an extension deadline of the end of March 2017. In March 2017, Scott Pruitt, head of the EPA under the new Trump administration, overturned the EPA's own decision to discontinue chlorpyrifos use. In April, environmental groups sued the EPA. Regulatory mechanisms must evolve to incorporate better shifting knowledge rather than be subject to the threat of ongoing litigation from advocacy groups to protect consumers. Widespread chlorpyrifos use also demonstrates the pitfalls of substitutions without adequate premarket testing. Chlorpyrifos' chemistry seemed an improvement over DDT, but there was little basis for this determination, a lesson learned through decades of scientific research and enormous financial and public health cost.

REFERENCES

Allen, P. 2008. Mining for justice in the food system: Perceptions, practices, and possibilities. *Agriculture and Human Values* 25(2):157–161. doi: 10.1007/s10460-008-9120-6.

Barr, D. B. and J. Angerer. 2006. Potential uses of biomonitoring data: A case study using the organophosphorus pesticides chlorpyrifos and malathion. *Environmental Health Perspectives* 114(11):1763–1769. doi: 10.1289/ehp.9062.

Bradman, A., B. Eskenazi, D. B. Barr, R. Bravo, R. Castorina, J. Chevrier, K. Kogut, M. E. Harnly, and T. E. McKone. 2005. Organophosphate urinary metabolite levels during pregnancy and after delivery in women living in an agricultural community. *Environmental Health Perspectives* 113(12):1802–1807.

Brown, D. and J. Warrick. 2000. EPA increases risk estimate of a pesticide. *The Washington Post*, June 1. https://www.washingtonpost.com/archive/politics/2000/06/01/epa-increases-risk-estimate-of-a-pesticide/94a6a7ba-2713-4e82-8369-ceb821c81050/

California Department of Pesticide Regulation. 2011. Pesticide Illness Surveillance Program. Accessed June 6, 2017. http://www.cdpr.ca.gov/docs/whs/pisp.htm

Carlton, E. J., H. L. Moats, M. Feinberg, P. Shepard, R. Garfinkel, R. Whyatt, and D. Evans. 2004. Pesticide sales in low-income, minority neighborhoods. *Journal of Community Health* 29(3):231–244.

Cashore, B. William, G. Auld, and D. Newsom. 2004. *Governing through Markets: Forest Certification and the Emergence of Non-State Authority*. New Haven, London: Yale University Press.

Casper, M. J. (ed.) 2003. Chemical matters. In *Synthetic Planet: Chemical Politics and the Hazards of Modern Life*, 1 ed. Introduction. New York: Routledge.

Centers for Disease Control and Prevention. 2009. *Fourth National Report on Human Exposure to Environmental Chemicals*. Department of Health and Human Services. http://www.cdc.gov/exposurereport/pdf/FourthReport.pdf

DeCaprio, A. P. 1997. Biomarkers: Coming of age for environmental health and risk assessment. *Environmental Science & Technology* 31(7):1837–1848. doi: 10.1021/es960920a.

Diamanti-Kandarakis, E., J.-P. Bourguignon, L. C. Giudice, R. Hauser, G. S. Prins, A. M. Soto, R. Thomas Zoeller, and A. C. Gore. 2009. Endocrine-disrupting chemicals: An endocrine society scientific statement. *Endocrine Reviews* 30(4):293–342. doi: 10.1210/er.2009-0002.

Doyle, J. 2004. *Trespass against Us: Dow Chemical & The Toxic Century*, 1st Ptg. edition. Monroe, ME: Common Courage Press.

Eskenazi, B., A. R. Marks, A. Bradman, K. Harley, D. B. Barr, C. Johnson, N. Morga, and N. P. Jewell. 2007. Organophosphate pesticide exposure and neurodevelopment in young Mexican-American children. *Environmental Health Perspectives* 115(5):792–798. doi: 10.1289/ehp.9828.

Fillmore, C. M. and J. E. Lessenger. 1993. A cholinesterase testing program for pesticide applicators. *Journal of Occupational Medicine: Official Publication of the Industrial Medical Association* 35(1):61–70.

Gottlieb, R. and A. Joshi. 2013. *Food Justice*: Reprint edition. Cambridge, MA: The MIT Press.

Guthman, J. 1998. Regulating meaning, appropriating nature: The codification of California organic agriculture. *Antipode* 30(2):135–154. doi:10.1111/1467-8330.00071.

Guthman, J. 2004. *Agrarian Dreams: The Paradox of Organic Farming in California (California Studies in Critical Human Geography)*, 1 ed. Berkeley, CA: University of California Press.

Harrison, J. 2008. Confronting invisibility: Reconstructing scale in California's pesticide drift conflict. In *Contentious Geographies: Environmental Knowledge, Meaning, and Scale*, M. T. Boykoff, M. K. Goodman, and K. T. Evered (eds.), Routledge Studies in Environmental Policy and Practice, Routledge. https://www.routledge.com/Contentious-Geographies-Environmental-Knowledge-Meaning-Scale/Boykoff-Goodman/p/book/9780754649717.

Harrison, J. L. 2006. 'Accidents' and invisibilities: Scaled discourse and the naturalization of regulatory neglect in California's pesticide drift conflict. *Political Geography* 25(5):506–529.

Haviland, J. A., D. E. Butz, and W. P. Porter. 2010. Long-term sex selective hormonal and behavior alterations in mice exposed to low doses of chlorpyrifos in Utero. *Reproductive Toxicology* 29(1):74–79. doi: 10.1016/j.reprotox.2009.10.008.

Kwong, T. C. 2002. Organophosphate pesticides: Biochemistry and clinical toxicology. *Therapeutic Drug Monitoring* 24(1):144–149.

Landrigan, P. J. and L. R. Goldman. 2011. Protecting children from pesticides and other toxic chemicals. *Journal of Exposure Science and Environmental Epidemiology* 21(2):119–120. doi: 10.1038/jes.2011.1.

Lessenger, J. E. 2005. Fifteen years of experience in cholinesterase monitoring of insecticide applicators. *Journal of Agromedicine* 10(3):49–56.

Lovasi, G. S., J. W. Quinn, V. A. Rauh, F. P. Perera, H. F. Andrews, R. Garfinkel, L. Hoepner, R. Whyatt, and A. Rundle. 2011. Chlorpyrifos exposure and urban residential environment characteristics as determinants of early childhood neurodevelopment. *American Journal of Public Health* 101(1):63–70. doi: 10.2105/AJPH.2009.168419.

Lu, C., K. Toepel, R. Irish, R. A. Fenske, D. B. Barr, and R. Bravo. 2006. Organic diets significantly lower children's dietary exposure to organophosphorus pesticides. *Environmental Health Perspectives* 114(2):260–263.

McWilliams, C. 1939. *California: The Great Exception*. Berkeley, CA: University of California Press.

Nash, L. 2004. The fruits of ill-health: Pesticides and workers' bodies in post-World War II California. *Osiris* 19:203–219. doi: 10.2307/3655240.

Norén, K. and D. Meironyté. 2000. Certain organochlorine and organobromine contaminants in Swedish human milk in perspective of past 20–30 Years. *Chemosphere* 40(9–11):1111–1123.

Parker-Pope, T. 2011. Pesticide exposure in womb affects I.Q. *Well*. April 21. http://well.blogs.nytimes.com/2011/04/21/pesticide-exposure-in-womb-affects-i-q/

Pesticide Action Network, North America. 2016. Chlorpyrifos | Pesticide Action Network. Accessed July 25. http://www.panna.org/resources/chlorpyrifos-0

Pulido, L. 1996. *Environmentalism and Economic Justice: Two Chicano Struggles in the Southwest*. Tucson: University of Arizona Press.

Pulido, L. and D. Peña. 1998. Environmentalism and positionality: The early pesticide campaign of the United Farm Workers' Organizing Committee, 1965–71. *Race, Gender & Class* 6(1):33–50.

Rauh, V. A., R. Garfinkel, F. P. Perera, H. F. Andrews, L. Hoepner, D. B. Barr, R. Whitehead, D. Tang, and R. W. Whyatt. 2006. Impact of prenatal chlorpyrifos exposure on neurodevelopment in the first 3 years of life among inner-city children. *Pediatrics* 118(6):e1845–e1859. doi: 10.1542/peds.2006-0338.

Richardson, R. J. 1995. Assessment of the neurotoxic potential of chlorpyrifos relative to other organophosphorus compounds: A critical review of the literature. *Journal of Toxicology and Environmental Health* 44(2):135–165. doi: 10.1080/15287399509531952.

Schafer, K. 2004. *Chemical Trespass: Pesticides in Our Bodies and Corporate Accountability.* Pesticide Action Network North America. http://www.panna.org/resources/publication-report/chemical-trespass.

Shamasunder, B. and R. Morello-Frosch. 2015. Scientific contestations over 'toxic Trespass': Health and regulatory implications of chemical biomonitoring. *Journal of Environmental Studies and Sciences* 1–13. doi: 10.1007/s13412-015-0233-0.

Szasz, A. 2007. *Shopping Our Way to Safety: How We Changed from Protecting the Environment to Protecting Ourselves.* Minneapolis, MN: University of Minnesota Press.

U.S. Court of Appeals for the Ninth Circuit. 2015. *Pesticide Action Network.* North America: Natural Resources Defense Council, Inc. v. U.S. Environmental Protection Agency.

U.S. Environmental Protection Agency (US EPA). 2016. Proposal to Revoke Chlorpyrifos Food Residue Tolerances. Overviews and Factsheets. Accessed July 21, 2016. https://archive.epa.gov/epa/ingredients-used-pesticide-products/proposal-revoke-chlorpyrifos-food-residue-tolerances.html

Viswanath, G., S. Chatterjee, S. Dabral, S. R. Nanguneri, G. Divya, and P. Roy. 2010. Anti-androgenic endocrine disrupting activities of chlorpyrifos and piperophos. *Journal of Steroid Biochemistry and Molecular Biology* 120(1):22–29. doi: 10.1016/j.jsbmb.2010.02.032.

Walker, R. 2004. *The Conquest of Bread: 150 Years of Agribusiness in California.* New York, NY: New Press: Distributed by Norton.

Whyatt, R. M. et al. 2003. Contemporary-use pesticides in personal air samples during pregnancy and blood samples at delivery among urban minority mothers and newborns. *Environmental Health Perspectives* 111(5):749–756.

Yiridoe, E. K., B.-A. Samuel, and C. M. Ralph. 2005. Comparison of Consumer Perceptions and Preference toward Organic versus Conventionally Produced Foods: A Review and Update of the Literature. *Renewable Agriculture and Food Systems* 20(4):193–205. doi:10.1079/RAF2005113.

8 On the front lines in school cafeterias

The trials and tribulations of food service directors

Michelle C. Pautz, John C. Jones, and A. Bryce Hoflund

As former First Lady Michelle Obama discovered, there is no shortage of assessments and prescriptions about school lunch programs in the United States. Some of those perceptions come from firsthand experiences with these programs—indeed, most of us can draw upon our own experiences as students to comment on the nature of these programs. However, our experiences in school cafeterias nationwide reflect only one side of the interaction. A population that is largely unheard from is the food service directors employed by more than 13,000 public school districts nationwide and tasked with front-line implementation of school food programs. Food service directors are responsible for implementing the National School Lunch Program (NSLP) and its companion breakfast program at the school district level. These professionals oversee all the school cafeterias and ensure compliance with state and federal requirements. Put simply, these individuals are the front lines of school food programs, yet their voices remain elusive in the conversation about these programs. In exploring policy implementation on the front lines, it is essential to include key actors in the process and, to date, the voices of food service directors are largely ignored.

This study endeavors to address this gap by culling the tales of food service directors in three metropolitan areas as a way to enrich and expand the discussions about school food programs through an understanding of the front lines. More specifically, this exploratory study reports on extensive semi-structured interviews with 16 food service directors in Dayton, Ohio; Omaha, Nebraska; and Newark, New Jersey, and their surrounding areas. In our effort to understand the trials and tribulations of these vital actors in implementing school food programs, we find, perhaps unsurprisingly, widely varied approaches to implementing these programs, particularly under the Healthy, Hunger Free Kids Act. With the federal structure in place in the United States, there is often more variation in program implementation than initial expectations might suggest. We are not in a position to make a judgment on this variability given our narrow study, but it does serve as a compelling research for more extensive research in this area. Additionally, our interviewees reveal that the complexities associated with program implementation continue to grow and, in some cases, prove quite burdensome to districts. Regardless, the insights and experiences of these front-line individuals bring a missing voice to the conversation about school food programs and other broader questions associated with food policy and politics.

However, before we share the stories of these individuals on the front lines of school food policy implementation, we begin by investigating the important efforts of front-line workers and overviewing the school food programs that food service directors implement nationwide. Next, we review our methodology and then discuss the findings from our interviews. Finally, we draw potential implications from this research and outline important next steps in cultivating a more comprehensive understanding of school food programs by focusing on this important population and their experiences.

Common perceptions about regulation and food policy

Perhaps the neglect of food service directors in the conversation about school food programs comes from fundamental assumptions about the nature of regulations and food policy more broadly. It is commonly presumed that once regulations are devised—in this case, surrounding the NSLP—implementation occurs without incident, as the difficult part of promulgating regulations is over. Even if that faulty presumption is acknowledged, the work and experiences of those individuals on the front lines are often overlooked, both in academic research and in the media, particularly with the tendency to take either extreme macro-levels or micro-levels of analysis. Put differently, a macro-level tendency keeps us focused on the mandates from the U.S. Department of Education or even the former First Lady's initiatives concerning healthy eating and childhood obesity, for example. Alternatively, the emphasis is on detailed histories of these programs (which are, of course, important for context; c.f. Levine 2008). The other overriding tendency related to school food research is micro-level case studies in which parents and students complain about this or that menu item or advocate trends, such as farm-to-school programs. Undoubtedly, these are important levels of analysis, but they omit a so-called "meso-level" and an ability to gain valuable insights from key stakeholders, such as food service directors. We endeavor to fill this gap at the meso-level and consider the work of those front-line civil servants tasked with implementing an elephantine system of regulations for school food programs while they are simultaneously the object of state and federal level oversight.

The role and significance of front-line workers

Before we discuss the work of food service directors, we first consider the roles and significance of front-line workers broadly and make the case to include food service directors among the usual populations of civil servants considered front-line workers. Political scientist Michael Lipsky was the first to focus academic attention on a population he termed "street-level bureaucrats" (Lipsky 1980). Subsequent research has tended to favor the term "front-line workers," however (c.f. Maynard-Moody and Musheno 2003). This group of individuals is defined as the "[p]ublic service workers who interact directly with citizens in the course of their jobs, and who have substantial discretion in the execution of their work" (Lipsky 1980, p. 3). Lipsky's (1980) classic text focuses on the work of teachers, police officers, legal aid attorneys, and social workers. Maynard-Moody and Musheno (2003) explore the stories of cops, teachers, and counselors. Pautz and Rinfret (2013) expand the definition of front-line workers to investigate the efforts of state environmental regulators and Oberfield (2014) focuses on cops and welfare caseworkers.

Front-line workers are critical public servants as they are the ones responsible for the interpretation and implementation of public policy. To successfully achieve their tasks, front-line workers exercise tremendous discretion in the day-to-day realities of their work. For example, police officers have to interpret city ordinances and welfare caseworkers make eligibility determinations regarding benefits. Environmental inspectors routinely interpret air quality regulations and make assessments regarding a firm's compliance with those regulations. Each interaction front-line workers have "...represents an instance of policy delivery" (Lipsky 1980, p. 3).

Perceptions abound regarding front-line workers and the nature of their work. Maynard-Moody and Musheno (2003) discuss the two most prevalent narratives surrounding front-line workers. The "state-agent narrative" is the most common narrative that emphasizes the rigid adherence to rules and procedures to ensure law abidance. This narrative holds that front-line workers should have their discretion curtailed and limited as much as possible. By contrast, the "citizen-agent narrative" encompasses the complexities and practices associated with the work of front-line workers where judgments and the exercise of discretion are commonplace, along with the need for flexibility. "The citizen agent narrative concentrates on the judgments that street-level workers make about the identities and moral character of the people encountered and the workers' assessment of how these people react during encounters" (Maynard-Moody and Musheno 2003, p. 9).

These competing narratives point to the various dimensions of front-line work that are relevant for our investigation of food service directors. First, front-line workers exercise discretion. Front-line workers "...have considerable discretion in determining the nature, amount, and quality of benefits and sanctions provided by their agencies" (Lipsky 1980, p. 13). One of the food service directors interviewed for this study reports blatant disregard for some rules that she—with her extensive training in nutrition—finds ridiculous. More on that example is to come. As a result of the nature of their work and the immediacy of their interactions with the public, the exercise of discretion is significant. Discretion makes them a target of political controversy. Maynard-Moody and Musheno maintain that discretion is essential given the impossible nature of their jobs and often, front-line workers encounter situations in which they deem the rules cannot and should not apply.

Second, with the exercise of discretion and other practical realities of working for government agencies, numerous conditions are imposed on front-line workers. More specifically, front-line workers face resource constraints, including lack of adequate information and training, burdensome caseloads, resource inadequacies, and the constant pressure to do more with less. As Lipsky (1980) notes, "[rules] may be so voluminous and contradictory that they can only be enforced or invoked selectively" (p. 14). Competing demands from public sector actors often result in goals that are ambiguous and in tension with one another. Demands for measured performance, often in a quantitative way, often accompany ambiguous goal setting. Further, front-line workers accomplish their tasks through routine interactions with the public who generally distrust government, can become frustrated navigating the byzantine bureaucracy, and who demand exceptions for themselves. Often front-line workers routinely interact with clients who are compelled, for a variety of reasons, to interact with a government official. Again, consider the work of food service directors. They are tasked with creating menus for school-aged kids with a range of palates, food cultural traditions, and appetites for just a few dollars per student, per meal, that also fit within the federal guidelines. Also, the regulations would seem to indicate that a school-sized diet Red Bull is acceptable to serve while a homemade vegetable barley soup is not.

Third, negative perceptions about the government are seemingly ubiquitous in American society and those perceptions extend to the tasks of front-line workers. These civil servants "...have considerable impact on people's lives" (Lipsky 1980, p. 3). As a result, the public frequently has a lot to say about food service directors' actions. For example, local news outlets routinely cover stories about what one school is serving in its cafeterias and how much plate waste is a problem, thereby wasting the hard-earned dollars of taxpayers. This results in a unique climate for food service directors to operate in as they are constantly defending their actions with little, if any, time for proactive nutritional education and programming.

Finally, in response to the previously discussed dimensions, many front-line workers develop patterns of practice, or coping mechanisms. These patterns enable them to cope with the often impossible nature of their jobs. As Lipsky (1980) notes, "...they develop patterns of practice that tend to limit demand, maximize the utilization of available resources, and obtain client compliance over and above the procedures developed by their agencies" (p. 83). Additionally, these workers "modify their concept of their jobs, so as to lower or otherwise restrict their objectives and thus reduce the gap between available resources and achieving objectives" (Lipsky 1980, p. 83). As we will soon discuss, these coping mechanisms are frequent in the work of food service directors. Their stories provide example after example of where they have to modify their work and their professional desires to meet with the constraints before them.

The foundation of front-line worker studies helps provide an important context for the work of school food service directors. As is the case with all front-line worker populations, it is vital to understand these populations in order to understand policy implementation and bureaucratic personalities (c.f. Oberfield 2014). Consequently, we argue that food service directors should be included among populations of front-line workers more typically studied. Food service directors are employed by the thousands of school districts across the United States and are tasked with implementing school food service programs. They are given the broad outlines of the requirements by the federal government and their state government and then have the difficult challenge of meeting both nutritional and financial requirements while also catering to the appetites of school-aged children and appeasing their parents and guardians. Additionally, they have routine interactions with the public in the course of their jobs. We contend that this work requires significant discretion. This environment creates challenges for any front-line worker. With this grounding, we turn next to contextualizing the work of front-line workers by reviewing the broad outlines of school food programs in the United States.

School food programs

Methodology

We collected data about food service directors in three metropolitan areas: Dayton, Ohio; Newark, New Jersey; and Omaha, Nebraska that oversee food service delivery in public schools. We compiled an initial list of food service directors in each municipal area. We conducted one-on-one, in-depth, open-ended interviews in person or via telephone with each food service director who agreed to participate and examined relevant written documents. A total of 16 food service directors (seven in Dayton, three in Newark, and six in Omaha) were interviewed. Getting food service directors to consent to an interview proved a bit more challenging than expected; however, there were also different responses in each of the three regions. In the greater Dayton area, the response rate was about 50% in terms of individuals who were contacted and those who agreed to an interview. The response rate to interview request in the greater Newark, New Jersey area was roughly 20%. The response rate in Omaha was 100%. In order to obtain candid responses to our questions, interviewees were guaranteed confidentiality. The interviews were not recorded; rather, extensive notes were taken during the interview and the notes were transcribed after each interview.

We asked a series of questions about their day-to-day job duties, including questions about how and why their jobs have changed over time, their relationships with stakeholders, their programs, and their interactions with state and federal regulators and agencies. The interviews were used in tandem with document analysis to determine whether they supported one another (Caudle 1994). From each interview, we gathered additional contacts using snowball or chain sampling, in which interviewees are asked to provide names of individuals who know about the issue (Caudle 1994). When interviews were completed, we compiled the interview notes and employed various qualitative techniques, including content analysis, to distill themes and other insights provided by interviewees.

There are limitations to this study. With a small sample size, we may have missed a perspective that is different from that of the individuals we interviewed.

However, using the snowball method helps to overcome this issue. Additionally, we observed a number of interview rejections due to the perceived political contention over NSLP programming despite our promise of respondent anonymity. We think it likely that other political contentions more broadly surrounding food in school may have led to our low response rate.

Findings

Three themes emerged from our interviews with school food service directors. The first is that our respondents noted some of the increasing complexities associated with implementing food regulations in schools. Next, we discuss the school food service directors' perceptions of regulatory interactions and oversight with the various federal and state agencies that oversee the implementation of school food programs. Finally, we outline the various coping mechanisms employed by school food service directors as they grapple with trying to meet the needs of the various stakeholders, from parents to school principals, to the various regulatory actors.

Increasing complexities associated with implementing regulations

The school food service directors that we interviewed mentioned that the implementation of regulations has become more complex over time in a number of ways. Most respondents mentioned that there are too many components and guidelines that they have to follow. Not only do they have to comply with the new nutritional guidelines recently enshrined by the Healthy, Hunger Free Kids Act (HHFK) in 2010, but they also have to make sure that they continue to comply with civil rights laws and equal opportunity employment. Several mentioned that they have to attend more training sessions now than in the past. Furthermore, the new guidelines have dramatically increased the amount of paperwork that school food service directors must deal with. One respondent estimates that 70% of her work day is engaged with paperwork of various types, which she maintains is a dramatic change from 5 to 10 years ago.

One respondent mentioned specifically that when the regulations were first proposed, she/he did not think it was going to be a big deal to implement them. However, this changed when both local and national media focused its attention on the revised guidelines. The media has produced numerous stories that maintain that children do not like the healthy foods and that waste has increased as a result of the new guidelines. The interviewee noted that, as a result of this attention, participation in the NSLP decreased, while breakfast was not impacted as much. Once the media storm passed, the interviewee noted that participation in the school breakfast and lunch programs increased dramatically.

Related to this, many maintained that the nutritional standards themselves leave much to be desired. One interviewee stated that they used to bake every day in their cafeteria, but once the new sodium guidelines were put into place by HHFK, baking was done away with. The whole grain requirements also presented numerous challenges for several respondents. First, several food service directors mentioned that parents complain about them, especially in light of increased awareness of celiac disease and gluten allergies. Furthermore, several mentioned that they have observed that children dislike the taste of whole grain products, but note that it is somewhat easier to change palates of younger children than those of older children. Others suggested specific strategies to obfuscate the conversion to whole grains, such as switching only after summer or winter breaks as to not offend their student's palates. A final complexity mentioned by interviewees is the prices that some vendors are charging for products. Specifically, they are increasingly confronted with vendors who increase the price for the products because they include "whole grains" or "reduced sodium."

Perceptions of regulatory interactions and oversight

When asked about their interactions with regulatory agencies at the state and federal levels, the overwhelming majority replied that their interactions vary significantly between the state and federal agencies, with the least amount of interaction occurring at the federal level. The various state agencies play a number of roles in the regulation and implementation of school food programs.

The majority of respondents indicated that, even though all the guidelines originate at the federal level, they have no or very limited interactions with agencies at the federal level. One interviewee mentioned that the most interaction she has with the federal agencies is that she receives memos. Several others mentioned that there is a huge disconnect between what is going on and what the feds think is going on, especially with regard to procurement rules and the 51% whole grain rules. One food service director wondered, "Why are they making this so hard?"

Interactions with state agencies are varied, but mostly center around audits and technical assistance. Several school food service directors mention that state agencies are supposed to provide audits of the school food programs (usually every 3–5 years). Usually, auditors give advance notice that they will be visiting the school district (some states even allow for the school food service directors to choose the dates for their visit) and, while there, examine production records and watch servers. School districts typically are required to provide items to the state agencies for review such as a sample of reduced lunch applications and a sample menu for a full month. Once the audit is completed, the auditors provide an exit review. Several interviewees mentioned that poor reviews could threaten school lunch reimbursement rates.

State agencies also provide technical assistance to school food service directors. The majority of our respondents mentioned that the state agencies provide important guidance on interpretation of the federal guidelines. The school food service directors that we spoke to, however, noted that there are some challenges to working with the state agencies. First, one interviewee mentioned that the state has so many unfunded mandates that they do not know what they are doing. They have too many reports to file and other things to do and there are not enough people to do them all. States are also burdened by the constant changes in and updates of regulations at the federal level. One interviewee mentioned that the state only passes the rules down from the federal government. Another said that if they had more time for technical assistance, their programs would be better.

Coping mechanisms employed by school food service directors

We asked how school food service directors cope with the challenges we noted previously. In terms of dealing with the media and resistance from parents and children, the school food service directors that we spoke to have dealt with the issue in a couple of ways. First, when bad media reports hit the airwaves (such as the pink slime scandal in 2012), several school food service directors mentioned that they reach out to parents and explain the school lunch program and the goals of the revised guidelines. One went so far as to form committees with kitchen manager and student focus groups about what they did or did not want to eat. This same school district is about to conduct a district-wide survey of parents on a variety of topics related to school lunch programs. Another school food service director says that she mostly hires mothers attempting to reenter the workforce to work in the cafeteria and constantly educates them about misperceptions.

Food service directors in other school districts indicated that they try to educate children how to cook. One school food service director noted that she constantly tries to find foods that are often "off the beaten track" and uses them to spark an interest in knowing more about the food and what they are eating generally. Another food service director mentioned that she taught students how to make crème fraiche for beef stroganoff. Still others mentioned that they try to use as much fresh and local ingredients as they can and introduce the children to the source of the ingredient.

With regard to dealing with the increasing number and complexity of nutrition guidelines, several said that they use some type of spreadsheet or nutrition software to help them plan the meals. Others buy preapproved food items and then print the nutritional information out to show children, parents, and other interested individuals. Initially, several school food service directors noted that they generated more waste from adherence to the new HHFK guidelines, but having software and learning more about the guidelines and products reduced the waste after the first year or so. Others are concerned about prices, and thus often work with vendors to determine whether they have items that they can sell at a reasonable price to the school district. One interviewee said that she shops for food from multiple vendors. When she wanted salmon, she talked to the fish supplier and told him about her philosophy and he sold her some salmon that the district could afford. The bottom line, as one respondent notes, is that, "As long as you use a little imagination and try, the new rules are workable." One interviewee, however, noted that implementing the new guidelines still presents challenges and, as a result, there are some guidelines that she does not follow because there are no penalties and she would rather have the children eat the meals. In order to continue to make headway on addressing the challenges, several school food service directors noted that they think it would be interesting to look at best practices from other districts.

Discussion and implications

Our findings suggested a number of significant implications. Acknowledging our small sample size, we believe our discussion here can serve as a jumping off point for additional exploration of food service directors.

Impact of Healthy, Hunger Free Kids Act

First, our data suggest a strong connection between the regulatory shift toward healthier school lunches under the HHFK umbrella and on-the-ground food service. Directors generally indicated an increased awareness and nutritional sensitivity to both healthier menu planning and the broad reduction of sodium use. However, this increased focus on healthy food service taxed the capacity of the respondents in other ways. These time consuming regulations create stress on directors for activities that are technically out of their administrative mission but still viewed as imperative. Examples of stressed activities included interactions with parents, nutritional education of students, interactions with principals and other district-level officials, and interactions with their counterparts in other districts. Interestingly, most respondent directors viewed this increased focus on healthier food service, along with an increased regulatory burden, in a positive light.

Dynamic implementation of Healthy, Hunger Free Kids Act

Second, our research uncovered evidence of dynamic implementation of HHFK across the districts sampled, rather than a uniform one-size-fits-all implementation of the new rules. Despite our small sample size, our respondents' districts displayed a wide variety of demographic and urban form characteristics. Each director surveyed reported their own novel way of implementing new rules and other actors in each corresponding district reacted differently to both the new rules and the food director's actions. Further, multistate sampling revealed differing state-level reporting requirements. This suggests nonuniform implementation of HHKF across the nation.

Alignment with broader front-line worker literature

Third, this evidence of dynamic implementation joins with other findings in support of our contention that food service directors are front-line workers. Additionally, we found that food service directors appeared to exist more within the "citizen-agent narrative" suggested by Maynard-Moody and Musheno (2003) and less in the "state-agent narrative." All of our respondents indicated that it was imperative that they serve food every day. Often, the desire to prevent students from going hungry required our respondents to engage in a variety of adaptive, strategic, and/or sufficing interventions to ensure continual food service. Respondents commonly suggested that they needed to adapt federal guidelines or, as one respondent suggested, "go insane." Examples of this adaptation included: engaging in salesmanship tactics to convince children to select healthy food over competing foods and flatly ignoring impractical rules, especially for short periods of time.

Further, we found evidence of a number of strategic interventions to serve as a coping mechanism for recent guidelines. These interventions directly echo the patterns of practice suggested by Lipsky (1980). Examples of strategic interventions include: introducing healthier menu items, such as whole grain pasta, after long school breaks; the creation of theme bars at high schools to provide students with more flexibility in their vegetable and fruit selection; the restriction of high school students who departed from the campus for lunch returning during the lunch period, as they commonly return with fast food for their friends. The introduction of in-classroom breakfast service also fits as a broad strategic intervention.

Finally, we also found evidence of a number of satisficing interventions designed to achieve the highest improvement possible, while still ensuring continual, daily food service delivery. Directors indicated that they would commonly submit a waiver request to the state auditors requesting the continued ability to serve menu items prepared the traditional way and with the traditional ingredients. Sodium requirements and white pasta were the two commonly cited waiver requests. Additionally, directors reported that the increased regulatory burden required them to hire new staff that they specifically designated to perform the nutritional documentation of their catalog of menu items. These employees rarely, if ever, participated in actual food preparation or service.

Conclusion

We hope our work can be viewed as a preliminary first step in research into the role that food service directors play in the implementation of daily food service to their districts. As part of this work, we sought to advance the idea that food service directors are part of a broader category of public administrator that works on the front line of interaction between the public sector and the citizenry. We found significant evidence to suggest that food service directors fit under the broad front-line worker umbrella as suggested by Lipsky and others.

Future research casting food service directors as front-line workers is needed. Our work should be used as a broad cut across potential food service director respondents. A logical next step in this research would be the creation of a quantitative survey instrument for mass distribution. However, through our research, we encountered several programs not supportive of using food service directors as research subjects. Any researchers interested in this arena should keep these challenges in mind. First, our rate of rejection was quite high, as discussed earlier. We believe this is due to the combination of spare availability of discretionary time to participate, as suggested by our findings above, and the desire to protect themselves and their districts from potential political fallout from the publication of research on this topic. This latter point is driven home by the sensitivity many respondents expressed over media coverage of their performance.

REFERENCES

Caudle, S. L. 1994. Using qualitative approaches. In *Handbook of Practical Program Evaluation*, edited by J. S. Wholey, H. P. Hatry, and K. E. Newcomer. San Francisco: Jossey-Bass Publishers, pp. 69–95.

Levine, S. 2008. *School Lunch Politics: The Surprising History of America's Favorite Welfare Program*. Princeton, NJ: Princeton University Press.

Lipsky, M. 1980. *Street-Level Bureaucracy: Dilemmas of the Individual in Public Services*. New York, NY: Russell Sage Foundation.

Maynard-Moody, S. and M. Musheno. 2003. *Cops, Teachers, and Counselors: Stories from the Front Lines of Public Service*. Ann Arbor, MI: The University of Michigan Press.

Oberfield, Z. W. 2014. *Becoming Bureaucrats: Socialization at the Front Lines of Government Service*. Philadelphia, PA: The University of Pennsylvania Press.

Pautz, M. C. and S. R. Rinfret. 2013. *The Lilliputians of Environmental Regulation: The Perspective of State Regulators*. New York, NY: Routledge.

9 GMOs

An examination of issues surrounding GMO regulations

Tania Calvao

The use of genetically modified organisms (GMOs) presents a number of uncertainties surrounding their effect on human health. At this stage, there is not enough scientific evidence of the long-term public health and environmental consequences of GMO use to provide definitive answers on their impact. The body of scientific evidence of the benefits and risks of GMO use has been marked by controversy and a lack of consensus in the scientific community. The need for more independent investigation to determine any risks to public health is clear. In the meantime, regulators can play an important oversight role to protect the public at large from harm while balancing the needs of various stakeholders such as producers, farmers, and consumers. What principles have been used in drafting regulatory frameworks and legislation? The history of public policy regarding GMOs in the United States and in Europe reveals two different sets of principles: one emphasizing speedy and comprehensive introduction of GMO products to the public marketplace, and the other more conservative. The European Commission has taken a precautionary approach toward GMO products and has permitted only limited varieties to be introduced in Europe; in the United States, regulatory principles have been established that seek to limit regulatory burdens with the rationale that the end product, rather than the process by which it is created, should be the focus of regulatory attention. Given the scientific uncertainty surrounding public health and the use of GMOs, the European approach of using a precautionary principle should be used as a general guide for future regulatory agencies while taking into account the needs of the various stakeholders. Although the application of a modified precautionary principle may place some additional burdens on the industry, it will enhance safety procedures and contain trade interests that may lead regulators to disregard risks associated with GMOs to human health and the environment.

Regulation in the United States

During the 1970s, genetic technologies started to be a cause of public concern. The development of recombinant DNA (rDNA) techniques posed questions in regard to possible harm caused by mutant organisms released into the environment. Some communities on the East Coast of the United States banned genetic research within their boundaries while protests and government discussions about the impact of the use of such technologies gained relevance. On the West coast of the United States, 140 members of the scientific community, biologists, lawyers, and physicians who supported genetic technologies convened in late February 1975 at Asilomar, Monterey Peninsula, California, in an attempt to introduce responsible self-regulation to counter the threat of local and national regulation Berg et al. 1975). Among other topics, strict safety research rules were discussed. The dialogue sparked by the Asilomar Conference led to the adoption of the guidelines by the National Institutes of Health (NIH) in 1976. The NIH is a research-funding arm of the U.S. government which plays a major role in the oversight of human gene therapy. Up to 1984, NIH guidelines were the standard for research in the United States (National Institute of Health Guidelines 1976).

As technology enabling the production of genetically modified (GM) products began to flourish in the 1980s, the U.S. President Reagan (1980–1988) administration was the first one to face the challenges posed by GMs on the regulatory front. In 1984, the Reagan administration created an interagency working group within the White House Office of Science and Technology Policy (OSTP) to draft a federal framework for food biotechnology, the Coordinated Framework for Regulation of Biotechnology. The Coordinated Framework set the tone for the U.S. regulatory framework which continues to the present: regulation of genetically engineered (GE) products should be issued only according to measurable risks. The approach has been to regulate products of biotechnology in the same way as conventional products under the existing web of federal statutory authority and regulation. The Coordinated Framework was submitted to the public for comments and opinions, and in 1986 the final version of the document was issued. The final policy document retained the reasoning of the initial draft version, stating that "existing statutes seem adequate to deal with the emerging processes and products [of genetic engineering]" (OSTP 1986). The Coordinated Framework also established broad outlines of the jurisdiction of the existing regulatory agencies over GM:

- The Food and Drug Administration (FDA) should be responsible for regulating food and feeds modified via genetic engineering (FDA 1992b).
- The United States Department of Agriculture—Animal and Plant Health Inspection Service (USDA-APHIS) should be responsible for regulating importation, interstate movement, and environmental release of transgenic plants with an aim of protecting existing crops from hazards.
- The Environmental Protection Agency (EPA) should be responsible for regulating microbial/plant pesticides, new uses of existing pesticides, and novel microorganisms. The EPA should promote reviews for safety for the environment, and the safety of new companion herbicides.

The FDA, since the advent of GMs, has been vigorously criticized in many instances for the way its approvals are granted. A peer-reviewed report released by EcoStrat (2000), an independent Swiss scientific assessment firm, indicated that the agency accepted inappropriate and scientifically questionable studies in approving the first Bt corn, a type of modified corn, for U.S. growers. In fact, the report states that studies submitted by the companies Novartis and Mycogen determining the effect of Bt corn on nontarget insects were so poorly designed that there was virtually no chance that adverse effects would be observed (p. 32). Nowadays, other federal departments and agencies have some role or interest in genetic engineering. These include the National Research Council, the Department of Health and Human Services (HHS) Center for Biotechnology Information, the Department of State's Office of International Information Programs, the Patent and Trademark Office, the Department of Commerce, the Federal Trade Commission, the Office of the U.S. Trade Representative, and the Customs Service.

In 1992, during the President George H.W. Bush administration, the OSTP released a new statement to provide ongoing direction to federal agencies. The document outlined the Principles of Regulatory Review, making clear that federal oversight under the Coordinated Framework should be limited to science-based risk assessment to "ensure the safety of planned introductions of organisms into the environment while not unduly inhibiting these introductions." It was emphasized that the end product would be the focus of regulatory attention, not the process in which such products are created. The rationale for this approach was that "products developed through biotechnology processes do not per se pose risks to human health and the environment; risk depends instead on the characteristics and use of the individual products." Another principle established that "when review is deemed necessary it should be designed to minimize regulatory burden while assuring protection of public health and welfare." The principles call for the government to "accommodate the rapid advances in biotechnology" (OSTP 1992).

In 1992, the FDA issued a Statement of Policy arguing that genes added to common food substances via genetic engineering are generally recognized as safe (GRAS) because the new food is largely the same as its conventional counterpart (FDA 1992b). The FDA also made a statement about labeling indicating that special labeling for GE foods is generally unnecessary because the agency has no evidence that GE foods are substantially different from other foods (Department of Health and Human Services, Food and Drug Administration 1992).

Toward the end of the President George H.W. Bush administration, the White House and the abovementioned agencies continued to work together on the division of authority. The Biotechnology Science Coordinating Committee (BSCC), an interagency committee responsible for coordination of science policy, working together with the agencies and OSTP, failed to establish consensus on which organisms would be subject to federal biotechnology oversight. Owing to the lack of consensus, the White House submitted the working material of the agencies and BSCC to the President's Council on Competitiveness, led by vice president Dan Quayle. The Council on Competitiveness's main purpose was the promotion of U.S. industry initiatives. It ended up defining the scope of federal biotechnology responsibility in a draft policy statement on GM foods entitled: "Exercise of Federal Oversight within Scope of Statutory Authority: Planned Introduction of Biotechnology Products into de Environment" (Exercise of Federal Oversight within Scope of Statutory Authority: Planned Introductions of Biotechnology Products into the Environment 1992).

In its "Principles of Regulatory Review," the President's Council on Competitiveness reiterated the Coordinated Framework tenet that federal oversight should be limited to science-based risk assessment. In broad lines, the four principles promulgated were

1. "[P]roducts developed through biotechnology process do not *per se* pose risks to human health and the environment; risk depends instead on the characteristics and use of the individual products"
2. Reviews should be designed to "minimize regulatory burden while assuring protection of public health and welfare"
3. Government should "accommodate the rapid advances in biotechnology"
4. Government should presume that the product poses minimal risk in the absence of any evidence to the contrary (FDA 1992a)

Considering the abovementioned principles, the existing FDA's statutory framework and the Federal Food, Drug and Cosmetic Act (FFDCA 2000), the FDA's approach for conventional foods, to be applied to GM cases, is that in the absence of identifiable risks, a manufacturer may place a product on the market, and the manufacturer is the one to bear responsibility for ensuring that a product is not adulterated or misbranded. The provisions related to adulteration and food additive provisions should be applied to GM, and an additional layer of review would be required when novel ingredients or components are added; therefore, existing ingredients added to conventional foods must be approved as food additives or GRAS.

At this stage, questions and critiques of the GM scientific community by the public and advocacy groups began to appear. In an effort to provide for a safeguard against erroneous GRAS presumptions, the FDA implemented a consultation program and in October 1997 issued a document entitled: "Guidance on Consultation Procedures for Food Derived from New Plant Varieties." Although under great pressure from public opinion at the time, no relevant changes were seen from the original regulatory framework. The document did little to change FDA policy; it merely clarified the agency's positioning and requirements (U.S. Food and Drug Administration Center for Food Safety and Applied Nutrition 1997). Since then, the FDA has faced strong legal challenges over the legitimacy of its policies and has also entered into numerous public consultations. However, there have been no indications to date that new policies or a different approach will be adopted in the near future by the agency.

In addition to the approval process, the labeling of GM products was also another important topic constantly discussed. The FDA's approach to labeling is in line with the product-based approach rather than the process-based approach. The FDA's position is that no specific label is needed for GM products considering that such products do not differ from conventionally produced counterparts. The authority for the FDA's labeling policy is found in (1) 21 U.S.C. § 343–1 and (2) 21 U.S.C. § 321(n) which state respectively that a food is misbranded if "its labeling is false or misleading in any particular," and labeling is misleading if it "fails to reveal all acts that are material in light of such representations or material with respect to consequences which may result from the use of the article to which the labeling relates." No further explanation in the statutes or legislative history of FFDCA reveals a clear explanation of what information would be material for the purpose of labeling. Although public pressure for mandatory labeling of GM products remains, the FDA's approach has not changed, and this approach has been upheld by the courts. In *Alliance for Bio-Integrity, et al. v. Shalala* (No. 98-1300 D.D.C.) on September 29, 2000, U.S. District Judge Colleen Kollar-Kotelly granted the government's motion for summary judgment and dismissed the challenge to the FDA's regulatory policies concerning GM food. Included in the challenges was one about mandatory labeling; the court affirmed the FDA's position and stated that consumer demand itself is not a basis for mandatory labeling.

The deferential role that the legislative and judicial branches have taken to industry objectives on labeling and fast-track introduction has also added to the controversies surrounding GMO regulation. There is no specific federal legislation regulating GMOs in the United States. Although insistently advocated by consumer groups and introduced in the last several congresses, federal legislation propositions, such as the Genetically Engineered Food Right-to-Know Act, mandating labeling of any GMO food or food with GM ingredients, have never advanced beyond the committee stage in either chamber. As for the judicial branch, the inclination has been to defer to the executive branch agencies' decisions.

Between 2012 and 2015, many states introduced bills or at least ballot initiatives to try to enable GMO labeling. In Maine, Vermont, and Connecticut, mandatory GMO labeling laws were even passed. All the pressure pushed GMO producers to seek protection from state legislation. GMO producers advocated for a GMO Protection Act that would preempt states' rights to regulate GMOS. The producers wanted to outlaw state GMO labeling and preempt legislative and judicial victories that would protect organic seed and community health and ban GMO crops. The early discussions on the so-called Farmer Assurance Provision began. The Farmer Assurance Provision (Section 733 of U.S. H.R. 933) Bill, more commonly known as the "Monsanto Protection Act," was passed by the Senate on March 20, 2013. The provision "tells USDA to ignore any judicial ruling regarding the planting of genetically modified crops" (H.R.933—Consolidated and Further Continuing Appropriations Act 2013, 113th Congress 2013–2014). This means that the USDA is authorized to grant "temporary" permission for GM crops to be planted even if the crops were not properly approved by a judge. On May 25, 2013, hundreds of thousands of protestors united to March against

Monsanto in response to the failure of California Proposition 37. These advocates oppose the "Monsanto Protection Act" and support the push toward mandatory labeling of GM foods. The marchers believed that consumption of these GMO foods plays a role in cancer, birth defects, and infertility. The new activist group has called themselves March against Monsanto and currently has over 244,500 members on Facebook. The Facebook page allows members to view videos about Monsanto, share information about brands and products to avoid, and also keeps members updated with current GMO news (Press Release n.d). After a lot of debate, a controversial provision which stripped federal courts of the authority to halt the sale and planting of potentially hazardous GE crops was removed from the government funding bill that was signed into law on October 16, 2013.

In 2015, the U.S. House of Representatives passed legislation that would block states from requiring the labeling of GM foods, a move that consumer rights groups decried as corporate power defeating consumers' right to know. The matter has moved to the U.S. Senate. As of today, as far as GMO regulation is concerned, EPA, the FDA, and the USDA are still the agencies involved in the regulation process in the United States.

To date, U.S. government regulatory agencies have supported the biotechnology industry's growth with a lack of stringent regulations and independent research. Although the agencies also have their own scientists, these scientists often serve as proxies for the GMO lobby who continuously repeat that the *lack of research* is *evidence of lack of adverse effects*. One of the largest players in GMO research and regulatory principles has been Monsanto.

Monsanto was founded in 1901 by a pharmacist named John Francis Queeny. The first product that the company produced was the artificial sweetener saccharin, Sweet & Low, in 1945. The company became the first to genetically modify a plant cell in 1982 and conducted its first field tests of GE crops 5 years later. After extensive research, development, and marketing of plant biotechnology, Monsanto has become the largest seed production company in the nation (Table 9.1).

The close relationship among GMO regulators and corporate producers poses ethical questions. "Revolving doors," the exchange of personnel between regulatory agencies and the GMO industry they oversee, is a key avenue of influence. Caplan and Spitzer (2001) cited several examples of such influence from Monsanto:

- Margaret Miller, former chemical lab chief at Monsanto, became an FDA deputy director
- Michael Taylor worked at the FDA in the late 1970s and early 1980s. He worked as an attorney for Monsanto, then returned to work for the FDA, and returned again to work as an attorney for Monsanto

As a major producer, Monsanto has a clear stake in seeing that the principles of U.S. regulatory action are based on accelerating the approval process of GMO products.

Table 9.1 Percent of Global Proprietary Seed Market by Company

Company—2007	% of Global Proprietary Seed Market
Monsanto (USA)	23%
DuPont (USA)	15%
Syngenta (Switzerland)	9%
Groupe Limagrain (France)	6%
Land O' Lakes (USA)	4%
KWS AG (Germany)	3%
Bayer Crop Science (Germany)	2%
Sakata (Japan)	<2%
DLF-Trifolium (Denmark)	<2%
Takii (Japan)	<2%
Top 10 Total	67% (of global proprietary seed market)

Source: Adapted from ETC Group (http://www.gmwatch.org/gm-firms/10558-the-worlds-top-ten-seed-companies-who-owns-nature Last visited March 12, 2016).

European oversight

In contrast to the U.S. regulatory emphasis on expediting approval, the European Commission has taken a precautionary approach toward GMO products and has permitted only limited varieties to be introduced in Europe. The precautionary-approach entails the identification of risk, scientific uncertainty, and ignorance. This principle states that, in the absence of scientific consensus, if an action or policy has a *suspected* risk of causing harm, no action can be taken until it is proven safe (Rio Declaration of 1992). In addition, the burden of proof that it is *not* harmful falls on those taking action. The Precautionary Principle is Principle 15 of the Rio Declaration (Rio Declaration of 1992). The Europeans have approached the regulation of GMs on the presumption that since the GMO process is new, it may have unintended or unproven hazardous consequences (European Parliament and the Council of the European Union, 2001) and regulations have been heavily based on the precautionary principle.

In Europe, as opposed to the United States, industry and government experts and policymakers seem to act in a more harmonic way, reaching consensus more frequently. European views on food safety and potential risks involving GMOs are framed by traumatic events such as mad cow disease, putting food safety as a priority of European public consciousness. Europeans learned with the mad cow disease episode that scientific knowledge is an inadequate guide to regulatory policy since even scientific knowledge has its own "limitations in providing appropriate information in good time" (Godard 1997). The use of the precautionary principle as a basis to regulate GMOs in Europe shows a decline in the role of existing scientific knowledge as the only guide to policymaking.

The European Union authorities created the EU's Biotechnology Steering Committee in 1984. In 1985, the Steering Committee established the Biotechnology Regulations Interservice Committee (BRIC), a technical committee serving as a forum to develop biotechnology regulations. The BRIC submitted a draft directive that was formally adopted by the European Council in 1990 as Directive 90/220/EED on the Deliberate Release of Genetically Modified Organisms. This directive called for extensive environmental risk assessments to be carried out by applicants applying to conduct field tests on GMOs. A subsequent Directive was adopted to require Member States to submit applications when they desired to market GM products (Lynch and Vogel 2001).

In 1996, the European Parliament and the Council of Ministers considered foods using GMOs as novelty foods and therefore requiring labeling. In 1997, the Novel Food Regulation established a second directive, amplifying the scope of the foods to be labeled and newly including GM soybeans and corn. Europeans have kept strengthening their regulations year by year, and in 2000 they put into place a very strict standard where food at least 1% of which was GM needed to be labeled.

In Britain, a cabinet-level committee was established to look carefully into the effects of so-called "Frankenstein foods," a nickname GMOs received from the British press during the late 1990s. One of the strongest opponents to GMOs in Britain was Prince Charles, who made a statement in 1998 expressing his concern about the long-term consequences of GMOs on the environment and public health. In this statement, he stated that GMO foods take mankind into "realms that belong to God and to God alone" (Charles 1998).

Scientific consensus and controversy

Advocates for GMOs claim several benefits from their use. As far as nutrition is concerned, GMOs may have the potential to reduce hunger and malnutrition, especially in developing countries. A deficiency of vitamin A is the primary cause of blindness in developing countries, and it is estimated that 500,000 children per year will become blind due to Vitamin A deficiency (Potrykus n.d.). Iron deficiency, which primarily affects women and children, is another concern. The nutritional quality of some products may be enhanced by adding micronutrients (Johnson 2002) such as vitamin A and iron. The Food and Agriculture Organization of the United Nations estimates that 842 million people experience hunger and malnutrition (Food and Agriculture Organization of the United Nations 2013). Improvement of the seed quality of some products may help communities in need fight these threats. However, there is controversy as to whether GMOs have or will make a significant impact on malnutrition compared to non-GMO crops of "substantial equivalence," according to a study by Pusztai. "If our future is dependent on an abundant food supply and more nutritiously enhanced 'biofortified' crops, then we still have to wait for science to tell us the truth about those products" (Pusztai 2001).

In regard to pesticides, some studies show that GMO seeds require fewer applications of pesticides and insecticides. In addition to killing the targeted insect, pesticides also kill useful insects such as the honeybee and ladybug (Kilman 1999). Since GMOs do not require as many pesticide applications, the threat of pesticide and insecticide-related illnesses is also reduced (Johnson 2002). As a result of GMO technology, global pesticide usage decreased by 9.1% from 1996 to 2010 (Brookes and Barfoot 2012a). Another safety benefit of GMOs is the ability to introduce pest and virus resistant traits into seeds such as corn, tomatoes, squash, plum, and papaya (Munkvold et al. 1999; Food and Drug Administration n.d.).

In addition to safety benefits, farmers proclaim that using GMO seeds has numerous economic benefits. A study of farmers using biotechnological manipulated cotton reported financial gains ranging from $25 per hectare in Argentina to $550 in China (James 2002). In 2010, the direct global financial impact from additional productivity and reduced production costs from GMO crops were $14 billion, with farmers in developing countries receiving about 55% of the direct financial benefits (Brookes and Barfoot 2012b). Additional factors contributing to the economic gains from GMO crops include a reduction in the length of time to grow GMO crops (Brookes and Barfoot 2012a,b), and a slower ripening process of perishable GMO produce (Falk et al. 2002).

The development of pest, disease, and drought resistant GMO crops has also resulted in higher yields. GMO cotton farmers in China increased their yields by 10% while Philippine farmers experienced increased yields of 20%–30% from GMO corn between 2003 and 2007 (Glick 2007). As a result of increased yields, farmers have more disposable income for necessities such as food as well as improvements to their farms and nonfarm enterprises (Mackey 2003).

In regard to the environmental impact, GMO supporters maintain that GMOs also protect the environment due to less tillage, a reduction in fuel usage, and lower emissions of greenhouse gases (Mackey 2003). Since GMOs require fewer applications of pesticides and tillage is reduced by herbicide-resistant crops, less fuel is used in the production of GMO crops. From 1996 to 2010, the use of GMO crops resulted in a global permanent reduction of 4582 million liters of fuel, and a reduction in carbon dioxide emissions equivalent to 760,000 cars (Brookes and Barfoot 2012a).

On the other hand, opponents of GMOs underscore that there is still uncertainty about the environmental impact and effects on human health in their use. If crops are treated with environmentally resistant genes, then they can potentially activate antibiotic resistant genes in humans (Antoniou, Robinson, and Fagan 2012). Animal studies have also found that the toxicity of GMO foods can lead to organ failure, infertility, and carcinomas. Additionally, herbicide resistant GMOs may be correlated to the emergence of pesticide resistance weeds and insects that may be contaminating other nontarget organisms and ecosystems (Armenakas 2013).

Studies show that biodiversity can be harmed by GMOs as well. GMOs have the potential to undermine biodiversity by creating invasive species that compete with native species. In the United States, 42% of the species that are threatened or endangered are at risk primarily due to nonindigenous species (Maghari and Ardekani 2011).

An increasing number of scientists are becoming concerned following the discovery that genes do not behave independently as originally suspected but instead are dynamic with one another (Lungbill and Knipler 2001). This means that one gene does not always represent just one trait. Targeting favorable traits in a single gene becomes difficult, resulting in imprecise engineering, as genes move and rearrange themselves after the initial injection (Mohajer 2004). Unfortunately, virus and bacterium genes also get injected into the new host during the process. Once GM, the genes are able to "jump-to" new species on their own. Additionally, the genetic engineering process may switch on mutations throughout the organism's DNA, creating proteins that can also cause allergic reactions in consumers (Surabhi, Singh, Mishra 2011). The current allergy assessment system is not reliable because it relies heavily on in vitro tests rather than detecting nutritional or toxicological effects of foods in humans and animals (Antoniou, Robinson, and Fagan 2012). At present, the only reliable approach to assess whether a new GMO crop is allergenic is through consumer consultation.

In October 2013, the European Network of Scientists for Social and Environmental Responsibility (ENSSER), led by European scientists questioning the safety of GMOs, released a statement that continues to be signed by scientists worldwide states that there is no scientific consensus on the safety of GMOs and advocating that "decisions on the future of our food and agriculture should not be based on misleading and misrepresentative claims that a 'scientific consensus' exists on GMO safety." Statistically significant effects found in tests carried out between 2007 and 2012 have been dismissed as not "biologically relevant" and scientifically indefensible because most trials were short term and did not thoroughly assess the safety of GMOs (Antoniou, Robinson, and Fagan 2012). The genetic engineers Dr. John Fagan and Dr. Michale Antoniou and researcher Claire Robinson issued the second edition of their article "Myths and Truths" in which they claim that "an increasing number of studies are showing problems with GMOs" and that "The GMO industry is built on myth" (ENSSER 2013).

Recommendations

The global demand for food production is estimated to increase by 70% by 2050 (Food and Agriculture Organization of the United Nations 2009). Proponents of GMOs view biotechnology as necessary to meet this demand. They argue that GMOs should be incorporated in agriculture, especially in developing countries (Food and Agriculture Organization of the United Nations 2009). However, consumers continue to be distrustful of GMO foods. With consumers insisting on non-GMO foods and full disclosure of food content, the agriculture industry will most likely continue to respond with organic non-GMO crops (Falk et al. 2002). Education of consumers is crucial as the debate continues. Proponents hope that consumer decisions will be based on factors such as nutrition, flavor, price, and safety (Falk et al. 2002) while opponents hope for a more cautious approach in the use of GMOs (Jefferson 2006).

The main difference between the United States and European regulations regarding GMOs involves the politics of risk and the way each one perceives and manages risks related to GMO. The European position seems to be much stricter, much more risk-averse than the American one. Although the European position cannot be considered perfect, it seems more protective of consumers and public health. Consumer and environmental interests seem to be more influential in the European Parliament than in the U.S. establishment. Standards aimed at better protecting public health and the environment are constantly issued in Europe in order to promptly attend to public demands and pressures. Considering all the uncertainties and unknown outcomes, it seems that a more rigorous approach, such as the one the Europeans are implementing, is a reasonable path. However, multiple cases of regulatory failure on both sides of the Atlantic can be still witnessed, most of them due to conflicts of interests among regulators and industry and unscientific procedures.

It took decades for the harmful effects of tobacco use to be acknowledged. It is possible that in the future scientists and health experts may discover that just like tobacco, GMOs do cause harm to our health and the environment, a harm that in some circumstances cannot be fixed. When assessing the existing evidence and controversies around GMOs and their use and development, regulators should use precaution. The goal should be to find a balance that can benefit both producers and consumers while protecting public health.

REFERENCES

Antoniou, M., C. Robinson, and J. Fagan. 2012. GMO myths and truths an evidence-based examination of the claims made for the safety and efficacy of genetically modified crops. Retrieved from Earth Open Source Website: www.earthopensource.org

Berg, P., D. Baltimore, S. Brenner, R. O. Roblin, and M. F. Singer. 1975. Summary statement of the Asilomar conference on recombinant DNA molecules. *Proceeding of the National Academy of the Sciences of the United States of America* 72(6):1981–1984.

Brookes, G. and P. Barfoot. 2012a. Global impact of biotech crops: Environmental effects, 1996–2010. *GM Crops & Food* 3(2):129–137. doi:10.4161/gmcr.20061.

Brookes, G. and P. Barfoot. 2012b. The income and production effects of biotech crops globally 1996–2010. *GM Crops & Food* 3(4):265–272. doi:10.4161/gmcr.20097.

Caplan, R. and S. Spitzer. 2001. Pesticide Action Network North America. *Regulation of genetically engineered crops and foods in the united state.* Retrieved from https://nativeseeds.org/pdf/GERegulations.pdf

Charles, P. 1998. *The Seeds of Disaster.* https://www.princeofwales.gov.uk/media/speeches/article-the-prince-of-wales-titled-the-seeds-of-disaster-the-daily-telegraph

Consolidated and Further Continuing Appropriations Act. 2013. 113th Congress (2013–2014). Retrieved from http://beta.congress.gov/bill/113th-congress/house-bill/933

Department of Health and Human Services. 1976. *National Agency of Health Guidelines.* Retrieved from website: http://oba.od.nih.gov/oba/rac/Guidelines/NIH_Guidelines.html

Department of Health and Human Services, Food and Drug Administration. 1992. *Premarket Notice Concerning Bioengineered Foods (Vol. 57).* Retrieved from Federal Register 22991 website: http://www.gpo.gov/fdsys/pkg/FR-2001-01-18/pdf/01-1046.pdf

Exercise of Federal Oversight within Scope of Statutory Authority. 1992. *Planned Introductions of Biotechnology Products into the Environment.* Federal Register. 57.27:6753, http://www.gpo.gov/fdsys/pkg/FR-2001-07-19/pdf/01-17981.pdf

Falk, M. C., B. M. Chassy, S. K. Harlander, T. J. Hoban, M. N. McGloughlin, and A. R. Akhlaghi. 2002. Food biotechnology: Benefits and concerns. *Journal of Nutrition* 132(6):1384–1390.

Federal Food, Drug and Cosmetic Act (FFDCA). 2000. *National Uniform Nutrition Labeling* U. S. Code, Title 21. Retrieved from website: http://www.fda.gov/food/guidanceregulation/guidancedocumentsregulatoryinformation/biotechnology/ucm096126.htm

Food and Agriculture Organization of the United Nations. 2009. *How to Feed the World in 2050.* Retrieved from http://www.fao.org/fileadmin/templates/wsfs/docs/expert_paper/How_to_Feed_the_World_in_2050.pdf

Food and Agriculture Organization of the United Nations. 2013. *The State of Food Insecurity in the World: The Multiple Dimensions of Food Security.* Retrieved from http://www.fao.org/docrep/018/i3434e/i3434e00.htm.

Food and Drug Administration. 1992a. *Principles for Federal Oversight of Biotechnology: Planned Introduction into the Environment of Organisms with Modified Hereditary Traits (1992.31118) Federal Register.*

Food and Drug Administration. 1992b. *Statement of Policy: Foods Derived from New Plant Varieties.* Retrieved from Federal Register Vol. 57, No. 104. website: http://www.gpo.gov/fdsys/pkg/FR-2001-07-19/pdf/01-17981.pdf

Food and Drug Administration Center for Food Safety and Applied Nutrition. 1997. *Guidance on Consultation Procedures: Foods Derived from New Plant Varieties.* Retrieved from website: http://www.fda.gov/food/guidanceregulation/guidancedocumentsregulatoryinformation/biotechnology/ucm096126.htm

Food and Drug Administration. n.d. *Completed Consultations on Bioengineered Foods.* Retrieved from http://www.accessdata.fda.gov/scripts/fcn

Glick, H. 2007. Plant biotechnology in Asia: Current benefits and future opportunities. *Asia Pacific Biotech News*, 11(4): 240–244.

Godard, O. 1997. Social decision-making under conditions of scientific controversy, expertise and the precautionary principle, integrating scientific expertise into decision making. In C. Joerges, K.-H. Ladeur, and E. Vos (eds.), *Integrating Scientific Expertise into Regulatory Decisionmaking - National Experiences and European Innovations*, Nomos Verlagsgesellschaft, pp. 39–73.

Hilbeck, A., M. Meier, and A. Raps. *Pesticide Action Network North America 2000.* Review on non-target organisms and transgenic Bt plants. Retrieved from EcoStrat GmbH Ecological Technology Assessment & Environmental Consulting website: http://www.greenpeace.org/international/Global/international/planet-2/report/2000/3/review-on-non-target-organisms.pdf

James, C. 2002. *Global Review of Commercialized Transgenic Crops: 2001 Feature: Bt Cotton. ISAAA Briefs No. 26.* Ithaca, NY: ISAAA.

Jefferson, V. 2006. The ethical dilemma of genetically modified food. *Journal of Environmental Health* 69(1):33–34.

Johnson, D. 2002. Biotechnology issues for developing economies. *Economic Development & Cultural Change* 51(1):1.

Kilman, S. 1999. Seeds of doubt: Once quick converts, farmers begin to lose faith in biotech crops—DuPont and others, mindful of their R&D billions, struggle to hold ground—prospects for labeling law? *Wall Street Journal* p.A, 1:6.

Lynch, D. and Vogel, D. Council of Foreign Relations. 2001. *The Regulation of GMO in Europe and United States: A Case-Study of Contemporary European Regulatory Politics.* Retrieved from http://www.cfr.org/agricultural-policy/regulation-gmos-europe-united-states-case-study-contemporary-european-regulatory-politics/p8688

Mackey, M. A. 2003. The developing world benefits from plant biotechnology. *Journal of Nutrition & Behavior* 35(4):210.

Munkvold, G., R. Hellmich, and L. Rice. 1999. Comparison of Fumonisin concentrations in kernels of transgenic Bt maize hybrids and nontransgenic hybrids. *Plant Disease* 83(2):130–138.

Office of Science and Technology Policy. 1986. *Coordinated Framework for Regulation of Biotechnology* (Vol. 62, No. 79, 19903). Retrieved from Federal Register website: http://www.gpo.gov/fdsys/pkg/FR-1997-04-24/pdf/97-10648.pdf

Potrykus, I. n.d. *The Golden Rice Tale.* Retrieved from http://www.agbioworld.org

The European Network of Scientists for Social and Environmental Responsibility (ENSSER). 2013.

Unknown. Press Release. n.d. March against Monsanto Official Website. Retrieved from http://www.march-against-monsanto.com/p/press-release.html

Part IV
Considering local food systems

10 From industrial food to local alternatives

A cultural food shift and new directions in public health

Alicia Andry

Introduction

Barry Popkin defines food systems as "the way we produce, transport, and distribute food" (2009, p. 22). The United States food system, based on an industrial model of production and distribution, has been the strongest influence in shaping the global food system as a whole (Albritton 2013, p. 343). In the industrial food model, consumers rarely have any contact with their immediate food source, are usually unaware of the energy inputs required to make the food, and may not even recognize the specific source from which their food originates. This leaves the average person with no concept of how their purchases impact the overall environment (Viljeon, Bohn, and Howe 2005, p. 41). In contrast to the industrial food model, local food systems are more intimate because consumers and producers often interact personally and are able to build a relationship as a result of their direct contact with each other (Nousiainen et al. 2009, p. 570). Face-to-face contact empowers both consumers and producers, and creates a fair and equitable distribution system in which the needs of all parties involved can be considered (Nousiainen et al. 2009, p. 590). Locally based food systems also make fresh produce more available in areas where it might be scarce, increasing the percentage of fruits and vegetables consumed (Miller 2013, p. 167) and potentially improving overall health.

More Americans are participating in local food options as a way to obtain healthier foods that do not bring into question the nutritional viability of food, damage to the environment, or the sustainability of our food system. What circumstances have shaped the modern industrial food system? What are the problems associated with the industrial food system that are prompting consumers to look for alternatives? What alternative food systems are available? Also, what is needed to encourage a societal shift from the industrial food system to more sustainable, local food systems? As emerging local food systems gain popularity, American society is moving to a more sustainable post-industrial food system, and public health administrators are in a position to play a role in the promotion of revised policies that support public health and in the education of the public to make choices that support individual and environmental health.

The making of an industry

Early policies that created the industrial food system

The twentieth century industrial model of agriculture looks much different from food production and distribution methods prior to that era. Before modern transportation and industrial food processing techniques, people consumed regionally grown and locally produced foods because of the short distance that food could travel from the point of production to the point of consumption without spoiling. The invention of modern transportation and advances in food science during the first half of the twentieth century paved the way for an industrial agricultural system that allowed consumers easy access to a wider variety of food items and convenience foods requiring less preparation. The use of machines and chemicals in agriculture became more prevalent, especially after WWII (Albritton 2013, p. 342). Simultaneously, populations began to shift from the central cities to the suburban outskirts (Fishman 2007, p. 70). The need for proximity to one's employment and access to city amenities via public transportation were traded for quick travel along more accessible roads in personal automobiles (Fishman 2007, pp. 74–75). This allowed families to relocate away from the populated and polluted central city to a single-family home in the suburbs (Fishman 74–75), while still maintaining a connection to city amenities. Increased transportation options and infrastructure also allowed companies to relocate from the central cities to the suburbs (Mieszkowski and Mills 1993, p. 136), which contributed to population decline, economic decline, and finally physical decline of downtown city areas (Fishman 2007, pp. 70–75). Many factors influenced these trends of suburbanization including "the abundance of land in the United States, greater reliance on the automobile, a more extensive system of freeways within urban areas, greater suburban fiscal autonomy, higher crime rates in central cities, and greater ethnic and social diversification in the United States" (Mieszkowski and Mills 1993, p. 141). All of these factors influenced the new urban landscape, structurally and socially, and created new requirements and opportunities for the industrial food system as it developed into what we know today.

This time period also saw an increase in food regulatory agencies, such as the United States Department of Agriculture (USDA), which introduced new agriculture and food regulations that had never been seen before in U.S. history. When the USDA was originally created in 1862 (Lusk 2016, p. 13), its two main objectives were to "ensure a sufficient and reliable food supply" and to provide the U.S. population with general information about topics related to agriculture (Nestle 2002, p. 33). The USDA's primary objective at that time was to provide U.S. citizens with general agricultural information and to obtain and distribute seeds (Lusk 2016, p. 13). In contrast, according to the 2016 USDA website, the USDA's current main objectives are to "provide leadership on food, agriculture, natural resources, rural development, nutrition, and related issues based on public policy, the best available science, and effective management" (United States Department of Agriculture 2016). These modern objectives are quite different from the objectives originally put forth by the organization at its conception.

According to the USDA Strategic Plan for 2014–2018, they now focus on rural repopulation, environmental conservation, increased agriculture and biotechnology production, and ensured food security and food access for U.S. children (United States Department of Agriculture 2014).

This drastic change in purpose occurred over a century of changing presidents, shifting social concerns, and new economic challenges. For example, the Great Depression prompted the creation of the Farm Board to monitor the prices of selected crops and purchase surplus from farmers when prices fell too low (Lusk 2016, p. 14). Later, the New Deal included the Agricultural Adjustment Act of 1933, which awarded government subsidies to farmers who restricted the amount and types of crops they grew (Lusk 2016, pp. 14–15). In 1964, President Johnson created the food stamp program and charged the USDA with feeding those who could not afford to feed themselves (Lusk 2016, p. 16). Each era in U.S. history added a new facet of regulation for the USDA to oversee. The organization is now made up of 17 agencies with a total of 18 offices, overseeing government regulation of "(1) natural resources and the environment; (2) farm and foreign agricultural services; (3) rural development; (4) food, nutrition, and consumer services; (5) food safety; (6) research, education, and economics; and (7) marketing and regulatory programs" (Lusk 2016, p. 16). The USDA has expanded over the years to cover many areas of agricultural, environmental, and economic regulation. Some of these areas overlap, creating the potential for confusion and contradiction within USDA policies and procedures (Lusk 2016, p. 27).

Originally created through the USDA, farm subsidies that support large monocrop production agriculture may have helped farmers a century ago, but the circumstances within American society have evolved. The current subsidies do little to help an imbalanced system and instead tend to enhance the "inefficiencies" of farming, promote "environmental degradation," and provide large sums of money to farmers who typically gross more income than the average farmer (Spruiell 2007, p. 44). For example, in 2005, the federal government subsidy program funneled more than $20 billion to agriculture (Albritton 2013, p. 342). To break this amount down, 46% was paid for corn, 23% was paid for cotton, 10% was paid for wheat, and 6% was paid for soybeans (Albritton 2013, pp. 342–343). Also in 2005, the top 10% of farms received 72% of the total subsidies, 60% of farms received no subsidies at all, and small and medium farms, along with fruit and vegetable crops, were completely omitted from this subsidy equation (Albritton 2013, p. 343). This policy system rewards a farmer for producing a subsidized crop that is then used to create an inexpensive processed food found on grocery store shelves but creates no incentive for a farmer who wishes to produce fresh fruits or vegetables. It also encourages monocrop development by rewarding the farmers who grow crops on a large scale (Lusk 2016, pp. 25–26). "The larger the farm and the higher the yield, the larger…the subsidy" (Albritton 2013, p. 342). This practice of monocrop farming was influenced by a number of factors including policies and government incentives, technological advances in farming, and market demand (Lusk 2016, p. 10), although one could argue that this is a false market demand created by early agricultural policies put into place starting in the era of the Great Depression (Lusk 2016, pp. 14–15). A discussion of the economic impacts and false market demand, however, is beyond the scope of this chapter.

Wheat, corn, and soybeans are currently the food crops most subsidized by the government and are therefore the crops most overproduced by farmers and most prolifically used in the industrialized food system (Koons Garcia 2009). "Agricultural researchers and the U.S. government worked very hard to develop these cash crops, to increase productivity, and to make them as inexpensive as possible" (Popkin 2009, p. 23). Large farms ultimately cater to large corporations by producing and supplying specific ingredients for them to create their food products (Albritton 2013, p. 342). As a result of a surplus of these cheap commodity crops, the food industry has had to invent new uses for them. These newly invented food products have become the basis of many processed foods found on grocery store shelves today (Koons Garcia 2009). Ingredients such as high-fructose corn syrup and corn starch can be found in many processed foods (Kenner 2009). In addition to foods, the promotion of corn-based ethanol through new government fuel mandates has added increased demand to an already over-produced corn supply (Spruiell 2007, p. 44). The entire industrial crop system was designed to enhance the production and distribution of just these few crops (Popkin 2009, p. 23). This focus on a few cash crops rather than on a large variety of foods has caused health problems for humans, animals, and the environment.

Problems created by the industrial food system

As the industrial food system became more prominent in the twentieth century, new environmental and human health concerns began to surface. Environmental concerns such as "groundwater contamination, soil erosion and degradation, chemical residues in food, and the demise of family and rural farms" over the past few decades have prompted people to look for alternatives that are potentially less detrimental to public health, the environment, and local economies (Beus and Dunlap 1990, p. 591). "While most critics recognize the benefits that stem from the current U.S. agricultural system, they also argue that when all of its hidden costs are considered, modern industrial agriculture is not the bargain it appears to be. Many critics see the problems of modern agriculture as fundamental flaws inherent in its structure, policies, and practices" (Beus and Dunlap 1990, p. 591). Modern fertilizer and pesticide usage has left land devoid of essential nutrients because the nutrients found in the soil are depleted faster than they can be replaced (Miller 2013, p. 35). Researchers in Switzerland have shown that farming methods that use synthetic fertilizers and other additives strip the soil of these essential nutrients when compared to alternative farming methods that do not rely on synthetic inputs and additives (Miller 2013, p. 38). By using farming methods that promote soil depletion and environmental degradation, future generations may face increased difficulty in cultivating their own food supply.

In addition to depletion of environmental resources, the industrial food production model has brought up questions regarding consumer health. In the early 1900s, the most prevalent causes of death were related to communicable diseases and infections (Nestle 2002, p. 31). As the century progressed and food systems shifted to the industrial model, these leading causes of death shifted to chronic diseases such as diabetes, coronary heart disease, cancers, and stroke (Nestle 2002, p. 31), all health issues related to and considered preventable with diet. Over a century ago, W. O. Atwater, a forerunner in modern nutrition and instigator of early food initiatives, warned of health issues that would arise from eating only a few, government-selected food items (Popkin 2009, pp. 24–25). The variety of food that our ancestors consumed is not the reality of the American diet today. As a result of this lack of variety, the health warning from Atwater over a century ago is now being realized. The industrial food system has given us an abundance of cheap food products but it has also created a system in which healthy foods such as fresh vegetables and fruits, with large amounts of essential micronutrients, are more expensive and more difficult (if not impossible) to come by in some areas (Popkin 2009, p. 24). Many studies have shown that diet, a lifestyle factor that can be controlled by individuals, is the largest influencing factor of our overall health (Albritton 2013, p. 342). More than two-thirds of the American population is now overweight, and those classified as very obese are the fastest-growing group within this overweight category (Albritton 2013, p. 344). While associated with diabetes, obesity is a risk factor for many other modern, common chronic diseases (Albritton 2013, p. 344). Diet affects health in many ways and therefore the industrial food system must be addressed when considering solutions to these health issues.

Toward a post-industrial food system

The U.S. is moving toward a post-industrial food system through the philosophical rejection of the industrial food system that dominates our society. The industrial food model was created as a result of a singular focus on economic growth (Beus and Dunlap 1990, p. 610). A post-industrial food system would essentially reject this singular focus on economic growth and reinvest in human and environmental health. This post-industrial food system might be related to pre-industrial food production techniques, but the scale of food production must match that of the industrial model in order to maintain the necessary amount of food to feed the current and growing population. It might look like a multifaceted system that provides local food in a variety of manners, through community gardens, backyard gardens, hydroponic and aquaponic food production, rooftop urban agriculture, local food cooperatives, community supported agriculture, farm-to-table programs, and vertical urban farm towers. This post-industrial food model would reject large inputs of chemicals and emphasize conservation of finite environmental resources. It would replace highly processed, calorie-dense food with less processed, nutrient-dense food. Also, it would supply food from many small sources using a variety of production methods instead of from a few large sources.

These changes are already occurring. Community gardens, farmers' markets, community supported agriculture, and even large-scale urban agricultural models are becoming more prominent in urban areas. This shift away from the industrial food model and toward more local alternative models is a rejection of modern agribusiness principles and an embrace of a "post-industrial, eco-agriculture" model (Beus and Dunlap 1990, p. 596), one that trades commodity crops, highly processed foods, and extensive food miles for biodiverse crops and whole foods that travel short distances from farm to table. Pre-industrial food production emphasized the production of food for survival while this new post-industrial food movement will emphasize food for human and ecological health. It is this ecological focus that sets the post-industrial alternative food movement apart from previous agricultural movements (Beus and Dunlap 1990, p. 600). This post-industrial food system expands beyond pre-industrial agricultural methods to large urban farm production that changes the landscape of cities as we know them today. This shift is already gaining momentum. It battles the principles of industrial agribusiness in a quest to gain a foothold in a healthier, more sustainable, and more robust future.

A return to local

Local food production alternatives

For hundreds of years prior to the current industrial food production model, humans produced and distributed food using other methods. So it should come as no surprise that there are modern alternatives to industrial agriculture. There are many approaches that one can take to create alternatives to the industrial food system (Beus and Dunlap 1990, p. 594), and many of these alternatives are based on models of food production used prior to the implementation of industrial methods. These different approaches share the common underlying philosophy of using fewer inputs to reduce energy usage and increase self-sustainability (Beus and Dunlap 1990, p. 594). Sometimes consumers sacrifice low costs for these positive benefits (Nousiainen et al. 2009, p. 572), but sometimes local alternatives cost less because inputs come in the form of personal time and labor rather than additives and fuel costs. Alternative food systems typically encourage food to be consumed as close as possible to its point of origin (Beus and Dunlap 1990, p. 601). Within these more simple and straightforward food systems, a domino effect can be observed in which one aspect is changed, and other aspects naturally follow. If one eats food that does not travel far, awareness of local food is increased, overall energy consumption is reduced, and that food system becomes less vulnerable to systemic breakdown (Beus and Dunlap 1990, p. 601). There are some negative aspects of relying only on local food production, such as an increased workload for producers and limitations to availability in local markets (Nousiainen et al. 2009, p. 578). Common alternatives to the industrial food production model, such as community gardening, urban farming, farmers' markets, and community supported agriculture, provide city residents access to foods that demonstrate both the positive and negative sides of local food production and distribution.

Community gardening and urban agriculture

In community gardening and large-scale urban agriculture models, food is produced in the same geographic area in which it is consumed. Community gardening became popular in the U.S. during the 1970s and was particularly appealing to urban dwellers in larger cities with very little green space access (Viljeon, Bohn, and Howe 2005, pp. 105–106). Gardens can be initiated by a number of different entities (churches, schools, etc.) but the common characteristic across the board is strong community involvement (Viljeon, Bohn, and Howe 2005, p. 83). These communal efforts can bring revitalization, a sense of security, and a decrease of crime in blighted areas (Viljeon, Bohn, and Howe 2005, p. 57). In addition, they can provide educational opportunities to youth through school-based and extracurricular programs for children and adults (Viljeon, Bohn, and Howe 2005, p. 58). Community gardens create a sense of collective efficacy among neighborhood residents by giving the residents a platform for shared time, shared meals, shared traditions, and an overall feeling of inclusiveness, both among the residents and between residents and local agencies (Miller 2013, p. 185). Community gardens can also increase residents' perceptions of beauty and safety within their surroundings, which encourages more time spent actively outdoors (Miller 2013, p. 186). The act of gardening itself can provide health benefits beyond just providing fresh produce. Community gardening, in particular, has been shown to raise the quality and quantity of an individual's connection to others, increase overall health through low-impact exercise, raise the levels of Vitamin D and serotonin which both act as natural antidepressants, and increase the amount of time an individual spends outside (Miller 2013, p. 51). Growing food takes time and effort, but the rewards of community gardening are multifaceted.

Urban agriculture is similar to community gardening in that food is grown in close proximity to its point of consumption, but it is grown on a much larger scale, and those who consume the food may not be directly involved in the production process. Like any other alternative agriculture practice, urban agricultural models can be designed differently to serve the specific need of the community. For example, Growing Power began in Milwaukee, Wisconsin as a nonprofit organization focused on helping urban youth, with the intention "to change the landscape of the north side of Milwaukee" (Growing Power 2014). Urban agriculture is one of the many areas of focus for this organization, and farms have now expanded outside of Milwaukee to include Madison, Wisconsin, and Chicago, Illinois (Growing Power 2014). In contrast to this nonprofit model, Gotham Greens in New York City is primarily an urban agriculture business that focuses on providing sustainably grown produce to "retail, restaurant and institutional customers" throughout the city (Gotham Greens 2016). They are committed to providing "hyper-local" produce that is grown in greenhouse structures on urban rooftops (Gotham Greens 2016). Although the missions of these urban agriculture models are very different, both challenge the way American society defines agriculture. There are countless numbers of organizations within the United States that work toward a similar cause of changing the urban landscape and redefining our food systems, but due to the limited scope of this chapter, only two examples can be provided.

Farmers' markets and community supported agriculture

Rather than producing food directly within the urban area, farmers' markets and community supported agriculture bring food into the city from nearby rural farms. These approaches eliminate the industrial middleman and put consumers directly into contact with farmers. Farmers' markets have become a booming market in the past decade (Viljeon, Bohn, and Howe 2005, p. 37). There was a 17% increase nationally in farmers' markets between 2010 and 2011 (Agriculture Marketing Service 2012), and as of 2015, the USDA has a listing that includes 8,476 farmers' markets nationwide (Agriculture Marketing Service 2016). Farmers' markets not only allow consumers to know the exact origin and production methods of their food, but also allow farmers to cultivate customer loyalty through direct contact with their consumers (Agriculture Marketing Service 2016). In more recent years, farmers' markets have begun to accept WIC dollars as well, in an attempt to encourage lower-income residents to shop at these markets where they will find fewer processed food items and more whole foods (Miller 2013, p. 179). One drawback to farmers' markets is that they are typically seasonal and affected by the regional climate, as are community supported agriculture efforts.

Like farmers' markets, community supported agriculture builds a direct relationship between farmer and consumer (Local Harvest 2016). Consumers (or members) pay a fee at the beginning of the growing season; farmers do the work of growing the food, and the resulting food is made available to members at regularly scheduled intervals throughout the growing season (Local Harvest 2016). According to the Local Harvest website, some advantages are that farmers can focus on tending crops during the growing season rather than selling their items at a market, food is very fresh when it reaches consumers, a variety of items are offered, and members usually have opportunities to visit the farm and see how the food is produced (2016). One potential disadvantage to community supported agriculture is "shared risk" (Local Harvest 2016). Members pay a flat fee before the growing season begins so if there is a problem with the harvest, members take the loss in the form of smaller shares during the growing season (Local Harvest 2016). Members also typically receive a predetermined variety of food, some of which they may not like or be familiar with, which differs from other alternative food production methods where the consumer can choose specifically either what items to grow or what items to purchase. Community supported agriculture is not as common as farmers' markets but both techniques of distribution source local, healthy foods to consumers with the goal of encouraging the positive aspects of eating local and discouraging the negative aspects of the industrial food system.

New directions in public health

A cultural food shift

Modern nutritional research has shown that the excessive consumption of sugar and refined grains found in most processed foods causes common chronic health issues such as obesity and diabetes, and yet the production of these products has been and continues to be subsidized by the U.S. government (Popkin 2009, p. 29). Not just one company, but many, carry the blame for the modern health epidemics that we are facing (Popkin 2009, p. 98). It is the collective food industry, from soft drink producers to fast food restaurant chains, meat production facilities to giant biotech companies, who make up the modern food production culture and who drive food consumption practices. A cultural shift in food consumption is needed, but in many cases it goes against the interests of large, powerful corporations that are vying for consumer loyalty in order to secure the company's financial success. To overcome the massive influence of the industrial food system, consumer education and policy changes are needed.

Education

Education can be a challenge and a roadblock when it comes to getting people to trade processed food products for unprocessed, fresh foods. Studies have shown that teaching youth about healthy eating habits can be one way to approach this problem. "One survey from the New York region showed that children are more than twice as likely to be avid veggie eaters if most of their meals are prepared at home and if their caregivers shop at a farm stand or farmers' market rather than a supermarket. For school-age children, farm-to-school programs, in which farm-fresh food is served in school lunches, and edible schoolyard curricula that teach students how to grow and prepare their food have also been shown to increase vegetable consumption" (Miller 2013, pp. 85–86). More schools are participating in farm-to-table lunch programs and initiating school gardens that are used as teaching tools to increase interest and exposure to fresh, unprocessed foods. Oftentimes, children will be more excited and willing to try new vegetables if they have a vested interest in growing those vegetables (Miller 2013, p. 182). In some cases, their enthusiasm can be contagious at home as well and spread to the adults in the family. A parent may not always know how to prepare a particular vegetable grown in a local garden, but educational outreach to them on cooking and food preparation could be a good starting point. Building general awareness of healthy eating through education is one place to start addressing this multifaceted issue of food and health, but unfortunately it is not the only thing needed to correct the problem.

Policies

Food policies have created and shaped modern foodscapes and eating habits for the past century. Policies created by the U.S. government support the industrial food system and large agribusiness, oftentimes to the detriment of small farmers, local food distribution efforts, and consumers. Food companies have helped shape the cultural attitudes about food and put these policies in place to serve the companies' best interests. One prominent soft drink manufacturer, in the face of research showing the detriments of consuming large amounts of sugar, was influential in shifting the focus from sugar consumption to lack of exercise as being the culprit behind metabolic-related illnesses (Popkin 2009, p. 125). Corporate food giants often play a direct role in shaping regulations and food norms. There are multiple examples of suggestions made by the World Health Organization that were contested by food corporations who were worried about losing profits, in which ultimately the corporations won (Albritton 2013, p. 345). This type of self-preservation is expected in a capitalistic system where companies rely on consumers to purchase their products, whether those products create health or illness.

The food industry includes a number of specialized organizations that influence food policy decisions, such as the International Life Science Institute, the American Diabetic Association and the American Heart Association, the American Beverage Association, and the Snack Food Association (Popkin 2009, pp. 125–132). These organizations were founded to positively advance the areas of food research and education, but unfortunately many of them are funded by large food companies who use these platforms as a promotional opportunity for their own products (Popkin 2009, p. 127). For example, the American Heart Association receives funding from the manufacturer of each product the organization endorses as "heart-healthy," and in these claims, the AHA often refers to industry-supported research but rarely includes independent studies that contradict the industry-supported research findings (Popkin 2009, p. 128). Researchers funded by groups with no affiliation to the manufacturer of the product being studied often find less-favorable results in comparison because independent researchers do not have a vested interest in promoting the product (Popkin 2009, p. 129). With this type of structure for policy making and food promotion, it is not surprising that food policy favors large companies over consumers and that consumers must decipher conflicting and confusing health information.

In some cases, people who are trying to make a positive difference in food-related health issues find themselves fighting against policies instead of being supported by them. For instance, supermarket representatives and dieticians may work together to encourage customers to purchase more fresh produce and unprocessed foods, but when these unsubsidized foods are the more expensive choices, it can be difficult to persuade customers to spend more money on the healthier options (Miller 2013, p. 165). A revision of policies that subsidize certain foods and not others could help close this price gap between processed and unprocessed foods (Popkin 2009, p. 169). Subsidies on fresh fruits and vegetables would bring prices down on these items and potentially make them more appealing to consumers, but this would require major federal food policy change.

Consumers also experience problems with location and accessibility when trying to purchase healthy food. Zoning ordinances in urbanized areas may restrict what types of businesses can operate within the city or how specific areas of land can be used. Residential zoning may prohibit the inclusion of a much-needed food market within a housing area. Also, a large grocery store that offers dietician consultations and cooking classes is of little help if the customer has no transportation to reach the store (Miller 2013, p. 166). Even more discouraging are recent studies about food accessibility and food deserts that show that making food accessible within a food desert does little to improve the dietary quality and fresh produce intake of the surrounding residents (Miller 2013, pp. 166–167). This factor alone may point to why both education and policy reform are needed when it comes to food. Educating people about healthy food choices does not help accessibility to healthy food, and making healthy food more easily accessible does not guarantee that healthy food choices will follow. Both aspects must be addressed simultaneously to encourage a cultural shift in food choices.

The role of public health administration

In the Western world, chronic health issues such as obesity, diabetes, and heart disease are typically found more predominantly among less affluent populations (Popkin 2009, p. 109). There are a number of possible reasons for this trend, including cheap, subsidized processed foods that contain large amounts of sugar and very few nutrients. Lifestyle changes have occurred in the past few decades to encourage these chronic health issues as well. Americans eat more and move less than they did in the mid-twentieth century and more fatty, sweet, processed foods are available now than ever before in human history (Popkin 2009, p. 119). These factors all contribute to the chronic diseases that have become more prevalent in American society over the past few decades. Public health administrators have an opportunity to be instrumental in instigating the cultural shift in how we educate and encourage people to practice lifestyle choices that will create better health.

Some experts in the areas of food and health are beginning to offer solutions to the issues discussed thus far. Popkin proposes an increase on taxes of processed, calorie-dense, nutrient-deficient foods in order to make these foods less appealing to consumers, as an increased tax on tobacco products helped motivate people to quit smoking (2009, p. 165). One problem with this idea is in determining what foods to include in the tax and what foods to exclude. Nutritional research has revealed a mix of conclusions about which foods are considered bad and which are considered good, and in many cases, new conclusions contradict previous findings. Sorting through the conflicting information to determine the ideal healthy diet could cause problems in identifying what foods to tax. A second problem with this idea is that the companies which manufacture the food items that are subject to additional tax may attempt to block the implementation of such a policy because it would ultimately affect their profits. If not, these companies may decide that they need to assert a high degree of influence in determining what items are subject to additional tax. Despite these uncertainties, Popkin is not the only one who has made this connection between the sugar and the tobacco industries. Albritton compares the two in his article, "Between Obesity and Hunger: The Capitalist Food Industry." The tobacco industry provides one example of how successful a higher tax and a well-planned long-term marketing campaign can be. Public health administrators could play the same role in fighting sugar addiction as they did in fighting tobacco addiction by encouraging healthy choices, educating the public, and supporting marketing efforts. Over time, society's food choices could shift in the same way that the culture shifted around tobacco products.

Conclusion

The Industrial Revolution, early twentieth century governmental policies, and a desire for economic efficiency in the face of urban sprawl helped shape the industrial food system. In the first half of the 1900s, cities served primarily as industrial centers, but toward the mid-1900s, the suburbs became the haven for the working man and the symbol of the American Dream. This was considered the ideal way of life, and the systems in place reflected that reality. The reality of the post-industrial age has reshaped our geography, and our needs are moving beyond a large one-size-fits-all industrial food system to a post-industrial multifaceted foodscape. Since 2002, some states have seen an increase in the number of smaller farms that produce food in an ecologically sustainable manner (Miller 2013, p. 12). More universities across the nation are adding programs to their curriculum that cover sustainable agriculture (Miller 2013, p. 12). A cultural shift has begun but completing the process takes time and effort from everyone involved. Public health administrators should lead this cultural shift by creating a structure that supports healthy food options, arms the public with knowledge and information about healthy food choices, and assists other health professionals in creating wellness in addition to treating illness.

REFERENCES

Agriculture Marketing Service. 2012. *Farmers' Markets and Direct-To-Consumer Marketing.* Accessed March 17, 2012. https:// www.ams.usda.gov/services/local-regional/farmers-markets-and-direct-consumer-marketing

Agriculture Marketing Service. 2016. *Farmers' Markets and Direct-To-Consumer Marketing.* Accessed May 24, 2016. https:// www.ams.usda.gov/services/local-regional/farmers-markets-and-direct-consumer-marketing

Albritton, R. 2013. Between obesity and hunger: The capitalist food industry. In *Food and Culture: A Reader*, 3rd ed., edited by C. Counihan and P. Van Esterik. New York: Taylor & Francis, pp. 342–352.

Beus, C. E. and R. E. Dunlap. 1990. Conventional versus alternative agriculture: The paradigmatic roots of the debate. *Rural Sociology* 55(4):590–616.

Fishman, R. 2007. Beyond Suburbia: The rise of the Technoburb. In *The City Reader*, 4th ed. edited by R. T. LeGates and F. Stout. New York: Routledge, pp. 69–77.

Gotham Greens. 2016. *Our Story.* Accessed May 14, 2016. http://gothamgreens.com/our-story/

Growing Power. 2014. *"About" and "History"*. Accessed May 14, 2016. http://www.growingpower.org/

Kenner, R. (director). 2009. *Food, Inc. 2008*. United States: Magnolia Pictures. [DVD].

Koons Garcia, D. (director). 2005. *The Future of Food. 2004*. United States: Cinema Libre Studio. [DVD].

Local Harvest. 2016. *Community Supported Agriculture*. Accessed May 24, 2016. http://www.localharvest.org/csa/

Lusk, J. L. 2016. *The Evolving Role of the USDA in the Food and Agricultural Economy*. Arlington, VA: Meractus Research, Mercatus Center at George Mason University (June), pp. 1–56. http://mercatus.org/publication/evolving-role-usda-food-and-agricultural-economy

Mieszkowski, P. and E. S. Mills. 1993. The causes of metropolitan suburbanization. *Journal of Economic Perspectives* 7(3):135–147.

Miller, D. 2013. *Farmacology: What Innovative Family Farming Can Teach Us about Health and Healing*. New York: HarperCollins Publishers.

Nestle, M. 2002. *Food Politics*. Berkeley and Los Angeles: University of California Press.

Nousiainen, M., P. Pylkkanen, F. Saunders, L. Seppanen, and K. Vesala, 2009. Are alternative food systems socially sustainable? A case study from Finland. *Journal of Sustainable Agriculture* 33(5):566–594.

Popkin, B. 2009. *The World is Fat*. New York: Penguin Books.

Spruiell, S. 2007. How do you keep them down on the farm if all they make is a lousy few mil? *National Review* 59(20):44–46.

United States Department of Agriculture. 2014. *USDA Strategic Plan FY 2014-2018*. Washington, D.C.: United States Department of Agriculture. Accessed January 24, 2016. http://www.usda.gov/documents/usda-strategic-plan-fy-2014-2018.pdf

United States Department of Agriculture. 2016. Accessed January 24, 2016. http://www.usda.gov/wps/portal/usda/usdahome

Viljeon, A., K. Bohn, and J. Howe (eds.) 2005. *Continuous Productive Urban Landscapes: Designing Urban Agriculture for Sustainable Cities*. Burlington, MA: Architectural Press.

11 An idealized conceptual framework for urban food system governance in postindustrial American cities

John C. Jones

Introduction

Today, American cities face a myriad of problems, including high rates of underutilized land, sustained unemployment and economic disinvestment, and high rates of dietary-related health morbidities, among many others. Many of the nation's postindustrial cities experience these problems more acutely than other communities. These problems are patterned and systemic. Piecemeal interventions are likely inadequate to address the scope of these problems. A growing number of scholars and urbanists suggest that growing the urban food system of these distressed communities may help to mitigate some of these problems (Kaufman and Bailkey 2000; Lawson 2005; American Planning Association 2007; Winne 2008; Nordahl 2009; Hodgson, Campbell, and Bailkey 2011; Cantrell et al. 2012). Absent from much of the expanding literature in this area is a discussion on the role that local governments should play in expanding the local food system of their community.

This research advances an idealized conceptual framework for governance of the urban food system borrowing from the partnership governance model suggested by Grossman and Holzer (2015). This framework is a synthesis of a broad examination of the following bodies of literature: local food systems and urban agriculture; postindustrial urban studies; urban public health; and public administration. A conceptual framework for the governance of the urban food system is necessary for two reasons. First, such a framework is important for communities around the country attempting to understand both (a) the characteristics of an effective urban local food system and (b) what steps are necessary to realize such a system. Second, for an urban food system rooted in partnership, governance is an essential response to sustained growth of neoliberalism across all levels of government in the United States. Without such a framework, interested local public officials may not realize the potential for an urban food system in which government actors view citizens and civil society organizations as partners and not as customers.*

---

* The creation of this framework is part of my preliminary work toward my doctoral dissertation that will examine local food enterprise expansion as an economic development tool in greater Newark, New Jersey and greater Dayton, Ohio.

The contested urban food system

The food system of twenty-first century urban America is defined by its connections with producers and distributors from across the nation and the world. Customers can, regardless of current season and home growth climate, find a wide variety of foods sourced from around the world at their local supermarket. Invisible to the average shopper is a robust, highly networked globalized production and distribution system that brings products from producers to supermarket shelves. This industrialized food system is a recent evolution in the history of humanity, only fully emerging in the second half of the twentieth century due to the convergence of the post-war wave of globalization, technological improvements in transportation and agriculture, and the relative peace of the post-war world (Norberg-Hodge, Merrifield, and Gorelick 2002).*

Current conflicts

The local food systems of many American cities are contested through a number of factors. First, sustained patterns of suburbanization throughout the second half of the twentieth century pulled many supermarkets away from central cities population centers and toward departing affluent consumers (Morland et al. 2002). This hollowing left only smaller corner stores and restaurants to provide food access points for many urban populations. Bereft of supermarkets, some scholars have suggested that many urban regions have become food deserts for their lack of affordable access to fresh fruits and vegetables (Shaw 2006). While Lucan et al. (2013) noted that food deserts are definitionally problematic, conceptually the idea of food deserts is linked to a negative externality of the industrialized food system. Some public health scholars suggested that this lack of access to healthy foods in urban areas may contribute to the expansion of the obesity and other dietary related morbidities (Morland, Roux, and Wing 2006; Giang et al. 2008).

Second, in recent years, some consumer desires have changed to reject certain aspects of the industrialized food system. Examples of this change are diverse, but Meyer et al. (2011) noted that demand has increased for locally produced foods. One example of this is the casual dining Mexican giant Chipotle recently pledged to source 10% of the food served from an individual store from local producers (Balakrishnan 2015). Reporting on the economic activity of locally produced foods is difficult due to the variety of distribution channels employed by local producers, but the U.S. Department of Agriculture (USDA) estimated $4.8 billion in local sales nationwide in 2008 (Low and Vogel 2011). As such, changing consumer desires in favor of local production may represent a paradigm shift

---

* Earlier industrialization of the urban food system occurred during the nineteenth century through the use of railroads, connecting rural producers with urban consumers. The use of a food-centric lens to examine Cronon's (1991) use of Von Thunen's central place theory in his discussion of Chicago's industrialization will provide an example of this.

in the national food system and consequently an opportunity for local producers to tap into increasing demand for locally produced foods.

Third, economic and built environment realities in many contemporary cities are quite different from the middle of the twentieth century. Nearly every major urban area in the United States has experienced some manifestation of postindustrial decline (Bowman and Pagano 2010). However, the former manufacturing centers of the Northeast and Midwest have experienced the problems of post-industrialism more acutely (Bluestone and Harrison 1982; Teaford 1993). In some cities, urban agriculture activities have reemerged. This reemergence of urban agriculture during a period of economic stress is consistent with the causal factors leading to other periods of urban agriculture in American cities (Lawson 2005; Pudup 2008). However, contemporary examples of urban agriculture remain largely at odds with existing land use and zoning policy regimes created by Modernist planners in the 1950s and 1960s (Pothukuchi 2000; Hodgson, Campbell, and Bailkey 2011). Often, the conflict manifests when local government officials seek a "higher and better use" for urban land (Hou, Johnson, and Lawson 2009) than that provided by urban agriculture. Despite this, given the sustained budgetary shortfalls faced by many distressed communities due to the combined effects of globalization, suburbanization, and retrenchment of federal spending on cities, some scholars have suggested that cities look to urban food system development as one method of fostering economic growth for these cities (Kaufman and Bailkey 2000; Hodgson, Campbell, and Bailkey 2011).

Urban food producers

Central to the idea of urban food system is the production of food. Urban food producers can take a number of distinct appearances and characteristics. Producers may be individuals or organized groups. Organized producers may be for-profit businesses or nonprofit organizations. Producers may consume their products themselves, donate them to others, or sell them commercially. Commercial sellers may engage in a number of different, potentially innovative, distribution models to local consumers. Some producers may distribute their products out of the region. Producers engage local spaces in their production efforts and may utilize local ingredients. Typically, producers are likely to engage in one or more of the following types of production.

- *Plant Cultivation*: Urban farmers' efforts can produce a wide variety of fruits and vegetables. Typically, urban farmers engage in a variety of innovative production techniques. Examples of such innovations include: raised bed farming on vacant lots; rooftop farming; indoor compost production; and hydroponic farming.
- *Animal Husbandry*: Animal husbandry includes the breeding, management, and harvest of animals and animal by-products. Examples of foods generated by animal husbandry include, but are not limited to, meat and milk from domesticated animals, fish, meat, eggs, and honey. Similar to plant

cultivation, urban farmers creatively engage urban space regarding the husbanding of animals. Examples of innovative husbandry techniques include aquaponic fish farming and rooftop beekeeping.

- *Value-Added Products*: Value-added products are food products that undergo at least a minimal manufacturing process. Often the exact manufacturing process may be the proprietary knowledge of the producer. Producers may describe these products as specialty, artisanal, or cottage. Examples of manufactured local foods might include, but are not limited to: breads; cheeses; candies; preserves and jellies; and salsas and hot sauces. Value-added products differ from the prepared food of restaurants and mobile food vending as value-added product manufacturers intend for their food to be stored, even for a limited amount of time, before consumption. Manufacturers may or may not utilize locally sourced ingredients.
- *Brewing and Distilling*: Brewing and distilling includes any manufacture of alcoholic beverages or spirits. Producers may either sell their product to local distributors and vendors for commercial sale, or sell directly to customers at or near their production site. Brewers and distillers may or may not utilize locally sourced ingredients.

Partnership governance

Grossman and Holzer (2015) described partnership governance as "multisectoral engagement," related to the progression of both citizen participation in a democratic system and a capacity of public administration and management. Partnership governance requires at least two partner actors and involves both the private and public spheres. Unlike New Public Management (NPM), as suggested by Osborne and Gaebler (1992), partnership governance rejects the view of citizens, businesses, and civil society organizations as customers. Instead, Grossman and Holzer suggest that public agencies should seek to collaborate with citizens, businesses, and civil society groups to form "transformational partnerships" that are better suited to addressing systemic problems. These partnerships are preferential to the more traditional principal-agent or "transactional" approach to public–private partnerships as supported by NPM, as principal-agent agreements specifically focus on a discrete set of deliverable goals stipulated by the contract.

The authors note that the development of a partnership governance system creates a new organizational *holon*. Holons are conceptual structures with the ability to affect change within their environment. Holons are often composed of smaller, individual, "part" holons that combine to compose a larger, "wholepart" holon. Larger holons are more capable of addressing problems than the independent subpart holons were previously unable or unwilling to address. For example, one way to conceptualize the "wholepart" holon of a municipal government would be the smaller "parts" represented by its various administrative departments. Given the existing problems with many distressed American cities, the existing urban socio-political structures in distressed communities are largely either unable or unwilling to address systemic postindustrial problems. Therefore, it is logical that a larger organizational holon develop to specifically address the complexity of the current urban food system in light of postindustrial challenges.

Forging partnership governance

Forging partnership governance with a specific goal is more complex than the perceptively simple contract-agent relationship advanced by NPM. Rather, Grossman and Holzer (2015) note that a community-level interorganizational structure is necessary to ensure that all participant organizations are collectively advancing the partnership's goals. Central to this structure is the need for trust and collaboration, without which partnership is impossible. The authors assert that public–private interactions regarding regional economic development generally follow this principal-agent structure, with public-private interaction appearing in support of a discrete goal. This may be effective for singular problems, but Grossman and Holzer believe that such a structure is poorly equipped to address systemic problems in the community.

Rather, the authors suggest a three-pronged structural model for partnership governance; agreement, management, and commitment. First, agreement requires all involved actors to map their organization's goals, values, and assets. Organizations then structure formal agreements with each other to achieve their collective and individual goals. Second, management requires oversight of the various interorganization agreements. Trained public administrators, especially government staffers, may be best suited to manage these agreements. Third and finally, organizations must abide by their commitments. This especially includes organizations providing funding or other resources to another organization within the broader partnership. Only through the proper administration of these prongs can trust and effective collaboration truly develop within the partnership.

Central to the development of partnership governance is the need for one or more public "intrapreneurs" to champion the partnership's mission. Such "intrapreneurs" are similar to their private sector entrepreneurial counterparts when pushing toward an objective. However, whereas a private sector entrepreneur might fully own and directly benefit from the success of their efforts, the public-sector "intrapreneur" will never fully own, nor fully benefit, from their efforts. Consequently, any benefits that accrue from their actions manifest outwardly as a public good as opposed to inwardly focused as an individual profit. A given partnership may benefit from multiple intrapreneurs either simultaneously or sequentially. Intrapreneurs might work for any organization within the larger partnership governance holon. Grossman and Holzer hold that government or quasi-governmental employees are the best positioned to be effective intrapreneurs. Government-employee intrapreneurs working toward local food systems development are often challenged as food system promotion is generally regarded as outside of the accepted powers and practices of local government in the United States (Castellanos et al. 2017).

Conceptual framework

Owing to the ongoing conflicts within the urban food system, community-wide coordination seems logical. However, attempts at forging community-wide partnerships have met with limited success due to limited resources, limited political and administrative capital from allied organizations, indistinct goals, and ineffective management (Winne 2008; Scherb et al. 2012; Castellanos et al. 2017). Applying the principles of partnership governance to the development of the urban food system is appropriate as it allows for the creation of a community-wide organizational holon capable of addressing the problems that its subordinate holon parts are either unwilling or unable to address individually. As such, an idealized conceptual framework addressing these factors is necessary for the development of an urban food system partnership governance holon. The framework is a seven-pronged model. The seven factors within the framework are as follows: regulation, finance, support, production, distribution, consumption, and waste disposal. Figure 11.1 provides a visual representation of the framework. Each factor will be addressed in detail below.

This framework is proscriptive in that it suggests that a community's food system should incorporate most, if not all, of these factors to approach an idealized level of governance of the food system. Nearly any given communities will likely have some elements of each of these factors present within its food system. Communities with developed food systems will likely have many elements of these factors within their system.

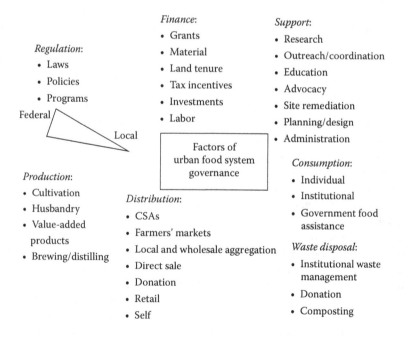

Figure 11.1 Factors of urban food system governance.

Organizations, either public or private, along with individuals may engage in discrete activities that encompass several factors listed in the model. Such activities are not mutually exclusive, and may occur either simultaneously or sequentially. The following two examples will illustrate this point. First, a municipal government may simultaneously engage in four discrete activities: regulation, finance, support, and waste disposal. Municipal laws and policies will exist that regulate aspects of the local food system. The city may provide a program which allows citizen groups to lease vacant city-owned lots for community gardening, a finance factor. The city's planning office may offer support to community gardens in the form of site planning assistance, a support factor. Finally, the city's waste management department collects waste from across the community and deposits it into a landfill. Second, a hospital may sequentially engage in two discrete activities: waste disposal and then consumption. First, the hospital may donate its kitchen's food scraps, a waste disposal factor, to a nearby commercial farm's composting program. Sometime later, perhaps after developing a deeper relationship with the farm through their donations, the hospital then decides to contract with the farm to provide food to the hospital's cafeteria service.

Factors affecting the urban food system

What follows is a brief overview of the seven factors of the conceptual framework, along with their subordinate aspects. When possible, examples of each subordinate aspect are provided. Each factor exists independently of the other factors. However, some cause and effect relationship exists between production, distribution, and consumption for obvious reasons. Organizations and individuals might engage in any number of factors or their subordinate aspects. Each factor is of relatively equal importance when considering the question of an idealized governance system. Consequently, factors are presented in no specific order.

Regulation

The regulation aspect is unique compared to the other aspects as, barring a very unusual situation, governments are the only organization with province over this aspect of the food system. Additionally, regulation is unique among the aspects as the full spectrum of laws from federal law down to municipal law potentially can impact the urban food system and its governance. I contend that local-level regulation has both (a) greater impact on the nature of a community's food system and (b) greater flexibility of action. Federal level regulation of the food system is largely tied to the highly contentious Farm Bill and the regulatory regimes of USDA and the Food and Drug Administration. Such national policies are highly entrenched and are unlikely to change due to local-level actions. Marion Nestle's work *Food Politics* (2002) provides an excellent overview of the national food system and its political undercurrents. Despite the entrenchment of national-level policies, local policymakers likely have significant flexibility to orient their community within the boundaries imposed by national policies. The desire for local sovereignty in policy direction, in spite of the boundaries created by national polices, may help explain the idea of an intellectual trap in local food research as suggested by Born and Purcell (2006).

- Laws relate to public laws and municipal ordinances that regulate the other aspects of the model. An example of a local level law impacting the food system is the regime of single-use zoning commonly used by municipal governments across the United States.
- Policies relate to the public position of government agencies regarding the implementation of existing laws. Often public documents are available which confirm an agency or government's position. A municipal comprehensive development plan is an example of a policy.
- Programs are the implementation of laws and policies. One example might be an adopt-a-lot program, in which a municipality will allow property owners to purchase a publicly owned vacant lot adjacent to the property owner's parcel for a nominal fee.

Financing

All aspects of financing involve the transmission of economic capital, generally money, material, or land, into and throughout a community's food system.

- Grants are awards of money, sometimes competitive in nature, to an organization or individual. Within the context of the food system, recipients of grants are generally community groups, for-profit farms, nonprofit organizations, and educational institutions.
- Materials are physical objects used in the various aspects of production or distribution. Material may either be used directly in the creation of food, such as food scraps converted into compost, or indirectly, such as scrap wood used in the construction of raised beds. Interested donors may provide this material in kind or it may be sold at a discount by an interested vendor.
- Tax Incentives are a government only aspect that involves the manipulation of various tax incentive programs to alter the cost–benefit ratio of local food production in favor of increased use. Examples might include reductions in real estate, business, or income taxes.
- Investment represents the injection of private capital into a local food system with the intention to develop or expand a commercial, profit-seeking enterprise. Investments may come from individual or established businesses or banks. An example of this is an investment bank's joint investment with a group of entrepreneurs to develop a hydroponic farm in an abandoned factory.
- Finally, Land Tenure describes the ability of interested parties to acquire land and/or buildings for use in food production or distribution. Producers will generally seek vacant, abandoned, or underutilized parcels. Parcels may be empty or may contain structures. Producers generally seek such land for economic reasons, although other factors such as location may play

into such decision-making. Producers may lease, purchase, or squat on land. Considering publicly controlled land, local governments may take an active role in leasing or selling vacant land to interested food system producers. However, a number of scholars have noted the tension between programs to encourage urban agriculture and the desire to see more traditional development occur on underutilized land (Hou, Johnson, and Lawson 2009; Hodgson, Campbell, and Bailkey 2011; Witt 2013). Commonly, local governments will offer short-term lease agreements for underutilized land to interested local food producers. Later, when local economic conditions change and the developers desire the land for traditional development, the local government will not renew the lease, thereby forcing the local producers to abandon the site.

- Labor can describe the trained employees of a revenue-seeking local food enterprise. Alternatively, it can also describe volunteers who supplement the efforts of an existent organization's employees or an informal group of neighbors at a community garden.

Support

Support of urban agriculture can take a variety of aspects.

- Education is the instruction of interested individuals for the technical skills necessary to participate in the urban foods system. This instruction potentially includes all aspects of production, as well as several aspects of the remaining factors. Educational actors may range from private individuals, to higher education faculty, to institutionally sponsored program staff like Cooperative Extension and the Master Gardener program, to profit-seeking schools or NGOs.
- Outreach/coordination fosters interaction between different actors within the community's food system. This aspect also serves as a major mechanism for increasing trust within the food system's governance. This aspect is performed across the spectrum of food system actors. Under a partnership governance model, some elements of this aspect should be centralized by an established organization(s) or government. A governing body, such as a food policy council, may also perform this centralized function.
- Advocacy is the application of political lobbying in favor of various aspects of the local food system. Generally, this function is performed by individuals and NGOs. Advocacy generally targets governments or business groups.
- Planning/design is the creation of tactics and strategies for the development of either a specific project of some aspect of the local food system or the community's larger strategic plan for the food system. Some level of this aspect is performed by any actor in the realization of a project; however, more specialized planning and design can be performed by trained professionals. These professionals may be employed in a private capacity, such as an architecture firm employed by a profit seeking development project, or may be government or higher education staff lending their time to a project.

- Administration is the management of either community's full food system governance structure or the management of some aspect or program. Trained public administrators, employed by government and/or NGOs, are likely the best suited to implement this aspect of support. Examples of this include the leaders of a community's food policy council or an NGO manager responsible for their organization's youth gardening program.
- Research is the empirical collection of information about the community's food system, as well as related data. Examples of related data might include, but is not limited to: land use and zoning; public health data, especially related to dietary morbidities; and market analysis. A combination of academics, NGO researchers, and government staffers might engage in research of the community's food system.

Production

Production can take four different aspects: cultivation, husbandry, value-added production, and brewing and distilling. Individual producers may employ any combination of the aspects.

- Cultivation is the farming of vegetable or fruit bearing plants. The method and location of cultivation can vary dramatically, from raised bed planters covered with plastic sheeting in a vacant lot to completely enclosed hydroponic growth in a converted industrial building.
- Husbandry encompasses all food derived from animals or their byproducts. Examples include, but are not limited to: meat from chickens, goats, pigs, etc.; the collection of eggs from chickens and other creatures; and honey harvested from urban beehives.
- Value-added production encompasses any handicraft or minimal manufacturing process involved in the creation of the end product. Value-added products may or may not use ingredients, in total or in part, created by other local producers. These components may be less chemically processed than similar food. Commonly, terms like "artisanal, gourmet, specialty, or cottage" may be used in the branding of value-added products.
- Brewing and distilling: Brewing and distilling includes any manufacture of alcoholic beverages or spirits. Producers may either sell their product to local distributors and vendors for commercial sale, or sell directly to customers at or near their production site. Examples might include beer, wine, and hard liquors.

Distribution

Distribution explains the mechanisms of exchange of harvested and/or produced food between local food producers and local consumers. Vendors may report these exchanges as taxable income, but others may conduct such exchanges informally. Distributors may seek to generate revenue for exchange, but others may not. However, seeking revenue is not always associated with seeking profit as nonprofit agencies with farms may seek to sell their product as a revenue generating mechanism.

- Direct Sale involves an immediate, face-to-face transaction between the producer and the customer. An example of this might be a vendor stand set up at a commercial urban farm.
- Self-distribution is transmission of food to its producer's own household. A backyard or community garden is the most common production site for such distribution.
- Community Supported Agriculture (CSA) allows customers to buy a share of a farmer's seasonal production. Farmers normally divide their harvest weekly or biweekly for delivery and/or collection by their customers. Customers normally pay a flat fee each week and may pay in full at the beginning of the growing season.
- Farmers' markets are gatherings of local producers where potential customers can visit multiple producers at once. Farmers' markets occur in a variety of spaces, both public and private. Markets may be largely impromptu with minimal external organization or they may be highly organized.
- Donation allows for the transmission of local production to needy members of the community. This could occur directly through hand-to-hand transfers, or through food assistance nonprofits, and religious organizations.
- Local Aggregation and Wholesale describes the sale of food by its producers to a middleman who will then sell the food to a direct retailer. Industrialization of the food system in the twentieth century pressured many local and regional level wholesalers out of business, in favor of national level distribution chains. The reemergence of local wholesale or aggregation points is necessary for a community's food system to sustain growth in the long term.
- Retail is the sale of local foods through a local business that purchased the food directly from its producer or from a wholesaler. This retailer may be a small business, like a healthy food store, or a major grocery store chain.

Consumption

Consumption is perhaps the most basic factor and is controlled by people or organizations who buy food from the local food system.

- Individuals are the most common consumer and are represented by the average person buying their weekly groceries.
- Institutions also purchase from local producers. Common examples of such institutions with food service operations include, but are not limited to: hospitals, schools and universities, and jails.
- Government subsidized food assistance programs, namely, the Supplemental Nutritional Assistance Program (SNAP) and the Special Supplemental

Nutritional Assistance Program for Women, Infants, and Children (WIC), are a noteworthy aspect of consumption as each program has specific requirements for both the individual recipients and the vendor. As such, program participants may find it difficult to redeem their benefits from vendors who lack the ability to process the redemptions.

Waste disposal

Finally, like consumption, waste disposal is a basic component of any food system.

- Institutionalized waste management is the traditional waste disposal regime managed by local governments that emerged in most communities in the twentieth century. Many communities likely collect and dispose of most food waste through this mechanism. While well entrenched in the day-to-day functions of businesses and households alike, waste disposal in this form can often disappear into the background of urban life. This form of disposal includes spoiled or otherwise undesirable foods, cooking scraps, and human bio-waste.
- Donation includes any contributions of food approaching their expiration dates by food vendors to needy individuals or charitable organizations. Vendors may formalize such donations by building relationships with a local food bank, pantry, or similar organization. Public health laws may exert regulatory oversight over such near or postexpiration donations.
- Composting is the use of nitrogen rich food waste in the creation of compost for later use as plant fertilizer. The collection of food waste for this purpose may be ad hoc or formalized. Additionally, the composter may range between an informal organization like a community garden and a formalized composting business or nonprofit.

Recommendations

Development of a partnership governance model to improve a community's urban food system requires the completion of a number of tasks to implement the suggested model. However, a broader change is also necessary to ensure that the community's political and governmental culture is supportive of partnership governance at the conceptual level.

Steps to implement urban food system partnership governance

For a community's food system to approach the idealized state of the conceptual model, the community's organizations must collectively provide mechanisms to address most, if not all, of the factors suggested in the conceptual model. For this to occur, the collection of public and private organizations interested in advancing their community's food system must implement the following steps:

1. Develop a partnership based on formal agreements that support most, if not all, of the factors of the conceptual model.
2. Centralize the overall management of the partnership's efforts to an individual or individuals with the skill sets, political capital, and positional longevity necessary to be effective leaders. This individual, or individuals, may be the partnership's main "intrapreneur(s)," but this is not necessarily required.
3. Members of the partnership must actively work toward the partnership's goals, fulfilling the commitments outlined within the partnership's formal agreements. Interorganizational trust will develop as organizations fulfill their commitments to each other over time and as the partnership's goals are advanced.

Growing a culture of partnership for the urban food system

In addition to the specific suggestions noted above, implementation of a partnership governance model for an urban food system likely requires a number of cultural developments to provide fertile ground from which a partnership governance model could take root.

Develop urban food system policy intrapreneurs

The existence of well-trained and socially networked intrapreneurs is of vital necessity to the development of partnership governance. Organizations interested in promoting their community's food system should find ways to encourage the developmental growth of such individuals. Grossman and Holzer believe that government staffers, given their training and position within the community's socio-political fabric, make superior intrapreneurs. Given the intersections of local food system conflicts, as noted above, and the purview of local governments, the authors' conclusion is logical and well-reasoned for this case. However, effective food system intrapreneurs might also come from well-developed civil society organizations with the political capital necessary to influence public decision makers. Regardless of the employment position of the intrapreneur, it is necessary for any potential intrapreneur to equip themselves with the knowledge of the public policy process as well as the administrative challenges inherent to public-private partnerships. Additionally, potential intrapreneurs should possess a developed understanding of the strengths and weaknesses, as well as the potential growth, of their community's food system.

Challenge modernist notions of urban space

Many of the laws, policies, and codes regulating the use of urban space find their roots in the Modernist theories of the mid-twentieth century (Hodgson, Campbell, and Bailkey 2011). This period aligns with the pinnacle of the development of the industrialized food system (Popkin 2007). As such, narratives of urban space reflect the economic realities of mid-century urban America. Chief among these realities is the highly industrialized American central city staffed by a highly paid workforce. As noted above, for many American cities, new macro-economic realities have created large amounts of abandoned urban space. Consequently, narratives and policies about the use of urban space should change to reflect current economic realities. Urban food system intrapreneurs, along with partnered organizations and producers, and the general public must petition their local governments to adapt policies to better reflect the economic realities of the early twenty-first century and not the mid-twentieth century.

Consider local food enterprise growth as economic development

Part of the Modernist rejection of urban agriculture stems from historical perceptions of the production capabilities of previous generations of urban farmers (Pothukuchi 2000). However, massive technological improvements in intensive farming in recent years may have changed the economic dynamics of urban agriculture to allow for sustained enterprise. An interesting example of this improvement in urban agriculture technology is Havana, Cuba. Before the fall of the Soviet Union, Cuba's agricultural industry was highly mechanized (Febles-Gonzalez et al. 2011). However, the fall of the Soviet Union ushered in a new era of gasoline austerity that compelled the Cuban government to develop an intensive urban agriculture policy as a means to shorten supply lines to population centers (Koont 2009). An increased focus on technological improvements and innovative techniques allowed urban agriculture in Havana to increase nearly ten-fold between 1997 and 2005, from 20,700 metric tons annually to 272,000 metric tons annually, respectively (Koont 2009).* Obviously, a whole host of factors separate conditions in Havana from that of American cities. Regardless of these factors, a radical increase in potential production seems agronomically possible. Consequently then, only economic, political, and administrative barriers remain to bar the expansion of urban agriculture in the United States. As such, local officials should tap into the growing demand for locally produced food by encouraging the development of intensive food production enterprises that use these new technologies in their communities.

REFERENCES

American Planning Association. 2007. *Policy Guide on Community and Regional Food Planning*. American Planning Association.
Balakrishnan, A. 2015. Local sourcing: Chipotle's double-edged sword? *CNBC*, 22 Dec 2015. http://www.cnbc.com/2015/12/22/local-sourcing-chipotles-double-edged-sword.html

---

* Other estimates vary; this is likely due to inconsistent measures, both by researchers and producers. See Febles-Gonzalez et al. (2011) and Cruz and Medina (2001) for other estimates.

Bluestone, B. and B. Harrison. 1982. *The Deindustrialization of America: Plant Closings, Community Abandonment, and the Dismantling of Basic Industry.* New York: Basic Books.

Born, B. and M. Purcell. 2006. Avoiding the local trap scale and food systems in planning research. *Journal of Planning Education and Research* 26(2):195–207.

Bowman, A.O'M and M. A. Pagano. 2010. *Terra Incognita: Vacant Land and Urban Strategies.* Washington, DC: Georgetown University Press.

Cantrell, P., K. Colasanti, L. Goddeeris, S. Lucas, and M. McCauley. 2012. *Food Innovation Districts: An Economic Gardening Tool.* Traverse City, MI: Northwest Michigan Council of Governments.

Castellanos, D. C., J. C. Jones, J. Christaldi, and K. Liutkus. 2017. *Perspectives on the Development of a Local Food System: The Case of Dayton, Ohio.* Agroecology and Sustainable Food Systems. (forthcoming)

Cronon, W. 1991. *Nature's Metropolis—Chicago and the Great West.* New York: W W Norton & Company.

Cruz, M. C. and R. S. Medina. 2001. *Agriculture in the City: A Key to Sustainability in Havana Cuba.* Kingston: Ian Randle Publishers.

Febles-Gonzalez, J. M., A. Tolon-Becerra, X. Lastra-Bravo, and X. Acosta-Valdes. 2011. Cuban agricultural policy in the last 25 years. From conventional to organic agriculture. *Land Use Policy* 28(4):723–735. doi: http://dx.doi.org/10.1016/j.landusepol.2010.12.008.

Giang, T., A. Karpyn, H. B. Laurison, A. Hillier, and R. D. Perry. 2008. Closing the grocery gap in underserved communities: The creation of the Pennsylvania Fresh Food Financing Initiative. *J Public Health Manag Pract* 14(3):272–279. doi: 10.1097/01. PHH.0000316486.57512.bf.

Grossman, S. A. and M. Holzer. 2015. *Partnership Governance in Public Management: A Public Solutions Handbook.* New York: Routledge.

Hodgson, K., M. C. Campbell, and M. Bailkey. 2011. *Urban Agriculture: Growing Healthy, Sustainable Places.* American Planning Association.

Hou, J., J. M. Johnson, and L. Lawson. 2009. *Greening Cities Growing Communities: Learning from Seattle's Urban Community Gardens.* Washington, DC: University of Washington Press.

Kaufman, J. and M. Bailkey. 2000. *Farming Inside Cities: Entrepreneurial Urban Agriculture in the United States.* Lincoln Institute of Land Policy.

Koont, S. 2009. The urban agriculture of Havana. *Monthly Review: An Independent Socialist Magazine* 60(8):44–63.

Lawson, L. 2005. *City Bountiful: A Century of Community Gardening in America.* Berkley, CA: University of California Press.

Low, S. A. and S. J. Vogel. 2011. Direct and intermediated marketing of local foods in the United States. USDA-ERS Economic Research Report (128).

Lucan, S. C., A. R. Maroko, J. Bumol, L. Torrens, M. Varona, and E. M. Berke. 2013. Business list vs ground observation for measuring a food environment: Saving time or waste of time (or worse)? *Journal of the Academy of Nutrition and Dietetics* 113(10):1332–1339.

Meyer, L., J. Hunter, A. Katchova, S. Lovett, D. Thilmany, M. Sullins, and A. Card. 2011. Approaching beginning farmers as a new stakeholder for extension. *Choices* 26(2):5.

Morland, K., A. V. Diez Roux, and S. Wing. 2006. Supermarkets, other food stores, and obesity: The atherosclerosis risk in communities study. *American Journal of Preventive Medicine* 30(4):333–339. http://dx.doi.org/10.1016/j.amepre.2005.11.003.

Morland, K., S. Wing, A. D. Roux, and C. Poole. 2002. Neighborhood characteristics associated with the location of food stores and food service places. *American Journal of Preventive Medicine* 22(1):23–29. http://dx.doi.org/10.1016/S0749-3797(01)00403-2

Nestle, M. 2002. *Food Politics.* Berkley, CA: University of California Press.

Norberg-Hodge, H., T. Merrifield, and S. Gorelick. 2002. *Bringing the Food Economy Home: Local Alternatives to Global Agribusiness.* Zed Books.

Nordahl, D. 2009. *Public Produce: The New Urban Agriculture.* Washington, D.C.: The Center for Economic Resources.

Osborne, D. and T. Gaebler. 1992. *Reinventing Government: How the Entrepreneurial Spirit is Transforming Government.* Reading, MA: Addison-Wesley Public Comp.

Popkin, B. M. 2007. The world is fat. *Scientific American* 297(3):88–95.

Pothukuchi, K. 2000. The food system: A stranger to the planning field. (Cover story). *Journal of the American Planning Association* 66(2):113.

Pudup, M. B. 2008. *It Takes a Garden: Cultivating Citizen-Subjects in Organized Garden Projects.* Pergamon-Elsevier Science Ltd.

Scherb, A., A. Palmer, S. Frattaroli, and K. Pollack. 2012. Exploring food system policy: A survey of food policy councils in the United States. *Journal of Agriculture, Food Systems, and Community Development* 2(4):3–14.

Shaw, H. J. 2006. Food deserts: Towards the development of a classification. *Geografiska Annaler: Series B, Human Geography* 88(2):231–247. doi: 10.1111/j.0435-3684.2006.00217.x.

Teaford, J. C. 1993. *The Twentieth-Century American City.* Johns Hopkins University Press.

Winne, M. 2008. *Closing the Food Gap: Resetting the Table in the Land of Plenty.* Boston: Beacon Press.

Witt, B. L. 2013. Urban agriculture and local government law: Promises realities, and solutions. *U. Pa. JL & Soc. Change* 16:221.

Part V

Missing connections in food, nutrition, and health policy

12 Beyond "Good Nutrition"

The ethical implications of public health nutrition policy

Adele Hite

As a registered dietitian, I was taught that individuals can exert considerable control over their future health outcomes, particularly those related to chronic disease, by simply following suggested dietary patterns. However, in my clinical experience, this did not always seem to be the case. Patients would report following standard nutrition recommendations for a reduced fat, plant-based, calorie-limited diet, yet were still struggling with chronic conditions this dietary pattern was supposed to prevent. It is possible that patients were lying about what and how much they were eating; this is a fairly common assumption in public health nutrition and in dietetics and one to which I will return. However, this perspective overlooks the history of controversy and the ongoing debate over the scientific basis for these recommendations. It also overlooks a paradoxical relationship between the standard nutrition recommendations that the patients I saw were trying to follow and diseases thought to be related to diet. Since the reduced-fat, plant-based, calorie-restricted diet paradigm to prevent chronic disease became institutionalized through federal dietary guidance in 1980—making it the accepted standard for what is considered a healthy diet—the rates of many chronic diseases have increased. Many experts have explained the failure of federal dietary guidance to prevent chronic disease by pointing out that, although there is some evidence that eating patterns of Americans have shifted toward recommended eating patterns, Americans have not been fully compliant with this guidance (Dietary Guidelines Advisory Committee [DGAC] 2010; Broad and Hite 2014). This narrative places the responsibility for the effectiveness of this public health intervention squarely on the shoulders of the population it is intended to assist, even as nutrition scientists continue to dispute the evidentiary basis for the intervention itself (Bahl 2015). Together, these issues raise questions about the ethics of current public health nutrition guidance, namely, "Who is responsible for the outcomes of a public health intervention?" and "What quality of evidence is needed to ethically implement a public health intervention, particularly in a nonemergency situation?"

Since evidence, effectiveness, and ethics are interconnected, a lack of effectiveness, coupled with concerns about standards of evidence, points to aspects of current public health nutrition guidance which are ethically problematic. Carter et al. (2011) have asserted, "evidence and ethics are implicitly related: evidence-based practice may be more ethical, and ethically sensitive practice more effective" (p. 465). This chapter will explore why the development of effective policy must begin with ethical considerations regarding what is considered sufficient evidence for a public health intervention directed at changing individual lifestyle behaviors. I begin by exploring a framework of standards for establishing an ethical foundation for public health prevention policies oriented at lifestyle choices. Next, an examination of the origins of U.S. federal public health nutrition guidance for prevention of chronic disease provides a background for recognizing ethical issues in current nutrition guidance. These ethical issues are summarized in two problematic assumptions foundational to current public health nutrition policy: that the scientific justification for federal dietary health recommendations is firmly established and that there are no potential drawbacks to implementing these recommendations as policy. This chapter ends with a rationale for developing ethically responsible public health nutrition policy.

Ethical rationale and standards of evidence for public health prevention policies

The primary ethical foundation of public health policy is the imperative to protect the health of the community as a whole, although this obligation often conflicts with the desires or rights of an individual (Bayer et al. 2007). A strong evidentiary base is needed to justify interventions that may impinge upon individual values or preferences. However, not all preventive measures are equally urgent. When the public's health is in imminent danger—due to outbreak of a contagious disease, food poisoning or contamination, or breakdown of sanitation infrastructure after a natural disaster—imposition on individual freedom may be ethically justified, even when evidence needed to address the situation is not fully established. However, these sorts of public health measures—quarantines and closed beaches—are infrequent. Nonemergency preventive health measures are far more common: seat belt laws, tobacco-free zones, vaccination programs, cancer screenings, and dietary recommendations. What criteria determine when it is permissible for public health officials to impact individual lives in nonemergency situations? Specifically, for an issue as central to life as food, under what conditions is it ethically justified to provide guidance for asymptomatic individuals to make dietary changes to prevent chronic disease (Malm 2002)?

Citing the relative dearth of work on bioethics of preventive medicine, philosopher and bioethicist Heidi Malm (2002) has taken up the particular ethical issues of common preventive practices, including "encouraging specific dietary changes as a means to avoid particular diseases" (p. 3). She has suggested that a possible explanation for this lack of attention is the mistaken assumption that preventive medicine practices are either not ethically problematic or not significantly different from traditional biomedical practices. Malm argues that preventive public health recommendations both warrant their own ethical examination and entail ethical issues requiring different evidentiary standards than those used in biomedicine. According to Malm, conditions under which it is ethical to provide preventive public health recommendations are when standards of evidence "beyond a reasonable doubt" demonstrate that unmistakably recommendations will provide an expected benefit to the individual, with minimal risk of harm (p. 5). In clinical medicine, the weaker standard of "preponderance of the available evidence" is considered to be adequate; however, preventive medicine must rest on a stronger standard. This stronger standard is related to two important differences in preventive public health measures compared to patient–provider interactions: with whom the interaction originates and the expected benefit to the individual (Malm 2002). In the first place, "our general theory of moral responsibility … entails that the more one is responsible for the occurrence of an event, the more one is responsible for the outcome of the event, and the medical imperative to do no harm" (p. 4). When a member of the public initiates an encounter with a health professional, the provider is obliged to offer the best information available, while the individual assumes a portion of responsibility for evaluating and enacting the information provided. Additionally, since preventive public health measures may in fact provide little, if any, benefit to a specific individual, the individual should also be exposed to little, if any, harm. With public health messages, experts— not the public—initiate the encounter between individual and information about behavior change and must assume responsibility for outcomes and be accountable for negative effects, though these may be unintended or unforeseen. In a public health emergency, it may be difficult to determine when providing potential benefit or ensuring no harm should take priority, and pragmatic concerns about expediency may trump evidentiary standards. However, when there is no emergency, there is no preexisting moral imperative that "something must be done." In this case, the principle of nonmalfeasance takes precedence: "… it is more important not to harm someone than it is to help them" (Holland 2015, p. 38), and a higher standard of evidence should prevail.

Historical context of public health nutrition guidance

To be clear, this critique is not directed at dietary guidance to prevent nutritional deficiencies in individuals, but at population-wide dietary health recommendations to prevent chronic diseases such as heart disease, cancer, and diabetes, as well as obesity, which is regarded as a disease in public health discourse. Prior to the creation of the Dietary Guidelines for Americans (DGA) in 1980, official federal dietary guidance was based primarily on assisting the public in choosing a varied diet that would prevent diseases of deficiency; importantly, no foods were singled out as uniquely healthful or harmful. In contrast, the DGA were the first public health nutrition recommendations to suggest that all Americans could use one dietary prescription to reduce the risk of a wide array of chronic diseases not specifically nutritional in nature. As the foundation of U.S. federal public health nutrition policy, the DGA provide the scientific rationale and policy basis for all government programs and practices related to nutrition, including research, public health promotion, and federally mandated food labels (United States 2010). The DGA also create a framework for beliefs and practices that drives consumer demand, shapes how food manufacturers formulate products, and directs the work of scientists, healthcare professionals, food system reformers, and the media. The DGA define a healthy diet as one that reduces or avoids certain food components—namely fat, saturated fat, cholesterol, and sodium—and increases others, such as carbohydrate, fiber, and polyunsaturated fats. In other words, good nutrition to prevent chronic disease means eating less meat and fewer whole fat animal products; avoiding processed foods high in trans fats, refined grains, or added sugars; and consuming more fruits, vegetables, whole grain products, and vegetable oil. Good nutrition also means balancing calories in with calories out to avoid weight gain. This recommended dietary pattern is thought to have beneficial effects on those biomarkers associated with chronic disease whose measurement and monitoring dominate interactions between patients and healthcare providers: weight, serum cholesterol, and blood pressure (Dietary Guidelines Advisory Committee [DGAC] 2015). Within the neoliberalist framework of "privatized market solutions to public problems" (Crawford 2006), the DGA provide a rationale for having individuals assume responsibility for their own health outcomes. By indicating which foods and dietary patterns will either prevent or contribute to the development of disease, the DGA are a measure by which food eaten by individuals—and indeed individuals themselves—may be judged relative to a standard endorsed by the federal government and promulgated by experts.

In this way, the DGA reflected a long tradition in America of nutrition guidance acting as an instrument of social management. Along with the information about how to avoid chronic disease, as established by the DGA, came the obligation for individuals to apply this guidance to their lives. Advice about "good nutrition" may reference nutrition science for its authority, but it has always come with a moral imperative to be a "good eater" (Biltekoff 2013). Although the DGA are treated as "simply a means of conveying facts of food and health" (Biltekoff 2012, p. 173), this guidance emerged from a complex interaction of social norms, historical context, and paradigmatic thinking that made following the precepts of "good nutrition" a moral obligation of good citizenship.

Senator George McGovern's Senate Select Committee on Nutrition and Human Needs, "began life as a soldier in the War on Poverty" (Oppenheimer and Benrubi 2013, p. 60). Formed in 1968 to address issues of malnutrition, the work of the Committee had been so successful in developing legislation that led to the creation of groundbreaking and highly praised hunger relief and food assistance programs that it shifted its attention to issues of "overnutrition" (Oppenheimer and Benrubi 2013). In 1977, the Committee issued a report called the *Dietary Goals for the United States* which tied an "epidemic" of killer diseases—obesity, diabetes, heart disease, stroke, and cancer—to changes in the American diet, specifically the increase in "fatty and cholesterol-rich foods" (Select Committee on Nutrition and Human Needs of the United States Senate 1977a, p. 3). However, many nutrition scientists saw the situation differently. Alfred Harper, the then chairman of the Food and Nutrition Board of the National Academy of Sciences, asserted that the apparent increase in chronic disease was related to the fact that

Americans were generally healthier and living longer; when adjusted for age, rates of many chronic diseases were actually decreasing: "A far stronger case can be made for concluding that the changes in our food supply during this century have been associated with improved rather than deteriorating health" (Broad 1979, p. 1061). Despite little evidence that the recommendations would be beneficial or were even needed, the suggested dietary modifications would become the basis for the first DGA and all that followed (Truswell 1987), but not because of uniformly convincing scientific evidence or a public health emergency. Rather, this guidance utilized nutrition science to respond to numerous social, political, and economic forces of the time.

In general, the shift in dietary guidance from acquiring adequate nutrition to preventing chronic disease supported a shift in thinking about public health that took place during the 1970s. During this decade, efforts to create a national health insurance plan lost momentum as inflation led to rising healthcare prices and a focus on cost control (Eisenberg 1977). In addition, after the successful eradication of many communicable diseases, cures for chronic diseases were elusive. Ideas about public health began to be reconceptualized around programs of prevention and individual responsibility. Federal dietary guidance to prevent chronic disease became central to the establishment of a neoliberal social order where individual responsibility for health, facilitated by products and services from the marketplace, replaced "collective responsibility for economic and social well-being" (Crawford 2006, p. 409). Pursuing good health through adherence to "good nutrition" became a central value in middle-class American life and a hallmark of responsible citizenship.

Specific recommendations to reduce the use of animal products were tied to these and a host of other cultural and political issues. During the energy crisis of the 1970s, food prices, especially for meat, shot up; housewives staged meatless Monday protests, not to promote vegetarianism, but to force meat producers to lower their prices. At the same time, droughts in Russia and Africa fueled predictions that the world might run out of food. America's ability to feed other nations had a myriad of political implications as well as humanitarian ones; at least theoretically, reducing meat consumption would divert grain fed to livestock to hungry populations across the globe. Meanwhile, since the 1960s, the American Heart Association (AHA) had been promoting a theory that eating less meat and animal fat could reduce the risk of heart disease. These events played out against a background of changes initiated by the Secretary of Agriculture Earl Butz in response to criticisms that the U.S. agricultural system was inefficient. Policies he instituted shifted land use to make room for additional corn, wheat, and soybean crops (Butz 1976). The dietary recommendations contained in McGovern's 1977 Senate report—which told the public to consume fewer animal products, eat more grain and cereal products, and to use corn and soybean oil instead of animal fats like butter and lard—fit neatly into the USDA's (United States Department of Agriculture) mandate to grow the agricultural economy. Typically, animal products undergo less processing after leaving the farm than corn, wheat, and soy products. Having consumers shift their purchases from less- to more-processed foods adds value to the agricultural economy through increased processing, marketing, and associated labor costs, without increasing production (Pyle 2005). Reformulating processed grain and cereal products to conform to DGA recommendations by replacing animal fats with corn and soybean oil would not only increase the amount of processing going into those foods, but also it would allow manufacturers to advertise these products as healthier alternatives to the original. At the same time, recommendations for a more plant-based diet supported progressive visions of conserving resources and feeding the hungry and addressed middle-class concerns with preventing disease and saving money on food.

Ethical issues in current public health nutrition guidance

In this regard, McGovern's 1977 report, which was to become the basis for the 1980 DGA, is an example of what Mayes and Thompson (2015) describe as "nutritional scientism," an appeal to nutrition science in order to justify cultural or ideological views about food and health (p. 593). McGovern's committee was sympathetic to progressive ideology related to reducing meat consumption; their report relied on studies of vegetarian populations and a vegetarian cookbook to make the case that meat and animal products were not only unhealthy but a waste of resources (Select Committee 1977a). They also knew how controversial dietary guidance to reduce meat, eggs, butter, and whole milk would be and they would have to present "the scientific integrity of the report" as "beyond question" (Austin and Hitt 1979, p. 326). However, scientific support for this dietary guidance was itself controversial and tended to fall along ideological lines. As Weed (1997) has noted, scientists may "hold different opinions about which scientific values are important to the assessment of evidence," and there are indications that extra-scientific values, not the least of which is the desire to have the correct hypothesis, influence how evidence is evaluated (p. 118). In general, scientists who supported the diet–heart hypothesis promoted by the AHA, which posited a causal link between animal fats in the diet and heart disease, felt that available evidence was adequate for creating national dietary guidelines; having their hypothesis ensconced as national policy would be a powerful endorsement of their view. In contrast, many scientists, including some who were also aligned with the diet–heart hypothesis, felt evidence was insufficient for population-wide guidance to be given (Select Committee on Nutrition and Human Needs, United States Senate 1977b). This conflict points to the ethical question implicit in long-term preventive public health guidance that Malm (2002) addresses: "What quality and quantity of evidence should be required before guidance to prevent chronic disease through lifestyle changes is given to the public?" This question cannot be answered by science or scientists but is rather a matter of public policy with significant ethical implications.

Early critics of the first federal dietary guidance for the prevention of chronic disease called attention to the moral dilemmas inherent in recommending long-term dietary changes without strong evidence. First, many felt it was inappropriate to offer one diet to reduce the risk of multiple diseases across an entire diverse population with evidence-based primarily on observational studies that could not establish cause–effect relationships (Select Committee 1977b, p. 705). Furthermore, scientists argued that without stronger forms of evidence and explicit testing of the proposed guidance, there was no guarantee that the recommended dietary changes would not cause harm (Select Committee 1977b, p. 666). Both of these concerns continue to haunt current federal dietary guidance, raising ethical issues related to quality and quantity of evidence needed to make recommendations and to uphold the directive to "first do no harm." Since DGA standards for "good nutrition" have become hegemonic, scientific uncertainties and limitations present at the start have become obscured.

Yet as the political power of the DGA has grown, so has the number of Americans designated as "unhealthy." The DGA standards for "good nutrition" have been widely accepted, but as a public health intervention, they have not been widely successful. Since the creation of the DGA in 1980, age-adjusted rates of diabetes in the United States have doubled (Centers for Disease Control and Prevention 2013). Age-adjusted incidence of all cancers has gone up (Siegel, Miller, and Jemal 2015, p. 12). Although cardiovascular disease mortality has decreased, incidence of heart disease, as indicated by hospital admission rates, has not (Cohen et al. 2015). Additionally, although body weight is not necessarily a measure of health, the prevalence of obesity in the United States has doubled (DGAC 2010). The failure of the DGA to help Americans prevent increases in chronic disease is typically seen as a problem of compliance (DGAC 2010), even though Americans appear to have made some efforts to shift their dietary intake toward DGA recommendations (Cohen et al. 2015). From this perspective, the effectiveness of the DGA has been limited due not to concerns regarding their evidentiary base or ethical implications, but to the failure of Americans to do as they have been told. This narrative of blame exempts the DGA from criticism, leaving intact two related assumptions regarding the scientific justification behind the DGA and the presumed outcomes of their implementation as policy: that nutrition science has reliably determined how food and health outcomes are related, and that there are no potential negative effects related to public health nutrition policies to prevent chronic disease and obesity. A reexamination of these assumptions suggests alternative explanations for the unfolding of negative consequences predicted by earlier critics and calls for a reexamination of the ethical and evidentiary concerns present when the DGA were first created.

Assumption: Nutrition science has determined what dietary patterns prevent chronic disease

The DGA were established under the assumption that nutrition science had provided policymakers with a consensus on how food and chronic disease are related. This view relied heavily on a relatively new field, nutritional epidemiology of chronic disease, whose methodology cannot be used to directly establish cause–effect relationships. As a result, causality must be established rhetorically, through "causal web" or "causal pie" models made up of "risk factors," which can ostensibly account for the multifactorial etiology of chronic disease. Nancy Krieger (2011) has written extensively about the lack of nonmethodological theory in epidemiology, a situation in which hypothesized causal factors may be treated as "self-evident, requiring no analysis, or else simply a matter of idiosyncratic inspiration (or ideological proclivities)" (p. 273). Since one of the primary conceptual commitments in epidemiology is to biologic causes of disease in individuals, investigations tend to be limited to factors that can be addressed through individual behavior change (Krieger 1994). In nutritional epidemiology, many environmental exposures that could affect food choice—such as dietary guidance given by authoritative organizations—are disregarded entirely. The paradoxical effect is that when data are collected from the American population, norms based on "good nutrition" guidance are part of the social context in which respondents live, but their potential influence on reported behavior is never acknowledged. For example, the educated healthcare professionals who constitute the datasets commonly used to examine diet–chronic disease relationships—such as Harvard's Nurses' Health Study and Health Professional's Follow-Up Study—would not only be familiar with DGA guidance, they would also be educated in the low-fat, heart-healthy paradigm of the AHA. They would be exposed to advertising and products proclaiming the health benefits of foods that conform to DGA and AHA recommendations. Whether or not they followed this advice, the participants in those studies would have known how a healthy diet was defined and what the "right" answers to the study questionnaires would be. Furthermore, these observational studies fail to account for the social pressures within the demographics typically surveyed to follow, or at least to agree with, "good nutrition" principles.

Influenced by guidance from the AHA and other groups, members of the middle and upper classes had begun to take up behaviors important to the pursuit of health, such as reducing fat in their diets and exercising, even before the DGA were created (Crawford 2006; Woolf and Nestle 2008). Nutritional observational studies conducted since the late 1960s would be informed by this social context, potentially confirming normative health behaviors as scientific findings. The "healthy user" or "healthy adherer" effect is a source of bias in observational studies that occurs when individuals who are more compliant with health-related directives have better health outcomes than individuals who are less compliant, even when "compliance" has no material effect on health. In randomized clinical trials, adherence to medication regimes appears to reduce risk of morbidity and mortality from causes not related to the medication's mechanism; for example, participants who take their assigned medication faithfully have better results than those who do not, even if their medication is a placebo (Simpson et al. 2006, p. 1). Compliant individuals are healthier than their noncompliant counterparts not because the therapy they are compliant with is necessarily effective—such as a placebo or a set of dietary rules—but because compliance is "a surrogate marker for overall healthy behavior" (Simpson et al. 2006, p. 5).

Nutritional epidemiology studies consistently demonstrate that those with better health outcomes are more likely not only to engage in many health-related behaviors, in addition to "good nutrition," but also to have higher education and income levels (Satia 2009); in other words, they are more likely to actively pursue health because they are more likely to have a stake in the moral valuation of its pursuit. In these studies, there is no way to differentiate between advantages that accompany the privileged class status of most "healthy adherers," their other health-related behaviors, and actual health effects of "good nutrition"; researchers simply attribute the better health outcomes of more privileged groups to their better dietary habits. A self-perpetuating "consensus" of findings results: people concerned about health eat a "healthy diet"; a "healthy diet" is one people concerned about health eat.

This tautology raises critical ethical issues when examining disparities between demographics of populations studied and those to which related policy is applied. The majority of studies produced in nutritional epidemiology are based on data drawn from white, middle-class, middle-aged professionals, such as the Nurses' Health Study and the Health Professionals Follow-up Study (Hite and Schoenfeld 2015). Yet it is exactly the populations not represented in these studies—older adults, young children, minority, and low-income populations—that are most likely to have their dietary patterns dictated at least in part by regulations drawn from the DGA. When more diverse populations are studied—minorities or low-income eaters, for example—a different picture of diet–chronic disease relationships emerges; in these populations, the DGA's version of "good nutrition" is less likely, not more likely, to be associated with good health (Zamora et al. 2010; Ben-Shalom et al. 2012).

This disconnect is tied to the logic of public health intervention as a matter of population, rather than individual, benefit. Associations are based on population averages, which only indicate when enough people benefit from a treatment or observed dietary pattern to create a statistically significant difference from a comparison group; when populations studied are largely homogeneous, differential outcomes in minority subgroups are undetectable (Kaput 2008). Furthermore, when a bell curve shifts due to a population intervention, there is no way to say whether any given individual or subgroup benefitted (Charlton 1995). In dietary studies, the size of associations between diet and chronic disease outcomes is so weak, with relative risks of the order of 0.8–1.2 (Potischman and Weed 1999), that it is clear that most people do not benefit at all. Nevertheless, when we "treat" an entire population in order to reduce risk for some members of that population, buy-in from individuals is often achieved through a rhetoric of risk: correlation in an observed population becomes causation for an individual; "reduces the population-level risk of a disease" becomes "prevents this disease for you as an individual." This type of persuasion is considered acceptable because it is accompanied by the assumption that there is little risk associated with recommendations to eat a reduced-fat, calorie-restricted, plant-based diet. However, prevention through the population strategy, as Paul Marantz (2010) has pointed out, is a double-edged sword. Small benefits may be magnified when applied to a population, but so may small harms. In fact, the assumption that there are no harms to population-based dietary recommendations for the prevention of chronic disease is an erroneous one.

Assumption: There are no risks related to public health nutrition recommendations

The second assumption foundational to the DGA is that highest standards of evidence were not necessary for providing population-wide dietary recommendations to prevent chronic disease because there were virtually no risks related to these recommendations. This argument appears to have been based primarily on the belief that Americans in the early twentieth century, along with many other populations across the globe, experienced no negative consequences by consuming a diet similar to the one recommended by federal dietary guidance to prevent chronic disease (Weil 1979). For example, early supporters of this guidance argued that at the beginning of the twentieth century, Americans ate more fruit, vegetables, and grain products and had less chronic disease (Select Committee 1977a, p. 1). At the same time, critics pointed out that, in the early 1900s, Americans had shorter life spans, which would preclude the development of chronic disease, and suffered more frequently from diseases of malnutrition (Select Committee 1977b). More importantly, other populations—including the American population of the past—were not only vastly different from the American population being addressed in the DGA, but had arrived at their presumably healthier dietary patterns through historical, geographical, sociocultural, and economic influences, not through public health directives. This points to a corollary assumption made by the creators of the first DGA: potential negative effects of the DGA would be essentially nonexistent because uptake would be voluntary. When the DGA were first being developed, they were directed at consumers, with the U.S. Surgeon General asserting, "Individuals have the right to make informed choices and the government has the responsibility to provide the best data for making good dietary decisions" (Richmond 1979, p. 2621). This rhetoric of choice failed to anticipate the exponential manner in which the influence of the DGA would expand; eventually, policy language would mandate the application of the DGA to all nutrition-related federal activities, including school lunches, labeling laws, and research agendas. The assumption that personal choice would remove any potential for harmful effects related to DGA guidance not only overlooks unanticipated risks associated with voluntary compliance but also fails to acknowledge risks associated with effects of dietary guidance that are beyond individual control. Acknowledgment of these previously unexamined risks indicates that failure of the DGA to achieve positive health outcomes is not due solely to lack of compliance.

A general risk associated with urging Americans to alter their dietary patterns is the risk of divergent food–health interactions: versions of "good nutrition" that may decrease the risk of one health concern may increase the risk of another. With heart disease being the leading cause of death in the United States, the science that formed the basis for the first DGA focused primarily on development of that disease. Supporters of the DGA point to a decrease in heart disease mortality that has occurred over the past 35 years, attributing it to dietary changes made in alignment with DGA recommendations: increased consumption of flour and cereal products and vegetable oils (Hu et al. 2000). Although scientists have also acknowledged that obesity rates climbed when Americans replaced dietary fat with starches and sugars (Dietary Guidelines Advisory Committee [DGAC] 2000), this has been attributed to Americans "overeating" rather than the nature of the recommendations. However, a good faith attempt to reduce dietary fat, saturated fat, and cholesterol does not necessarily mean that the recommended nutrient targets will be reached. Increased hunger and decreased satiety that might result from changing dietary patterns could also lead to consumption of more overall calories (Cohen et al. 2015). Early critics of population-wide guidance to prevent chronic disease pointed to both risk of malnutrition associated with a reduced intake of animal products and risk of health problems associated with foods recommended to replace them (Select Committee 1977b). Now, over 40% of the population has inadequate protein intake, and adolescent and premenopausal women, particularly from minority populations, are at risk for iron deficiency anemia; animal products and meat in particular, foods the DGA say should be limited, are rich sources of both nutrients (U.S. Department of Health and Human Services and U.S. Department of Agriculture 2016). Vegetable oils may decrease cholesterol levels—and thus lower the risk of heart disease—but might increase the risk of cancer (National Research Council Committee on Diet and Health 1989); for individuals with a family history of diabetes, replacing fat with carbohydrate might increase the risk of chronic disease, rather than lower it (Reaven 1986).

Loss of traditional foods that do not "fit" DGA recommendations is another risk. Under "good nutrition" principles, foods that are both culturally and nutritionally valuable are often stigmatized as dangerously unhealthy unless prudently modified. However, some traditional foods are the way they are for a reason. In Southern soul food cooking, salt pork cuts the bitter taste of greens, while fatback provides a vehicle for flavor as well as fat-soluble vitamins. Greens made with little or no salt or fat do not taste "right" to many people, and as a dietitian, I found that Southerners who were told to give up salt pork and fatback used to cook greens were likely to give up greens altogether. In my dietetics training, I was taught to respect the values of those who, for cultural, religious, or personal reasons, consumed vegetarian or vegan diets. Similarly, many individuals value animal products as a central part of their food heritage: sausages of Eastern Europe and China; ghee, or clarified butter, of India; chorizo and eggs of Latin America. Although the DGA have paid lip service to the notion that diets from all cultural traditions can be part of "good nutrition," when it comes to animal products, dietitians are trained to engage in what I call "pork-shaming"—counseling people how to eliminate, limit, or modify use of traditional animal-based foods in order to avoid saturated fat and cholesterol. In this way, the DGA work to discourage many aspects of ethnic diets in favor of a normative standard based on Anglo-Saxon food habits. To be "multiculturally competent" as a dietitian is to ensure that "clients' traditional health beliefs and diet are being balanced with healthy American food choices" (Holli et al. 2009, p. 169).

The previous risks assume that individuals make some effort to follow the dietary guidance they have been given, an assumption few public health experts endorse. However, the DGA reach far beyond individual "choice" about what to eat. The U.S. food system and healthcare system are complex, vast, and interconnected. The DGA affect how healthcare professionals are trained in nutrition, what goes into food products and how they are labeled, and what consumers come to believe about diet and disease relationships and about themselves, now and in the future, as the DGA also influence nutrition research agendas and the education of scientists. Thus, since the responsibility for limiting harmful "lifestyle" exposures has increasingly been laid on the individual, environmental levels of an exposure with its own set of risks have increased, namely dietary health recommendations based on populations rather than individuals. Even a determined individual with adequate resources who asks a healthcare provider for an individualized diet to address health concerns runs the risk of being unwittingly exposed to DGA influence. Once normative "good nutrition" principles have been established through acceptance of nutritional epidemiology methods, and these preventive dietary health recommendations are taught as part of health professionals' education, there is a very real risk that a clinician may end up treating individual patients using a public health "lens." Before even meeting the patient, outlines for intervention are clearly indicated and healthcare providers may fail to consider—or even be aware of the existence of—alternative paths to dietary health.

The DGA not only affect nutrition education of healthcare professionals but also they produce widespread uniform changes throughout the food supply. Since consumers are taught to reject certain food components as "unhealthy," novel ingredients introduced into the food supply to replace them may create new health risks. Shortly after the first DGA warned Americans to limit their intake of foods containing saturated fat and cholesterol, a public health advocacy group, Center for Science in the Public Interest, began a successful campaign to have food manufacturers use hydrogenated vegetable oils to replace ingredients like butter and lard, insisting that *trans* fats posed no health risks: "Nearly all targeted firms responded by replacing saturated fats with *trans* fats" (Schleifer 2012). Sixteen years later, the same group began a campaign to have *trans* fats removed from the food supply due to concerns about their association with heart disease. High fructose corn syrup also offered a cheap, plentiful replacement for saturated fats in manufactured foods, and it also is now considered to pose its own risks to health (Lustig 2013).

The DGA's presumption that science has adequately determined which foods should or should not be eaten in order to reduce risk of disease leads to the inevitable conclusion that individuals should be able to control health outcomes through the "right" food choices, but in fact the influence of the DGA on the food–health environment makes notions of individual agency, willpower, and "food choice" problematic with regard to dietary health. Nevertheless, "'healthy' food choice has become an ethical act expected of all rational individuals" (Mayes and Thompson 2014, p. 159). One of the risks associated with this assumption is creation of a population of "worried well," whose attention is focused on preventing illness, rather than enjoying the health they have. Food may come to be viewed as a magic talisman, warding off or inviting evil in the form of chronic disease, and health may be seen as an "end in itself," one which reveals the moral worth of those who possess it (Crawford 1980; Harper 1988). However, one of the most serious risks of this assumption is that it permits evaluation of anyone whose health or body size seems to indicate violations of the dietary-moral code as somehow inferior or abnormal. For example, the 2010 DGA recognize a discrepancy similar to the one which I noted at the beginning of this chapter, observing that average caloric intakes recorded from national data "do not appear to be excessive, [but] the numbers are difficult to interpret because survey respondents, *especially individuals who are overweight or obese,* often underreport dietary intake" (emphasis added; U.S. Department of Agriculture and U.S. Department of Health and Human Services 2011). In other words, the official conclusion is that people who are overweight and obese are likely to lie about how much they eat when asked. The ethical implications of linking body size with moral character are clearly problematic. Beyond that, it is unclear what public health purpose is served by an enterprise that assumes or compels deception on the part of the population it means to assist and doubts the character of individuals before doubting the appropriateness of the advice dispensed.

Finally, the DGA present broad risks to public health more generally. Early critics of federal dietary guidance for the prevention of chronic disease suggested that a focus on individual responsibility for prevention would result in "trivial and superficial approaches to health promotion" and shift attention away from the government's responsibility to improve economic, environmental, and social conditions related to health (Eisenberg 1977, p. 1232). Public health campaigns and research agendas based on the DGA represent money and effort diverted from public health endeavors which may have proved more effective in safeguarding health. Importantly, basing widely promoted public health directives on insufficient evidence presents a risk of misuse of public health authority and loss of trust when better evidence contradicts original guidance or when promised results do not materialize (Harper 1988). Also, when evidentiary and ethical considerations are not addressed at the creation of preventive public health policies, such reversals and failures are inevitable.

Toward the creation of ethical public health nutrition policy

To be sure, these are not a full accounting of the potential risks associated with population-wide dietary guidance based on limited evidence (see Charlton 1995; Malm 2002; Mayes and Thompson 2014); however, those risks outlined above, as well as others, relate on the whole to the issue of scientific uncertainty. As Sheila Jasanoff (2003) has pointed out, "To date, the unknown, unspecified, and indeterminate aspects of scientific and technological development remain largely unaccounted for in policy-making" (pp. 239–240). This is particularly true in public health nutrition policy making, where methodologies available for ascertaining links between diet and chronic disease all have distinct limitations, and an evidentiary standard of "beyond a reasonable doubt" may be difficult to reach in many cases. Employing Jasanoff's (2003) "technologies of humility"—which call for admitting uncertainties and risks, revealing the normative within the scientific, and acknowledging the diversity of bodies and values served by public health nutrition policies—would be a move toward development of more ethical public health nutrition policy.

When public health officials encourage asymptomatic individuals to change their lifestyle habits in order to prevent diseases which may or may not develop in a given individual regardless of behavior, it is imperative that the principle of nonmalfeasance be openly addressed. When unambiguous evidence is unlikely to be forthcoming, as is the case with nutrition, uncertainties and risks should be evaluated with input from bioethicists and experts in policy development, not just nutrition scientists. Furthermore, policymakers should recognize that generation of nutrition knowledge is in and of itself a normative practice. Population-level aggregate data may not adequately address differences—genetic, economic, social—that impact health in ways separate from and overlapping with diet. At the very least, populations observed should be commensurate with populations to which a policy will be applied. In addition, public health nutrition policy must be developed with an awareness of the diversity of meanings and values surrounding both food and health. Mayes and Thompson (2014) argue, "those who use nutrition evidence to command individual food choices have an ethical burden to articulate why the biomedical value of food should be prioritized over and perhaps to the exclusion of values such as pleasure, comfort, belonging or well-being" (p. 159). This ethical burden is heightened when there is an honest acknowledgment of limitations of that evidence.

The above approaches may serve to ameliorate public health nutrition policy already in place, as the DGA are revised, expanded, and further implemented; however, they do not fully address a central ethical issue tied to current narratives of responsibility surrounding the DGA. Public health nutritionists have maintained that deciding "whether the evidence is good enough to recommend population-based dietary changes comes down to a matter of subjective judgment" (Woolf and Nestle 2008, p. 263). However, outside of public health emergencies, it is not the case that recommendations have to be made at all. When a decision is not morally imperative and evidence linking diet and chronic disease is unclear enough to render its evaluation "a matter of subjective judgment," whose judgment prevails and whose values are represented are issues of politics, power, and privilege, not issues of science or public health. In those cases, when what is truly needed is "less advice and more information" (Reaven 1986), the ethical burden for the outcome of a policy lies with those who insist it is necessary.

REFERENCES

Austin, J. E. and C. Hitt. 1979. *Nutrition Intervention in the United States: Cases and Concepts.* Cambridge, MA: Ballinger Publishing Co.

Bahl, R. 2015. The evidence base for fat guidelines: A balanced diet. *Open Heart* 2(1). doi: 10.1136/openhrt-2014-000229.

Bayer, R., L. O. Gostin, B. Jennings, and B. Steinbock (eds.). 2007. *Public Health Ethics: Theory, Policy, and Practice*, 1st ed. New York: Oxford University Press.

Ben-Shalom, Y., M. K. Fox, and P. K. Newby. 2012. *Characteristics and Dietary Patterns of Healthy and Less-Healthy Eaters in the Low-Income Population*. Alexandria, VA: U.S. Department of Agriculture, Food and Nutrition Service, Office of Research and Analysis.

Biltekoff, C. 2012. Critical nutrition studies. In *The Oxford Handbook of Food History*, edited by J. M. Pilcher. New York: Oxford University Press, pp. 172–190.

Biltekoff, C. 2013. *Eating Right in America: The Cultural Politics of Food and Health*. Durham: Duke University Press.

Broad, W. 1979. Jump in funding feeds research on nutrition. *Science* 204(4397):1060–1061. doi: 10.1126/science.451549.

Broad, G. and A. Hite. 2014. Nutrition troubles. *Gastronomica: Journal of Food and Culture* 14(3):5–16. doi: 10.1525/gfc.2014.14.3.5

Butz, E. L. 1976. An emerging, market-oriented food and agricultural policy. *Public Administration Review* 36(2):137. doi: 10.2307/975128.

Carter, S. M., L. Rychetnik, B. Lloyd, I. H. Kerridge, L. Baur, A. Bauman, C. Hooker, and A. Zask. 2011. Evidence, ethics, and values: A framework for health promotion. *American Journal of Public Health* 101(3):465–472. doi: 10.2105/AJPH.2010.195545.

Centers for Disease Control and Prevention. 2013. *Number (In Millions) of Civilian, Noninstitutionalized Persons with Diagnosed Diabetes, United States, 1980–2011*. National Center for Health Statistics, Division of Health Interview Statistics. National Center for Chronic Disease Prevention and Health Promotion, Division of Diabetes Translation. http://www.cdc.gov/diabetes/statistics/prev/national/figpersons.htm

Charlton, B. G. 1995. A critique of Geoffrey Rose's 'Population Strategy' for preventive medicine. *Journal of the Royal Society of Medicine* 88(11):607–610.

Cohen, E., M. Cragg, J. de Fonseka, A. Hite, M. Rosenberg, and B. Zhou. 2015. Statistical review of U.S. Macronutrient Consumption Data, 1965–2011: Americans have been following dietary guidelines, coincident with the rise in obesity. *Nutrition (Burbank, Los Angeles County, Calif.)* 31(5):727–732. doi: 10.1016/j.nut.2015.02.007.

Crawford, R. 1980. Healthism and the medicalization of everyday life. *International Journal of Health Services: Planning, Administration, Evaluation* 10(3):365–388.

Crawford, R. 2006. Health as a meaningful social practice. *Health* 10(4):401–420. doi: 10.1177/1363459306067310.

Dietary Guidelines Advisory Committee (DGAC). 2000. *Report of the Dietary Guidelines Advisory Committee on the Dietary Guidelines for Americans, 2000*. Washington, DC: U.S. Department of Agriculture and U.S. Department of Health and Human Services. http://www.health.gov/dietaryguidelines/dgac/pdf/dgac_ful.pdf

Dietary Guidelines Advisory Committee (DGAC). 2010. *Report of the Dietary Guidelines Advisory Committee on the Dietary Guidelines for Americans, 2010*. Washington, DC: U.S. Department of Agriculture and U.S. Department of Health and Human Services. http://www.cnpp.usda.gov/sites/default/files/dietary_guidelines_for_americans/2010DGACReport-camera-ready-Jan11-11.pdf

Dietary Guidelines Advisory Committee (DGAC). 2015. *Scientific Report of the 2015 Dietary Guidelines Advisory Committee*. Washington, DC: U.S. Department of Health and Human Services and U.S. Department of Agriculture.

Eisenberg, L. 1977. The perils of prevention: A cautionary note. *New England Journal of Medicine* 297(22):1230–1232. doi: 10.1056/nejm197712012972210.

Harper, A. E. 1988. Killer French fries. *Sciences* 28:21–27.

Hite, A. H. and P. Schoenfeld. 2015. Open letter to the secretaries of the U.S. Departments of Agriculture and Health and Human Services on the Creation of the 2015 Dietary Guidelines for Americans. *Nutrition (Burbank, Los Angeles County, Calif.)* 31(5):776–779. doi: 10.1016/j.nut.2014.12.019.

Holland, S. 2015. *Public Health Ethics*, 2nd ed. Malden, MA: Polity Press.

Holli, B. B., J. O. Maillet, J. A. Beto, and R. J. Calabrese (eds.). 2009. *Communication and Education Skills for Dietetics Professionals*, 5th ed. Philadelphia: Wolter Kluwer Health/Lippincott Williams & Wilkins.

Hu, F. B., M. J. Stampfer, J. E. Manson, F. Grodstein, G. A. Colditz, F. E. Speizer, and W. C. Willett. 2000. Trends in the incidence of coronary heart disease and changes in diet and lifestyle in women. *New England Journal of Medicine* 343(8):530–537. doi: 10.1056/nejm200008243430802.

Jasanoff, S. 2003. Technologies of humility: Citizen participation in governing science. *Minerva* 41(3):223–244. doi: 10.1023/A:1025557512320.

Kaput, J. 2008. Nutrigenomics research for personalized nutrition and medicine. *Current Opinion in Biotechnology* 19(2):110–120. doi: 10.1016/j.copbio.2008.02.005.

Krieger, N. 1994. Epidemiology and the web of causation: Has anyone seen the spider? *Social Science & Medicine* 39(7):887–903.

Krieger, N. 2011. *Epidemiology and the People's Health Theory and Context.* New York: Oxford University Press.

Lustig, R. H. 2013. Fructose: It's 'Alcohol without the buzz'. *Advances in Nutrition: An International Review Journal* 4(2):226–235. doi: 10.3945/an.112.002998.

Malm, H. 2002. 'Do this, it could save your life!' and other problematic claims in preventive medicine. *Newsletter on Philosophy and Medicine/American Philosophical Association* 1(2 Revised):3–9.

Marantz, P. R. 2010. Rethinking dietary guidelines. *Critical Reviews in Food Science and Nutrition* 50(s1):17–18. doi: 10.1080/10408398.2010.526846.

Mayes, C. R. and D. B. Thompson. 2014. Is nutritional advocacy morally indigestible? A critical analysis of the scientific and ethical implications of 'healthy' food choice discourse in liberal societies. *Public Health Ethics* 7(2):158–169. doi: 10.1093/phe/phu013.

Mayes, C. R. and D. B. Thompson. 2015. What should we eat? Biopolitics, ethics, and nutritional scientism. *Journal of Bioethical Inquiry* 12(4):587–599. doi: 10.1007/s11673-015-9670-4.

National Research Council Committee on Diet and Health. 1989. *Diet and Health: Implications for Reducing Chronic Disease Risk.* Washington, DC: National Academies Press (US). http://www.ncbi.nlm.nih.gov/books/NBK218743/

Oppenheimer, G. M. and I. D. Benrubi. 2013. McGovern's Senate Select Committee on Nutrition and Human Needs Versus the Meat Industry on the Diet-Heart Question (1976–1977). *American Journal of Public Health* 104(1):59–69. doi: 10.2105/ajph.2013.301464.

Potischman, N. and D. L. Weed. 1999. Causal Criteria in Nutritional Epidemiology. *American Journal of Clinical Nutrition* 69(6):1309s–1314s.

Pyle, G. 2005. *Raising Less Corn, More Hell: The Case for the Independent Farm and against Industrial Food.* New York: PublicAffairs.

Reaven, G. M. 1986. Effect of dietary carbohydrate on the metabolism of patients with non-insulin dependent diabetes mellitus. *Nutrition Reviews* 44(2):65–73. doi: 10.1111/j.1753-4887.1986.tb07589.x.

Richmond, J. B. 1979. Foreword. *American Journal of Clinical Nutrition* 32(12):2621–22.

Satia, J. A. 2009. Diet-related disparities: Understanding the problem and accelerating solutions. *Journal of the American Dietetic Association* 109(4):610–615. doi: 10.1016/j.jada.2008.12.019.

Schleifer, D. 2012. The perfect solution. How trans fats became the healthy replacement for saturated fats. *Technology and Culture* 53(1):94–119.

Select Committee on Nutrition and Human Needs of the United States Senate. 1977a. *Dietary Goals for the United States*, 2nd ed. Washington: U.S. Government Printing Office. http://catalog.hathitrust.org/Record/000325810

Select Committee on Nutrition and Human Needs, United States Senate. 1977b. *Dietary Goals for the United States: Supplemental Views*. Washington, DC: U.S. Government Printing Office. https://babel.hathitrust.org/cgi/pt?id=umn.31951d00283417h;view=1up;seq=1

Siegel, R. L., K. D. Miller, and A. Jemal. 2015. Cancer statistics, 2015. *CA: A Cancer Journal for Clinicians* 65(1):5–29. doi: 10.3322/caac.21254.

Simpson, S. H., D. T. Eurich, S. R. Majumdar, R. S. Padwal, R. T. Tsuyuki, J. Varney, and J. A. Johnson. 2006. A meta-analysis of the association between adherence to drug therapy and mortality. *BMJ* 333(7557):1–6. doi: 10.1136/bmj.38875.675486.55.

Truswell, A. S. 1987. Evolution of dietary recommendations, goals, and guidelines. *American Journal of Clinical Nutrition* 45(5):1060–1072.

United States. 2010. *2010 Dietary Guidelines for Americans: Backgrounder, History and Process*. Washington, DC: U.S. Department of Agriculture. http://purl.fdlp.gov/GPO/gpo4085

U.S. Department of Agriculture and U.S. Department of Health and Human Services. 2011. *Dietary Guidelines for Americans, 2010*. 7th ed. Washington, DC: U.S. Government Printing Office. http://www.cnpp.usda.gov/DGAs2010-PolicyDocument.htm

U.S. Department of Health and Human Services and U.S. Department of Agriculture. 2016. *Dietary Guidelines for Americans, 2015–2020*, 8th ed. Available at http://health.gov/dietaryguidelines/2015/guidelines/

Weed, D. L. 1997. Underdetermination and incommensurability in contemporary epidemiology. *Kennedy Institute of Ethics Journal* 7(2):107–127.

Weil, W. B. Jr. 1979. National dietary goals. Are they justified at this time? *American Journal of Diseases of Children (1960)* 133(4):368–370.

Woolf, S. H. and M. Nestle. 2008. Do dietary guidelines explain the obesity epidemic? *American Journal of Preventive Medicine* 34(3):263–65. doi: 10.1016/j.amepre.2007.12.002.

Zamora, D., P. Gordon-Larsen, D. R. Jacobs Jr., and B. M. Popkin. 2010. Diet quality and weight gain among black and white young adults: The Coronary Artery Risk Development in Young Adults (CARDIA) study (1985–2005). *American Journal of Clinical Nutrition* 92(4):784–793. doi: 10.3945/ajcn.2010.29161.

13 Framing food within a health policy system

Health in all policies

Sabrina Neeley

Health is often equated with access to healthcare; however, health is a broader concept, determined by the interaction of multiple modifiable and nonmodifiable factors both internal and external to an individual. Over the years, numerous researchers have weighted the relative contribution that various factors make to the health of an individual; depending on the source, behavior accounts for 30%–50% of health, social and environmental factors contribute 20%–50%, genetics contributes 20%–30%, and medical care accounts for 10%–20% (McGinnis, Williams-Russo, and Knickman 2002; Booske et al. 2010; McGovern, Miller, and Hughes-Cromwick 2014).

The greatest impact toward improving the health of individuals and populations can be achieved by addressing the social factors, hereafter referred to as Social Determinants of Health, which encourage or impede health-related behaviors. These improvements require interventions at the community or society level, typically with public policy tools. Food policy often addresses concerns about the production, distribution, pricing, and availability of particular items in order to regulate supply and/or demand of certain food items. A different approach to policy development is the Health in All Policies (HiAP) approach, which encourages decision-making about food as a social determinant of health for individuals and populations.

Social determinants of health

Social determinants of health are the factors external to an individual (i.e., food, housing, transportation, economics, culture, etc.) that enable or inhibit that person's achievement of good health. These are factors that lie outside the healthcare system, are based in the communities in which people live, work, and play, and reflect policy decisions about the distribution of resources, money, and power (Stahl et al. 2006; Newman et al. 2014; Bliss et al. 2016). Structural or systemic differences in social determinants of health create health inequities (Wernham and Teutsch 2015; WHO 2016c).

Traditionally, societies have attempted to address health disparities and inequities by focusing on changing the way individuals behave, or how they make decisions about their health. This focus on the individual often fails because of lack of consideration of capabilities, motivations, and opportunities external to the individual that enable or block desired behaviors (Hendriks et al. 2013). Simply telling individuals that they need to eat healthier food in order to reduce their risk of disease will not be successful if those individuals do not have access to healthy food. Unhealthy communities and systems result in unhealthy behaviors and interventions that do not consider social determinants and health equity may actually increase disparities (Hall, Graffunder, and Metzler 2016). Building a farmers' market in a wealthy neighborhood may likely result in residents of that neighborhood eating more fresh produce, but may actually contribute to increasing the disparities in consumption of healthy foods for the entire community if similar efforts are not made in poor neighborhoods. Health promotion creates supportive environments that enable people to control and improve their health and well-being, in order to increase health equity (WHO).

The role of government policy in health

The government should be concerned about advancing the health of its citizens; individuals who possess good health are better students and more productive workers; they incur lower direct and indirect healthcare costs, and they contribute to economic stability and growth (Stahl et al. 2006; Kickbusch 2010). Societies are evaluated on health indicators, and health is a key factor in development and security (Kickbusch 2010; Krech 2011). As rates of chronic disease rise worldwide and governments are faced with rapidly increasing costs of healthcare, attention must turn to addressing the factors that contribute to health.

Thomas Frieden, director of the U.S. Centers for Disease Control and Prevention (CDC), has explicitly stated the role of government in relation to the health of its citizens, "Government has a responsibility to implement effective public health measures that increase the information available to the public and decision makers, protect people from harm, promote health, and create environments that support healthy behaviors" (Frieden 2013, p. 1859).

In the 2015 Shattuck Lecture, Frieden presented the Public Health Pyramid, a framework for identifying the areas of public health within which interventions can achieve the greatest impact (p. 1749). The base of the 5-level pyramid, where the greatest number of people can benefit, is addressing "socioeconomic factors." One level up is "changing the context to make individuals' default decisions healthy." According to Frieden, addressing these two factors would have the biggest impact on the health of a population, more so than the top three levels of the pyramid (long-lasting protective interventions, clinical interventions, and counseling and education).

Priorities and policies concerning food and nutrition

Globally, governmental bodies issue health-related goals and strategies to frame the conversation around where policy decisions should be made, and resources should be channeled. Concerns about hunger, malnutrition, and access to healthy and safe foods typically garner high priority in many societies. Since these issues are often highly correlated with poverty and health inequities, successful interventions must go beyond just provision of food, to establishing systems that allow people to grow, transport, sell, and purchase nutritious foods for themselves and their families.

Policy initiatives are required to address the social determinants that directly increase or decrease health equity. Addressing structural determinants such as the political context, socioeconomic position, as well as intermediary and cross-cutting determinants such as living and working conditions, food, social and environmental factors, social cohesion, and even the health system must be a priority if a community wants to advance health equity (Hall, Graffunder, and Metzler 2016). Policies that do not have an explicit health focus may disproportionately disadvantage those who already face inequities (Gelormino et al. 2015).

The *United Nations 17 Sustainable Development Goals* set priorities for attention and resource allocation worldwide. The goals related to food and nutrition include: (1) no poverty, (2) zero hunger, (3) good health and well-being, (6) clean water and sanitation, (10) reduced inequalities, (14) life below water, and (15) life on land (United Nations 2016).

In the United States, the *National Prevention Strategy* was released in June 2011, under the direction of the U.S. Surgeon General (www.surgeongeneral.gov). This strategy outlined a set of national goals for improving health and quality of life for everyone in the United States. Healthy eating was identified as one of the seven priorities for targeted action. Recommendations for food and nutrition include the following (http://www.surgeongeneral.gov/priorities/prevention/strategy/healthy-eating.html):

- Increase access to healthy and affordable foods in communities
- Implement organizational and programmatic nutrition standards and policies
- Improve nutritional quality of the food supply
- Help people recognize and make healthy food and beverage choices
- Support policies and programs that promote breastfeeding
- Enhance food safety

For the past 30 years, *Healthy People*, an initiative of the U.S. Department of Health and Human Services' Office of Disease Prevention and Health Promotion, has defined a set of evidence-based 10-year objectives for improving the health of Americans. The *Healthy People* (2020) objectives related to social determinants of health, food, and nutrition include the following (https://www.healthypeople.gov/2020/topics-objectives):

- Create social and physical environments that promote good health for all
- Promote health and reduce chronic disease through the consumption of healthful diets and achievement and maintenance of healthy body weights

- Separate goals for reducing diabetes, cancer, chronic kidney disease, heart disease, and stroke
- Reduce foodborne illnesses in the United States by improving food safety-related behaviors and practices

Over the past 40 years, international organizations have advocated for the move toward development of priorities and policies that promote and provide health benefits, an HiAP approach.

Health in all policies

The development of HiAP began in 1978 when The International Conference on Primary Health Care composed the *Declaration of Alma-Ata* (1978) to express the need for urgency by all public sectors to address the health of all people. The subsequent Ottawa Charter for Health Promotion (WHO 2016a) identified the fundamental conditions and resources for health and advocated for the use of legislation, taxation, and other fiscal measures, and organizational change as health promotion policy tools to improve safety, health, and equity and the participants at the conference pledged a political commitment to health and equity. The WHO initiated the link between health and urban planning in 1998 through its European Healthy Cities Program, which focused on healthy public policy and healthy urban planning and included 12 objectives related to promoting healthy lifestyles, social cohesion, equity and social capital, safety and security, and conservation, in addition to employment, good quality housing, educational, cultural, and healthcare facilities, air and water quality, and encouraging local food production and access to healthy food (Barton and Grant 2001, p. S132). The European Healthy Cities Program grew out of the advocacy specified in the *Ottawa Charter* and was at the forefront of the evolution to the HiAP framework (De Leeuw et al. 2015).

The WHO defines *Health in All Policies* (HiAP) as "an approach to public policies across sectors that systematically takes into account the health implications of decisions, seeks synergies, and avoids harmful health impacts in order to improve population health and health equity" (WHO 2013a, p. i19). HiAP addresses social determinants of health by focusing policy action in sectors that have an effect on health but are not primarily concerned with health, such as housing and transportation (Stahl et al. 2006; Baum et al. 2014). The goal of HiAP is to identify the root causes of ill health and health inequities, and develop policy initiatives that improve these conditions, in order to create healthy communities that embrace a "culture of health," where health implications are considered in all decision-making (Bostic et al. 2012; Wernham and Teutsch 2015; Bliss et al. 2016). HiAP is the outcome of joining global health and justice; it develops and implements policies that help vulnerable populations overcome barriers to health (Friedman and Gostin 2015).

The Adelaide Statement on Health in All Policies (2010) was written by the participants of the April 2010 Health in All Policies International Meeting in

Adelaide. The purpose of the statement was to engage leaders at all levels by promoting the role of inter-sectoral collaboration and "joined up" government to address the inequalities that contribute to ill health in a community. As it states, "Good health enhances quality of life, improves workforce productivity, increases the capacity for learning, strengthens families and communities, supports sustainable habitats and environments, and contributes to security, poverty reduction, and social inclusion" (*Adelaide Statement on Health in All Policies* 2010, p. 258). The statement encourages government leaders at the local, regional, national, and international levels to identify common goals and to consider health, well-being, and equity in all policy decision-making. "Government objectives are best achieved when all sectors include health and well-being as a key component of policy development because the causes of health and well-being lie outside the health sector and are socially and economically formed" (p. 1).

In 2013, participants at the 8th Global Conference on Health Promotion wrote the *Helsinki Statement on Health in All Policies* to reiterate the position that "governments have a responsibility for the health of their people and that equity in health is an expression of social justice" (World Health Organization 2013b, p. i17). The group advocated for governments' use of an HiAP approach as a means to achieve the United Nations' Millennium Development Goals (now Sustainable Development Goals), through "prioritizing health and health equity, building institutional capacity, and establishing the structures, processes, and resources necessary to achieve implementation" (World Health Organization 2013b, p. i18).

Successful HiAP initiatives create supportive environments that make the healthy choice the easiest or most convenient choice (Baum and Sanders 2011; Carey et al. 2014; Carrera 2014; Holt et al. 2016). HiAP initiatives encourage policy development that advances the health equity of traditionally disadvantaged groups while also improving the health of the general population (Corburn et al. 2014; Hall, Graffunder, and Metzler 2016).

HiAP and food

In addition to promoting inter-sectoral collaboration in policy-making, the *Adelaide Statement on Health in All Policies* (2010) also addressed concerns about improving food security and safety by advocating for sustainable agriculture policies that consider health in food production, distribution, and marketing. Baum and Sanders (2011) argue that the global food supply is dominated by transnational corporations that grow, produce, process, manufacture, distribute, and market food. These authors believe that more regulation of these companies is needed to improve the security and safety of the food supply, and also to address concerns about targeting consumers with unhealthy foods that contribute to ill health and chronic disease.

Utilization of an HiAP framework would be appropriate when considering policy development related to access to safe, nutritious, and affordable food, land use and sustainable economic development, climate change, food marketing and farm-to-school initiatives, to name a few (Collins and Koplan 2009; Baum and

Sanders 2011). The health of individuals and populations is directly affected by policies related to urban design and land use (Gelormino et al. 2015). Gelormino and colleagues advocate for the use of a framework that examines the impact of urban policies on the relationships between the urban environment and health through the pathways of nature, social context, and behavior while being attuned to health inequities (Gelormino et al. 2015, p. 739). Studies that use an equity lens to examine outcomes of urban policies in a variety of cities and countries demonstrate that inequities are directly related to poor urban design for green space, public gardens, availability of healthy food options, air quality, and other built environmental conditions that lead to poor health. Health inequities perpetuate poor environments that lead to poor health outcomes.

Urban planning can substantially increase or decrease risks to human health through decisions related to land and water use, natural habitat, air and water quality, and the location of commercial buildings, greenspaces, housing, and transportation (Barton and Grant 2001; Krech 2011). Bentley (2013) proposes an ecological public health model that recognizes the interdependencies between urban environments, social equity, and public health; humans as part of the ecosystem. This perspective requires recognition of, and attention to, the principles of conviviality ("living with"), equity, sustainability, and global responsibility.

Achieving success with a HiAP approach

The WHO identified six key components to the successful implementation of an HiAP Framework (World Health Organization 2013a, p. i22):

1. Establish the need and priorities for HiAP
2. Frame planned action
3. Identify supportive structures and processes
4. Facilitate assessment and engagement
5. Ensuring monitoring, evaluation, and reporting
6. Build capacity

Other researchers and policy professionals have evaluated the use of an HiAP approach in multiple initiatives across several locations. Gase, Pennotti, and Smith's (2013) review of the literature and case studies related to HiAP implementation in the United States identified seven key strategies and provided numerous examples of successful strategies and tactics at the local, state, and national levels. These authors also highlight important challenges to successful HiAP implementation, not the least of which is the conflict between the resource-intensive nature of inter-sectoral collaboration and diminishing budgets.

Numerous researchers have examined HiAP planning and implementation at the local, state or territorial, and national level and identified the following elements as essential for success, as well as those elements that pose challenges to the success of the policy implementation (see Table 13.1).

Table 13.1 Conditions for, and Barriers to, Successful Implementation of an HiAP approach

Conditions for Successful Implementation	Barriers to Successful Implementation
A clear government mandate (Adelaide Statement on HiAP 2010; Rantala, Bortz, and Armada 2014; Delany et al. 2015; Wernham and Teutsch 2015) and leadership (Greer and Lillvis 2014; Bliss et al. 2016)	Political opposition (Bostic et al. 2012) or changes in political leadership (Greaves and Bialystock 2011; Rantala, Bortz, and Armada 2014; Wernham and Teutsch 2015)
Practical cross-sector initiatives and concrete plans for addressing health concerns (Adelaide Statement on HiAP 2010; Gase, Pennotti, and Smith 2013; Hofstad 2016)	Lack of clear operationalization of "integrated" public health policy (Hendriks et al. 2014)
Provision of resources (Delany et al. 2015)	Lack of support and/or adequate resources (Delany et al. 2015; Hendriks et al. 2013; Rantala, Bortz, Armada 2014; Wernham and Teutsch 2015)
Adequate and appropriate framing of health problems and causes (Holt et al. 2016)	Root causes may not be considered (Holt et al. 2016)
Community involvement/engagement with stakeholders outside of government (Adelaide Statement on HiAP 2010; Pool and Stratton 2015; Wernham and Teutsch 2015)	Complex nature of multiple-sector collaboration and different perspectives (Greaves and Bialystock 2011; Baum et al. 2014; Corburn et al. 2014; Greer and Lillvis 2014; Bert et al. 2015; Hofstad 2016)
Long project duration (Delany et al. 2015)	Local policies tend to focus on small, specific projects rather than broader strategic goals (Barton and Grant 2001; Greer, Lillvis 2014)
Shared understanding of, and alignment with, goals and work of the different sectors (Freiler et al. 2013; Gase, Pennotti, and Smith 2013; Baum et al. 2014; Greer and Lillvis 2014; Rantala, Bortz, and Armada 2014; Delany et al. 2015; Wernham and Teutsch 2015)	Lack of quality and quantity of evidence-based data related to outcomes (Freiler et al. 2013; Carey et al. 2014; Rantala, Bortz, and Armada 2014; Bert et al. 2015; Wernham and Teutsch 2015)
Shared value in the approach (De Leeuw and Peters 2014)	Perceived abstract nature of public health to nonhealth officials (Hendriks et al. 2013)
Use of a "win–win" strategy (Molnar et al. 2016)	Lack of economic models (Greaves and Bialystock 2011)
Systematic processes (Adelaide Statement on HiAP 2010), timelines, and milestones (Delany et al. 2015)	Complex program evaluation (Bauman, King, and Nutbeam 2014)
Trust and credibility of all participants and stakeholders (Delany et al. 2015)	
Accountability and transparency (Adelaide Statement on HiAP 2010)	

Tools for HiAP development and evaluation

Selecting and using an evidence-based tool for HiAP development and evaluation can address some of the challenges and concerns with bringing multiple stakeholders together to identify values, align goals, and select appropriate intersectoral initiatives and outcome measures. As noted in Delany et al. (2014), the *Health Lens Analysis* (HLA) tool was developed by the Centre for Health Equity Training, Research, and Evaluation at the University of New South Wales, and has been used for collaborations between the university, the government, and nongovernmental organizations since 2003. The HLA is a valuable tool for determining the "practical processes for undertaking inter-sectoral policy making" (Delany et al. 2014, p. 5). This tool can be used during the early agenda-setting stage, as well as the later stages, of policy development, because it helps identify connections between health and other sectors (Delany et al. 2014, 2015).

Health Impact Assessment (HIA) is a broader approach that provides a set of procedures and methods that can be used to systematically assess the impact of a policy on health (Collinsand Koplan 2009; Sukkumnoed and Reukpompipat 2010; Wismer and Ernst 2010; Delany et al. 2014; Mattig et al. 2015; Wernham and Teutsch 2015; Molnar et al. 2016). It is similar to the more commonly known Environmental Impact Assessment (EIA). Some advocates argue moving a step further to the use of a *Health Equity Impact Assessment* (HEIA) that not only evaluates the impact of policies on health but also provides a measurement of how a policy could differentially impact various groups of individuals and overall health equity (Hall, Graffunder, and Metzler 2016).

HIA can be used to facilitate collaboration between individuals and organizations inside and outside government once an issue is identified, as is the case in New South Wales (Delany et al. 2014). Use of an HIA creates greater opportunity to identify health opportunities in policy development (Greer and Lillvis 2014). Simos and colleagues evaluated 10 case studies from five European countries and provide details about the nature of the problems and projects, details about how an HIA was used in the process, and information about the nature of political prioritization, among other characteristics. The authors also summarized the factors impacting the main policy outcomes of acceptability, feasibility, and sustainability (Simos et al. 2015).

The Sustainable Communities Index (Wernham and Teutsch 2015) provides a "set of indicators for livable, equitable, and prosperous cities," as well as guidelines and tools for communities that want to use these measures (Sustainable Communities Collective 2016). One measure, "Neighborhood completeness" includes the indicators of distance to, and availability of, products in supermarkets and other food outlets that offer fresh fruits and vegetables, acceptance of food benefits, access to farmers' markets, and access to community gardens, all factors which impact the health and well-being of citizens.

Numerous case studies and best practices guides have also been created to assist communities in the development and implementation of HiAP initiatives. In conjunction with the 2010 Adelaide Health in All Policies Meeting, the

Government of South Australia produced a guide to HiAP implementation that provides an overview of the history and evolution of HiAP, as well as examples of how the framework has been used (Kickbusch and Bucketts 2010). In 2012, The European Observatory on Health Systems and Policies published a guide for inter-sectoral collaboration, providing advice and case studies for WHO Member States interested in working together to implement HiAP initiatives (McQueen et al. 2012).

In the United States, the American Public Health Association (APHA) collaborated with the Public Health Institute and the California Department of Health (CDPH), with funding from the U.S. CDC and The California Endowment, to publish the *Health in All Policies* framework (Rudolph et al. 2013). This handbook provides a set of guidelines for state and local governments to incorporate health considerations when engaging in decision-making around social and environmental factors that contribute to improved health and well-being for all citizens and promote health equity. The health of a city is measured by the health of its citizens, so although it is challenging, improving the health of the citizens should be a priority for local government (Wernham and Teutsch 2015).

Examples of successful HiAP implementation

HiAP has been implemented in numerous countries in western Asia, Europe, and South America, as well as in Australia, New Zealand, and Canada (Kickbusch and Bucketts 2010; World Health Organization 2013a; Simos et al. 2015) and was the focus of the Finnish European Union (EU) Presidency in 2006 (Stahl et al. 2006). In Iran, the recent adoption of an HiAP approach has prompted the government to create Councils of Health and Food Security and provincial Health Master Plans (Khayatzadeh-Mahani et al. 2015).

In Norway, the 2011 Public Health Act and an HiAP perspective epitomize the tradition of reducing health disparities through policy-making around social determinants and by explicitly stating that population health is the responsibility of the local government (Hagen et al. 2015; Hofstad 2016). Within this system, a Public Health Coordinator (PHC) is charged with facilitating vertical and horizontal collaboration for HiAP initiatives, since public health responsibility lies with local governments, utilizing flow-through funding from the central government. The organizational structure, particularly the proximity of the PHC to decision-making powers, is strongly associated with success.

In South Australia, an HiAP approach to policy-making was adopted in 2008, has been used to coordinate government initiatives in a variety of policy areas, and was linked to the Seven Strategic Priorities of Government in 2012 and 2013 (Delany et al. 2014, 2015). An HiAP Unit was formed within the government to facilitate action (Delany et al. 2015). This state uses a *HLA* process to guide intersectoral collaboration (Baum et al. 2014; Delany et al. 2014). Newman and colleagues (2014) identified potential policies related to the promotion and marketing of healthy food, as well as zoning that limits fast food penetration. A logic model provided by these authors outlines a framework for examining the factors that

Table 13.2 Examples of HiAP Implementation in the United States

Community/State	Organizations Involved	Action	Citation
Los Angeles, CA	County Board of Supervisors' workgroup	Developed and implemented policies around active transportation that served a dual purpose of increasing access to gardens and farmers' markets	Wernham and Teutsch (2015)
Richmond, CA	Created the Richmond Health Equity Partnership (RHEP)	Community forums of residents and government officials collaboratively defined health and health equity and identified contributing to health inequities in the neighborhoods Intervention reduced toxic stressors through multiple sectors; zoning regulations encourage development of healthy food stores that promote food access	Corburn et al. (2014)
San Francisco, CA	Program on health, equity, and sustainability	Implemented programs to increase access to healthy food	Wernham and Teutsch (2015)
Detroit, MI		Detroit Future City plan laid foundation for urban revitalization efforts, including long-term goals for vacant land use for food and energy production and food security New hospital in the Henry Ford Health System contains a community center and café open to the public that provides freshly grown produce and is overseen by a farmer	Pool and Stratton (2015)
Seattle/King County, WA		All county activities are judged against a set of 14 determinants of equity and health, including access to healthy affordable food	Hall, Graffunder, and Metzler (2016)
Washington, DC		Sustainability plan included improving access to nutritious food and decreasing food insecurity	Wernham and Teutsch (2015)
The State of California	California Strategic Growth Council's HiAP Task Force	Defined and described a healthy community Requires focus on populations that have traditionally faced disadvantage and injustice; seeks to identify initiatives that would address disparities and inequities through policy efforts Creation of the Farm-to-Fork Office	Wernham and Teutsch (2015), Hall, Graffunder, and Metzler (2016)
The State of Minnesota	MN Department of Health and Healthy Minnesota Partnership Created the Council on Institutional Collaboration	Shifts focus away from healthcare and influencing health behavior change in individuals to addressing community-level factors that contribute to or detract from, achieving health and health equity	Bliss et al. (2016)

influence healthy eating, the policy areas related to food and drink production, distribution, preparation, and consumption, as well as opportunities to address social determinants that are related to obesity (Newman et al. 2014, p. 47). The goal of this logic model is to assist nonhealth sector officials in identifying areas that could be addressed through an HiAP approach, while also benefiting the other agencies. The HiAP Unit developed individual plans for each collaborating department that included details about how policy development could be coordinated. For example, green space allocation and water tanks for gardening could be added to new housing policy initiatives, which would benefit the individuals needing better access to healthy food options, while also increasing social connections among residents.

The United States tends to lag behind other countries in adoption of an HiAP approach and the use of tools such as the *HLA* or *HIA* (Collins and Koplan 2009), although both the U.S. Association of State and Territorial Health Officers (ASTHO) and the National Association of County and City Health Officials (NACCHO) advocate for this approach (Pool and Stratton 2015). At the federal level, the U.S. Department of Housing and Urban Development has adopted a HiAP approach to policy-making after the Obama administration implemented "place-based budgeting" that requires consideration of geography when determining fiscal priorities (Bostic et al. 2012). HUD's efforts at neighborhood revitalization recognize that urban areas with concentrated poverty often lack access to healthy food, safe public spaces, and transportation, which create challenges to healthy eating and physical activity and may decrease the health of these populations. Several authors provide examples of successful implementation of HiAP in the United States, along with an overview of funding, tools, and processes (see Table 13.2).

Conclusion

An HiAP approach to policy development provides added value through its focus on inter-sectoral collaboration of traditional policy-making entities. Rather than focusing exclusively on regulating the factors that affect supply and demand of certain foods, this approach addresses food as a social determinant of health and utilizes tools that identify opportunities to improve the health and health equity of communities by creating environments that make healthy choices easy and convenient.

REFERENCES

Adelaide Statement on Health in All Policies. 2010. Adelaide: World Health Organization and Government of South Australia. http://www.who.int/social_determinants/hiap_statement_who_sa_final.pdf

Barton, H. and M. Grant. 2001. Urban planning for healthy cities: A review of the progress of the European healthy cities programme. *Journal of Urban Health: Bulletin of the New York Academy of Medicine* 90(Suppl. 1):S129–S141.

Baum, F. E. and D. M. Sanders. 2011. Ottawa 25 years on: A more radical agenda for health equity is still required. *Health Promotion International* 26(S2):ii253–ii257.

Baum, F. et al. 2014. Evaluation of health in all policies: Concept, theory and application. *Health Promotion International* 29(S1):i130–i142.

Bauman, A. E., L. King, and D. Nutbeam. 2014. Rethinking the evaluation and measurement of health in all policies. *Health Promotion International* 29(S1):i143–i151.

Bentley, M. 2013. An ecological public health approach to understanding the relationships between sustainable urban environments, public health and social equity. *Health Promotion International* 29(3):528–537.

Bert, F., G. Scaioli, M. R. Gualano, and R. Siliquini. 2015. How can we bring public health in all policies? Strategies for healthy societies. *Journal of Public Health Research* 4(393):43–46.

Bliss, D., M. Mishra, J. Ayers, and M. V. Lupi, M. Valdes. 2016. Cross-sectoral collaboration: The state health official's role in elevating and promoting health equity in all policies in Minnesota. *Journal of Public Health Management Practice* 22(Suppl. 1):S87–S93.

Booske, B. C., J. K. Athens, D. A. Kindig, H. Park, and P. L. Remington. 2010. *County Health Rankings Working Paper: Different Perspectives for Assigning Weights to Determinants of Health.* Madison, WI: University of Wisconsin Population Health Institute.   http://www.countyhealthrankings.org/sites/default/files/differentPerspectivesForAssigningWeightsToDeterminantsOfHealth.pdf

Bostic, R. W., R. L. J. Thornton, E. C. Rudd, and M. J. Sternthal. 2012. Health in all policies: The role of the U.S. department of housing and urban development and present and future challenges. *Health Affairs* 31(9):2130–2137.

Carey, G., B. Crammond, and R. Keast. 2014. Creating change in government to address the social determinants of health: How can efforts be improved? *BMC Public Health* 14:1087.

Carrera, P. M. 2014. The difficulty of making healthy choices and 'Health in all policies.' *Bulletin of the World Health Organization* 92(1154):154.

Collins, J. and J. P. Koplan. 2009. Health impact assessment: A step toward health in all policies. *Journal of the American Medical Association* 302(3):315–17.

Corburn, J., S. Curl, and G. Arredondo. 2014. A health-in-all-policies approach addresses many of Richmond, California's place-based hazards, stressors. *Health Affairs* 33(11):1905–1913.

Corburn, J., S. Curl, G. Arredondo, and J. Malagon. 2014. Health in all urban policy: City services through the prism of health. *Journal of Urban Health* 91(4):623–636.

Declaration of Alma-Ata. 1978. *International Conference on Primary Health Care.* Alma-Ata, USSR. September 6–12. http://www.who.int/publications/almaata_declaration_en.pdf

Delany, T. et al. 2014. Health impact assessment in New South Wales and health in all policies in South Australia: Differences, similarities and connections. *BMC Public Health* 14:699.

Delany, T., A. Lawless, F. Baum, J. Popay, L. Jones, D. McDermott, E. Harris, D. Broderick, and M. Marmot. 2015. Health in all policies in South Australia: What has supported early implementation? *Health Promotion International Advance Access* 1–11.

De Leeuw, E., G. Green, L. Spanswick, and N. Palmer. 2015. Policymaking in European Cities. *Health Promotion International* 30(S1):i18–i31.

De Leeuw, E. and D. Peters. 2014. Nine questions to guide development and implementation of health in all policies. *Health Promotion International* 30(4):987–997.

Freiler, A., C. Muntaner, K. Shankardass, C. L. Mah, A. Molnar, E. Renahy, and P. O'Campo. 2013. Glossary for the implementation of health in all policies (HiAP). *Journal of Epidemiology Community Health* 67:1068–1072.

Frieden, T. R. 2013. Government's role in protecting health and safety. *New England Journal of Medicine* 368:1857–1859.

Frieden, T. R. 2015. The future of public health. *New England Journal of Medicine* 373:1748–1754.

Friedman, E. A. and L. O. Gostin. 2015. Imagining global health with justice: In defense of the right to health. *Health Care Analysis* 23:308–329.

Gase, L. N., R. Pennotti, and K. D. Smith. 2013. 'Health in all policies': Taking stock of emerging practices to incorporate health in decision making in the United States. *Journal of Public Health Management Practice* 19(6):529–540.

Gelormino, E., G. Melis, C. Marietta, and G. Costa. 2015. From built environment to health inequalities: An explanatory framework based on evidence. *Preventive Medicine Reports* 2:737–745.

Greaves, L. J. and L. R. Bialystock. 2011. Health in all policies—All talk and little action? *Canadian Journal of Public Health* 102(6):407–409.

Greer, S. L. and D. F. Lillvis. 2014. Beyond leadership: Political strategies for coordination in health policies. *Health Policy* 116:12–17.

Hagen, S., M. Helgesen, S. Torp, and E. Fosse. 2015. Health in all policies: A cross-sectional study of the public health coordinators' role in Norwegian municipalities. *Scandinavian Journal of Public Health* 43:597–605.

Hall, M., C. Graffunder, and M. Metzler. 2016. Policy approaches to advancing health equity. *Journal of Public Health Management Practice* 22(1 Suppl):S50–S59.

Healthy People. 2020. Washington, DC: U.S. Department of Health and Human Services. Accessed April 25, 2016. https://www.healthypeople.gov

Hendriks, A.-M., J. Habraken, M. W. J. Jansen, J. S. Gubbels, N. K. de Vries, H. Van Oers, S. Michie, L. Atkins, and S. P. J. Kremers. 2014. Are we there yet? *Operationalizing the Concept of Integrated Public Health Policies Health Policy* 114:174–182. doi:10.1016/j.healthpol.2013.10.004.

Hendriks, A.-M., S. P. J. Kremers, J. S. Gubbels, H. Raat, N. K. de Vries, and M. W. J. Jansen. 2013. Towards health in all policies for childhood obesity prevention. *Journal of Obesity* 632540:1–12. doi:10.1155/2013/632540.

Hofstad, H. 2016. The ambition of health in all policies in Norway: The role of political leadership and bureaucratic change. *Health Policy* Article in Press. doi:10.1016/j.healthpol.2016.03.001.

Holt, D. H., K. L. Frohlich, T. Tjornhoj-Thomsen, and C. Clavier. 2016. Intersectoriality in Danish municipalities: Corrupting the social determinants of health? *Health Promotion International Advance Access* 1–10. doi: 10.1093/heapro/daw020.

Khayatzadeh-Mahani, A., Z. Sedoghi, M. Mehrolhassani, and V. Yazdi-Feyzabadi. 2015. How health in all policies are developed and implemented in a developing country? A case study of a HiAP initiative in Iran. *Health Promotion International Advance Access*, 1–13. doi: 10.1093/heapro/dav062.

Kickbusch, I. 2010. Editorial: Health in all policies: Where to from here? *Health Promotion International* 25(3):261–264. doi: 10.1093/heapro/daq055.

Kickbusch, I. and K. Bucketts (eds.) 2010. *Implementing Health in All Policies: Adelaide 2010*. Adelaide, South Australia: Department of Health, Government of South Australia.

Krech, R. 2011. Healthy public policies: Looking ahead. *Health Promotion International* 26(S2):ii268–ii272. doi:10.1093/heapro/dar066.

Mattig, T., N. Cantoreggi, J. Simos, C. F. Kruit, and D. P. T. H. Christie. 2015. HIA in Switzerland: Strategies for achieving health in all policies. *Health Promotion International Advance Access* 1–8. doi:10.1093/heapro/dav087.

McGinnis, J. M., P. Williams-Russo, and J. R. Knickman 2002. The case for more active policy attention to health promotion. *Health Affairs* 21(2):78–93. doi: 10.1377/hlthaff.21.2.78.

McGovern, L., G. Miller, and P. Hughes-Cromwick. 2014. *Health Policy Brief: The Relative Contribution of Multiple Determinants to Health Outcomes*. Robert Wood Johnson Foundation and Health Affairs. August 21:1–9. http://healthaffairs.org/health-policybriefs/brief_pdfs/healthpolicybrief_123.pdf

McQueen, D. V., M. Wismar, V. Lin, C. M. Jones, and M. Davies (eds.) 2012. *Intersectional Governance for Health in All Policies: Structures, Actions and Experiences*. Copenhagen: European Observatory on Health Systems and Policies.

Molnar, A., E. Renahy, P. O'Campo, C. Muntaner, A. Freiler, and K. Shankardass. 2016. Using win-win strategies to implement health in all policies: A cross-case analysis. *PLoS ONE* 11(2):e0147003. doi:10.1371/journal.pone.0147003.

Newman, L., I. Ludford, C. Williams, and M. Herriot. 2014. Applying health in all policies to obesity in South Australia. *Health Promotion International* 31(1): 44–58.

Pool, R. and K. Stratton. 2015. *Bringing Public Health into Urban Revitalization: Workshop Summary*. Washington DC: National Academies Press. doi:10.17226/21831.

Rantala, R., M. Bortz, and F. Armada. 2014. Intersectoral action: Local governments promoting health. *Health Promotion International* 29(S1):i92–102.

Rudolph, L., J. Caplan, K. Ben-Moshe, and L. Dillon. 2013. *Health in All Policies: A Guide for State and Local Governments*. Washington, DC and Oakland, CA: American Public Health Association and Public Health Institute.

Simos, J., L. Spanswick, N. Palmer, and D. Christie. 2015. The role of health impact assessment in phase V of the healthy cities European network. *Health Promotion International* 30(S1):i71–85.

Stahl, T., M. Wismar, E. Ollila, E. Lahtinen, and K. Leppo (eds.) 2006. *Health in All Policies: Prospects and Pitfalls*. Finland: Ministry of Social Affairs and Health.

Sukkumnoed, D. and K. Reukpompipat 2010. Chapter 5. Health impact assessment in Thailand: A learning tool for addressing health in all policies. In *Implementing Health In All Policies: Adelaide 2010*, edited by I. Kickbusch and K. Buckets. Adelaide, South Australia Department of Health, Government of South Australia, pp. 65–70.

SurgeonGeneral.gov. 2016. *National Prevention Strategy*. Washington, DC: U.S. Department of Health and Human Services. Accessed April 25, 2016. http://www.surgeongeneral.gov/priorities/prevention/strategy/

Sustainable Communities Collective. 2016. *Sustainable Communities Index*. Accessed April 30, 2016. http://www.sustainablecommunitiesindex.org

United Nations. 2016. *Sustainable Development Goals*. New York. Accessed April 25, 2016. http://www.un.org/sustainabledevelopment/blog/2015/12/sustainable-development-goals-kick-off-with-start-of-new-year/

Wernham, A. and S. M. Teutsch. 2015. Commentary: Health in all policies for big cities. *Journal of Public Health Management Practice* 21(1 Suppl):S56–65.

Wismer, M. and K. Ernst. 2010. Chapter 4. Health in all policies in Europe. In *Implementing Health in All Policies: Adelaide 2010*, edited by I. Kickbusch and K. Buckets. Adelaide, South Australia: Department of Health, Government of South Australia, pp. 53–64.

World Health Organization. 2013a. Health in all policies (HiAP) framework for country action. *Health Promotion International* 29(S1):i19–i28. doi:10.1093/heapro/dau035.

World Health Organization. 2013b. The Helsinki statement on health in all policies. *Health Promotion International* 29(S1):i17–i18. doi:10.1093/heapro/dau036.

World Health Organization. 2016a. *Health Promotion: The Ottawa Charter for Health Promotion*, November 21, 1986. Geneva. Accessed April 5, 2016. http://www.who.int/healthpromotion/conferences/previous/ottawa.en/

World Health Organization. 2016b. *Health Promotion*. Geneva. Accessed April 25, 2016. http://www.who.int/topics/health_promotion/en/

World Health Organization. 2016c. *Social Determinants of Health*. Geneva. Accessed April 25, 2016. http://www.who.int/topics/social_determinants/en/

World Health Organization. 2016d. *The Control of Neglected Zoonotic Diseases*. Geneva. Accessed May 23, 2016. http://www.who.int/zoonoses/control_neglected_zoonoses/en/

14 Framing food within a health policy system

One health

Sabrina Neeley

One health

Old ideas about the connections between the health of humans and animals that formed the foundation of both human and veterinary medicine have reemerged in response to the rapid rise of global health emergencies due to outbreaks of infectious diseases that are spread from animals to humans through domestic pets, wildlife, insects, and contaminants in the food and water supply. The security of the global food supply, and its ability to sustain human populations is dependent upon the safety of the global food supply.

One approach to understanding and improving the interface between humans, animals, and the environment is *One Health*. The *One Health Initiative* (www.onehealthinitiative.com) is a collaboration between the following human and animal health organizations (Bokma et al. 2008; Corning 2014; Glynn and Brink 2014):

- American Medical Association (AMA)
- American Veterinary Medical Association (AVMA—www.onehealthcommission.org)
- World Organization for Animal Health (OIE)
- American Association of Pediatrics (AAP)
- American Nurses Association (ANA)
- American Association of Public Health Physicians (AAPHP)
- American Society of Tropic Medicine and Hygiene (ASTMH)
- U.S. Centers for Disease Control and Prevention (CDC)
- U.S. Department of Agriculture (USDA)
- U.S. National Environmental Health Association (NEHA)

This collaboration emphasizes the interconnectedness of the health of humans, animals, and the environment (Shomaker, Green, and Yandow 2013). Attention to the relationships between environmental health, ecology, veterinary medicine, public health, human medicine, molecular biology, and health economics, particularly at the system level, is critical to understanding how to address emerging hazards and consequential disease. Animals and humans are susceptible to environmental hazards that may ultimately affect the food supply and food safety. The goal is to find a balance between a sustainable food production system that nourishes populations and the ability to monitor and control the spread of infectious disease that threatens humans and animals (McMahon et al. 2015).

The Manhattan Principles developed at the Wildlife Conservation Society's 2004 meeting on "One World, One Health" (www.oneworldonehealth.org) define and outline the goals of a One Health approach to disease prevention and control (Jeggo and Mackenzie 2014). These goals include the following:

- Recognition of the link between human health, animal health, and biodiversity
- Recognition of threats to health from land and water use
- Advocacy for innovation in prevention, surveillance, monitoring, and control of disease
- Better protection of wildlife and biodiversity
- Increased investment and collaboration among various stakeholders

One Health changes the approach to disease, moving from simply treating human disease to an environmental surveillance—prediction—prevention approach, that addresses the systems and upstream factors that caused or contributed to the disease (Conrad, Meek, and Dumit 2013; Heymann and Dixon 2013; Atlas and Maloy 2014). "One Health is gaining recognition nationally and internationally as a practical and innovative approach to global health challenges that recognizes the interconnectedness among humans, animals, and their shared environment as well as the economic, cultural and physical factors that influence health" (Conrad, Meek, and Dumit 2013, p. 211).

The inclusion of not only human, veterinary, and environmental health professionals and scientists, but also public health, social science, and policy professionals, allows for knowledge generation and evidence that can inform policy, improve training, and address sustainability challenges (Barrett and Bouley 2015, p. 218)."Good policy must be based on objective scientific studies that integrate epidemiology, ecology, microbiology, social science, and economics to balance the expectation of safe and nutritious food with the need for efficient and profitable production, and sustained environmental health" (Cardona et al. 2015, p. 51).

Zoonotic disease and risks to the food supply

The World Health Organization (WHO 2006) defines zoonoses as "diseases and infections that are naturally transmitted between vertebrate animals and humans" and estimates that zoonoses constitute 61% of all known human infectious diseases, and represent 75% of emerging diseases (WHO 2006). The WHO estimates that, worldwide, almost 1 in 10 people every year are sickened from foodborne disease, resulting in 420,000 deaths (mostly in children under the age of 5) and 33 million healthy life years lost (WHO 2015). Asokan, Fedorowicz, and Tharyan (2011) suggest that 90% of human foodborne illness is zoonotic in origin, making the global burden of foodborne illness an issue of high priority. A better understanding of zoonotic disease is critical for increasing food safety, as is understanding the environmental hazards that may contaminate drinking water or enter the food supply through the contamination of agricultural food crops.

The safety of the food supply has long been recognized as a key function of public health. Public health agencies worldwide are strategically involved in monitoring and responding to food safety crises, in order to maintain food security and prevent hunger. In 2014, the WHO outlined a decade-long set of priorities related to food safety (*Advancing Food Safety Initiatives*). The Food and Agriculture Organization of the United Nations (FAO 2016), in its *Rome Declaration on Nutrition* and *Framework for Action* (2014), declared the "right of everyone to have access to safe, sufficient and nutritious food" and advocated for government's responsibility in addressing concerns about nutrition. In the United States, the CDC partners with the U.S. Food and Drug Administration (FDA) and the USDA Food Safety and Inspection Service, as well as state and local public health departments, to monitor and respond to food safety concerns.

Public health agencies and researchers have expressed concerns about factors that increase the risks to food safety and food security, including the rapid growth in the global population and demand for food, the health of the ecosystem and the effects of climate change, and technology advances that have led to global travel and transportation of food. These threats to food safety and food security underscore the need to understand, and simultaneously improve, the human–animal–environment interface (Barrett and Bouley 2015).

Increasing global population and demand for animal-based protein

"The global human population, now over seven billion, places unprecedented pressure on the planet" (Shomaker, Green, and Yandow 2013, p. 50). The United Nations (2016) estimates that the world's population will reach 8.5 billion by 2030, and that this growing population will require more food. Much of the population growth is taking place in developing countries that may not have a well-established food system or sustainable food supply, and in countries that often face geopolitical destabilization, conflict, and natural disasters. Even in countries that do not regularly face food shortages, average per capita calorie consumption, consumption of animal protein sources, and year-round demand for nonlocal foods have increased over time, stressing the global food system (WHO 2003).

This increasing population creates serious challenges to food safety and security. Increased demand for animal-based protein has resulted in significant changes to meat production. In many countries, animals intended for food supply are now housed, slaughtered, and processed in large-scale production facilities. In these facilities, animal crowding increases the risk of disease spread from animal to animal, and the potential risk of disease spread from animals to humans. Infectious microbes can be introduced at any point along the food supply chain from "feed to fork"—farm, slaughter, processing, storage, shipment, distribution, preparation, and consumption (Coker et al. 2011; Choffnes et al. 2012; Conrad, Meek, and Dumit 2013; Heymann and Dixon 2013; Cantas and Suer 2014; Wall 2014; Wielinga and Schlundt 2013).

Ecosystem health

Animal health (and ultimately human health) is impacted not only by the production systems we have created to meet the demand for food, but is also impacted by habitat destruction, and the degradation and contamination of the ecosystem (Arambulo 2011; Asokan, Asokan, and Tharyan 2011). Since animal habitats are destroyed or are breached by human development, the intermingling of wildlife and domesticated food animals increases, along with the risk of zoonoses.

In addition to the loss of animal habitats, production of plants for both human and animal food depletes soil and water resources (Angelos et al. 2016). Deforestation clears land for farming and animal production; overplanting degrades the land, and runoff from agricultural and commercial operations pollutes the water supply. "The world's human population is altering the global ecosystem through mechanisms such as climate change, biodiversity loss, land degradation and deforestation, and marine pollution." (Shomaker, Green, and Yandow 2013, p. 51). Changes to the ecosystem increase the risk of disease development and disease spread (Coker et al. 2011; Heymann and Dixon 2013) and researchers have expressed grave concerns that the changes being made to increase food production and decrease hunger today may have serious negative implications on health in the future (Cardona et al. 2015, p. 52).

The risk of zoonotic disease due to declines in ecosystem health is exacerbated by climate change, "a change of climate attributed directly or indirectly to human activity that alters the composition of the global atmosphere and oceans" (Black and Butler 2014, p. 466). Climate change affects food security and food safety because it is a contributing factor in drought, crop failure, and decreases in the food and water supply (Shomaker, Green, and Yandow 2013), in production of feed and livestock (Black and Butler 2014), in increased vectorborne and foodborne zoonotic disease (Ahmed, Sparagano, and Seitzer 2010), and in increased risk of chemical contamination of food and feed from agents such as mycotoxins and pesticide residue (Black and Butler 2014). Climate change can also multiply the threats to human health by directly and indirectly exacerbating the risks from food production, food safety, food security, poverty, and disease (Black and Butler 2014, p. 465). Human health is tied to biodiversity and health of the ecosystem (Cleaveland, Borner, and Gislason 2014; Jeggo and Mackenzie 2014).

Globalization and travel

Technology advances have made it easier than ever for humans to travel globally, creating additional risks of disease spread, and increasing the speed with which diseases may be transmitted (Jeggo and Mackenzie 2014; Shomaker, Green, and Yandow 2013, p. 51). Asymptomatic individuals traveling from areas where diseases such as cholera (from food and water contamination) are endemic can introduce or spread the disease to areas where it is not endemic, as was alleged in the 2010 outbreak in Haiti (Transnational Development Clinic et al. 2013). The transcontinental and intercontinental transportation of animals and vegetation also poses a threat to human and animal health (Shomaker, Green, and Yandow 2013, p. 51).

Choffnes et al. (2012) provide a very thorough overview of the concerns about safety in the U.S. food supply, given the global scope of food sources, distribution, and production. Globalization increases the risks of foodborne pathogens and threats to human health. These authors cite studies suggesting that in the United States alone, 48 million illnesses, 128,000 hospitalizations, and 3000 deaths are caused by foodborne disease every year (Choffnes et al. 2012, p. 3).

One health and food safety

Many cases of zoonotic disease originate in animals bred for food purposes (Wielinga and Schlundt 2013, p. 7). Food and food safety is the key connection between human and animal health, so a *One Health* approach centers around agriculture, livestock production, and food safety in order to prevent and control disease (Arambulo 2011; Bidaisee and Macpherson 2014; Wielinga and Schlundt 2013; Lammie and Hughes 2016). "Food-borne zoonoses are an important public health concern worldwide and every year a large number of people are affected by diseases due to contaminated animal-originated food consumption...Prevention of food-borne zoonoses must begin at the farm level with the concept of 'One Health'" (Cantas and Suer 2014, p. 5). In addition, a collaboration between human and animal health can speed response and control when an outbreak occurs (Wielinga and Schlundt 2013). Animals can also serve as sentinels for environmental exposure or contamination (Buttke 2011; Hilborn and Beasley 2015).

One example of a common foodborne pathogen is *Salmonella*. Humans and many animals are susceptible to this organism, and it can also harbor in plants, soil, and water. Most humans are easily infected with *Salmonella* through consumption of infected or contaminated meat or plants, although it can also be spread from animals to humans through direct contact. Understanding the human, animal, and environmental reservoirs of the infection, how to reduce the risk of infection in animals, and how to prevent environmental transmission is critical to the control of the disease (Silva, Calva, and Maloy 2014).

Individuals and communities in under-resourced areas often bear a higher burden from foodborne zoonotic disease and water contamination. Disease in food animals can not only cause human disease, but can result in the destruction of a significant portion of the food supply and contribute to waste of food resources in areas and populations that already suffer from hunger and malnutrition (Ahmed, Sparagano, and Seitzer 2010; Asokan, Asokan, and Tharyan 2011; Wielinga and Schlundt 2013).

Multiple foodborne outbreaks in the early 2000s motivated the Institute of Medicine's Forum on Microbial Threats to host a 2011 workshop on *Improving Food Safety through a One Health Approach*. Choffnes et al. (2012) provides thorough details about these outbreaks, as well as a summary of the workshop that brought together experts to examine current evidence and propose interventions to address threats to the global food system and food supply.

The greatest risks of foodborne illness come from animal proteins, vegetation and soil contamination, and water contamination (see Table 14.1).

Benefits of a one health approach

According to Grace (2014), utilizing a *One Health* approach adds value and reduces costs through resource sharing between human and veterinary medicine, controlling zoonoses, early detection and response, pandemic prevention, and research and development. Grace estimates that the annual costs for zoonotic diseases worldwide are at least $50 billion in human illness and deaths and $25 billion in lost livestock and also argues that the cost of control of zoonotic diseases is approximately one-fourth the cost that is currently borne from human and livestock illness and death. Disease control in animals is more cost-effective than disease control once it crosses over to humans (Arambulo 2011). The culling of livestock herds in the United Kingdom following the identification of Mad Cow/Creutzfeldt–Jakob disease was estimated to cost $5.75 billion, with additional losses in exports. The H5N1 outbreak in 2003–2004 resulted in large-scale slaughter of poultry in Asia, costing the average family more than twice their monthly income (Heymann and Dixon 2013).

Studies in New Zealand found that control of *Campylobacter* in poultry is more cost-effective and has a larger public health impact when interventions take place at the farm, although later measures at the point of slaughter, processing, postharvest decontamination, and food preparation are necessary as well (Golz et al. 2014).

Adopting a one health approach

Numerous researchers have provided examples of the use of a *One Health* approach in responding to and reducing the risk of disease outbreaks. While many examples address risks of nonfoodborne zoonotic and vector disease, the successful implementation of this approach transcends the type of disease and the transmission method. Researchers have identified the following conditions as essential for success, as well as challenges to the success of a *One Health* approach (see Table 14.2).

Cross-disciplinary knowledge and coordination is essential for the overall success of a *One Health* approach, disease reduction, and improved food security. Angelos and colleagues (2016) suggest that "the ability of modern societies to adequately address these and other food-related problems will require an educated workforce trained not only in traditional food safety, security, and public

Table 14.1 Common Sources of Risks for Foodborne Illness

Source	Pathogen/Disease/Risk	Citation
Animal proteins		
Meat	*Escherichia coli* O157 Salmonellosis Campylobacteriosis "mad cow"/ Creutzfeldt–Jakob	Cantas and Suer (2014), Coker et al. (2011), Garcia, Fox, and Besser (2010), Golz et al. (2014), Currier and Steele (2011), and Hope (2013)
Eggs	*Escherichia coli* O157 Salmonellosis Campylobacteriosis	Cantas and Suer (2014), Coker et al. (2011), Garcia, Fox, and Besser (2010), and Golz et al. (2014)
Milk	Brucellosis Q Fever	Cantas and Suer (2014), Godfroid et al. (2013), and Lee and Brumme (2013)
Ice cream	Listeriosis	CDC (2015)
Poultry	H5N1 (Avian influenza)	Coker et al. (2011)
Fruit bats	Ebola	Cardona et al. (2015)
Multiple sources contaminated through feed and water	methyl mercury melamine	Buttke (2011)
Multiple sources	Antimicrobial resistance	Asokan, Asokan, and Tharyan (2011), Cantas and Suer (2014), Currier and Steele (2011), Collignon (2013), Heymann and Dixon (2013), Infectious Diseases Society of America (2016), Lammie and Hughes (2016), and Wielinga and Schlundt (2013)
Vegetation and soil contamination		
Salad greens and other vegetables	Salmonella Listeria Cyclospora	CDC *List of Selected Multistate Foodborne Outbreak Investigations* (CDC 2016)
Nuts and nut butters	Salmonella	CDC *List of Selected Multistate Foodborne Outbreak Investigations*
Sprouts	*Escherichia coli* O157	CDC *List of Selected Multistate Foodborne Outbreak Investigations*
Pomegranate seeds	Hepatitis A	CDC *List of Selected Multistate Foodborne Outbreak Investigations*
Cantaloupe	Listeria	Shomaker, Green, and Yandow (2013)
Water contamination		
Drinking and irrigation water	Multiple pathogens and chemicals	Cantas and Suer (2014), Courtenay et al. (2015), Garcia, Fox, and Besser (2010), and Hilborn and Beasley (2015)
Runoff from dairy cow waste	Nitrates	Courtenay et al. (2015)
Human and animal waste Agricultural fertilizer	Algal blooms Cyanobacteria	Hillborn and Beasley (2015)

Table 14.2 Conditions for, and Barriers to, the Success of a *One Health* Approach

Conditions for Success	Barriers to Success
Increased awareness of One Health and an interdisciplinary approach to disease reduction (Ahmed, Sparagano, and Seitzer 2010)	Overlapping jurisdictions and mandates (Leung, Middleton, and Morrison 2012; Lee and Brumme 2013)
Sense of urgency and common purpose (Rubin, Dunham, and Sleeman 2014) Rapid response (Askoan, Asokan, and Tharyan 2011; Lammie and Hughes 2016)	Lack of urgency (Leung, Middleton, and Morrison 2012)
Shared conceptual frameworks (Min, Allen-Scott, and Buntain 2013)	Lack of clear, shared definition of *One Health* (Leung, Middleton, and Morrison 2012; Lee and Brumme 2013)
Effective cross-sector communication (Asokan, Asokan, and Tharyan 2011; Min, Allen-Scott, and Buntain 2013)	Communicating goals, objectives, and success (Leung, Middleton, and Morrison 2012)
Adequate funding and resources (Grace 2014; Min, Allen-Scott, and Buntain 2013)	Lack of specific metrics for overall or combined benefit and value make it difficult to obtain adequate governmental support, funding and resource allocation (Hueston et al. 2013; Hasler et al. 2014; Jeggo and Mackenzie 2014)
Effective surveillance and risk assessment for both humans and animals (Ahmed, Sparagano, and Seitzer 2010; Asokan, Asokan, and Tharyan 2011; Ayudhya, Assavacheep, and Thanawongnuwech 2012; Heymann and Dixon 2013; Grace 2014; Wall 2014; Lammie and Hughes 2016)	Perceived barriers to obtaining adequate evidence and support for the approach because of difficulty doing comparative research (Lee and Brumme 2013)
Improved investigation and control measures (Ahmed, Sparagano, and Seitzer 2010; Lammie and Hughes 2016)	Difficulty directly linking success to the implementation of a *One Health* perspective (Godfroid et al. 2013)
Effective community and stakeholder engagement (Asokan, Asokan, and Tharyan 2011; Conrad, Meek, and Dumit 2013; Min, Allen-Scott, and Buntain 2013)	Resistance to policy implementation if companies believe their benefits or profits are at stake through increased regulation, fees, or financial penalties (Heymann and Dixon 2013)
Appropriate and judicious use of antimicrobials and antibiotics (Asokan, Asokan, and Tharyan 2011; Currier and Steele 2011; Collignon 2013; Wielinga and Schlundt 2013; Lammie and Hughes 2016)	
Effective vaccination campaigns (Asokan, Asokan, and Tharyan 2011; Ayudhya, Assavacheep, and Thanawongnuwech 2012; Collignon 2013; Godfroid et al. 2013; Lammie and Hughes 2016)	
Innovation in new diagnostic tests, therapies, and vaccines (Lammie and Hughes 2016)	

(Continued)

Table 14.2 (Continued) Conditions for, and Barriers to, the Success of a *One Health* Approach

Conditions for Success	*Barriers to Success*
Increased education, training, and capacity building (Min, Allen-Scott, and Buntain 2013; Jeggo and Mackenzie 2014; Lammie and Hughes 2016)	
Robust food safety management systems, especially for sanitation, hygiene, waste management, and safe food handling (Wall 2014)	

health, but also in other areas including food production, sustainable practices, and ecosystem health" (p. 29).

Researchers and policy makers have developed guidelines for the successful use of a *One Health* approach for reducing disease, informing policy, and for education and training. Heymann and Dixon (2013) provide a detailed framework for understanding and addressing the determinants of emerging zoonotic diseases. Coker and colleagues (2011) propose a conceptual framework for *One Health* research that can inform policy. Their framework includes opportunities for examining contexts, inputs, interventions, mechanisms, and outputs (p. 329). Angelos and colleagues (2016) outline a curricular framework for food safety and security education and training that includes a *One Health* approach. The curriculum includes foundations in (1) local and global food and feed supply and safety, (2) food and waterborne illnesses, (3) food security, (4) food production, and (5) the ecosystem. These educators also advocate for coursework and training that expounds upon the interlinkages between food and feed, agriculture and ecosystem, and food and society. Approximately 20 universities worldwide offer graduate-level coursework in *One Health* (Grace 2014).

The European Cooperation in Science and Technology (COST) network has recently formed the Network for Evaluation of One Health (NEOH), which is working to develop a methodological framework and evaluation tools to determine cost-effectiveness of a *One Health* approach, in order to provide evidence for policy decision-making (Haxton, Sinigoj, and Riviere-Cinnamond 2015).

Some researchers, however, have criticized the current *One Health* framework as being too narrow and suggest that the environmental/ecosystem and wildlife perspectives have not been included to the extent needed, particularly when domestic food animals interact with the environment and wildlife (Hueston et al. 2013; Rubin, Dunham, and Sleeman 2014; Barrett and Bouley 2015; McMahon et al. 2015). Others criticize the *One Health* approach for its lack of consideration of the benefits that social scientists could bring to the discussion. Lapinski, Funk, and Moccia (2015) propose a complex systems framework through which adding knowledge of communication, human behavior, and economics could increase the effectiveness of response to health threats.

Examples of successful implementation of a one health approach

The use of a One Health approach in various countries throughout the world provides numerous examples in a diversity of geographic areas and governmental structures. Since the late 1990s, several outbreaks of Avian Influenza H5N1 in Asian poultry have sickened over 600 people, killed more than 300 people, resulted in the slaughter of at least 400 million poultry, and have cost an estimated $20 billion (U.S.) in economic loss. A rapid, coordinated global system, set up during the first outbreak in 1997, addresses each new case with increased surveillance, research, and communication to provide quick response (Rubin, Dunham, and Sleeman 2014).

In New South Wales, Australia, animal diseases that pose a risk to human health (zoonoses) are monitored and addressed through a series of policies and procedures within a coordinated system of human and animal health sectors. Surveillance for waterborne diseases affecting both human and animal health, as well as avian influenza, is also included in this coordinated system (Adamson, Marich, and Roth 2011). Detection of a foodborne disease in humans prompts not only investigation by the human health authorities but also the NSW Food Authority and a possible response by the animal health authorities to check the source of animal feed.

In Europe, the increased risk of foodborne disease through meat consumption is addressed through an integrated "feed to food" surveillance and inspection process (Blaha 2012, p. 3; Lammie and Hughes 2016). This process includes increased responsibility for food safety from all persons involved in the production of food from animal origin; continuous process-optimization at the farm to insure prevention of disease when meat is consumed; examination and use of compliance data to promote continuous improvement in inspection. This system also combines infection data from humans, animals, and food, in order to identify and monitor common agents and sources.

In 2006, an outbreak of *Escherichia coli* 0157:H7 linked to contaminated bagged spinach sickened 199 people across the United States. A One Health approach broadened the scope of the investigation and microbes were isolated in pigs, cattle, surface water, sediment, and soil in the farm areas where the spinach was grown (Garcia, Fox, and Besser 2010). In the United States, surveillance and monitoring of infectious agents is conducted by a combination of FoodNet (Foodborne Diseases Active Surveillance Network), the National Animal Health Monitoring System (NAHMS), the National Antimicrobial Resistance Monitoring System for Enteric Bacteria (NARMS), and PulseNet, the national foodborne outbreak tracking system (Choffnes et al. 2012; Lammie and Hughes 2016).

In 2012–2013, eight outbreaks in 24 states of human salmonellosis linked to poultry sickened over 500 people. Most of the time, *Salmonella* is spread through foodborne sources, although humans can be infected through direct contact with animals. As part of the investigation, specimens from ill humans were serotyped and subtyped by state public health laboratories, sent to PulseNet, and added to the national database. PulseNet personnel identified a disease cluster, which prompted further case definition and interviewing of sick individuals for common exposures. Mail-order hatcheries were identified as the source of infection and a single hatchery that shipped baby poultry around the country for backyard flocks was implicated in the outbreak. Environmental sampling from crickets and the floor of the poultry house at this hatchery confirmed the *Salmonella* strain. The hatchery implemented improved sanitation, disinfection, insect eradication, and vaccination programs, as well as periodic sampling and monitoring by public health authorities, resulting in eradication of the pathogen (Nakao et al. 2015)

As examples of successful implementation of a One Health approach are published, and as better outcome measures are developed, wider use of this approach is expected. In 2014, the WHO *Global Report on Surveillance* (WHO 2014) called for coordinated surveillance, sampling, and testing from humans, foods, food animals, environmental sources, along with consideration of antibiotic-resistance organisms, when investigating foodborne infection (Lammie and Hughes 2016).

Conclusion

One Health provides a collaborative, interdisciplinary approach to surveillance, outbreak investigation, and implementation of best practices to improve the health and wellness of individuals, populations, and the ecosystem. This perspective broadens the approach to policy development around the food supply and food safety by considering the interconnectedness of human, animal, and ecosystem health. *One Health* advocates for the inclusion of a broader set of stakeholders and partners, as well as the development of a broader set of desired impacts and outcomes, with the overarching goal of balancing a sustainable food production system with the ability to more quickly and effectively monitor and control the spread of infectious disease that threatens humans and animals (McMahon et al. 2015).

REFERENCES

Adamson, S., A. Marich, and I. Roth. 2011. One Health in NSW: Coordination of human and animal health sector management of Zoonoses of public health significance. *NSW Public Health Bulletin* 22(56):105–112.

Ahmed, J. S., O. Sparagano, and U. Seitzer. 2010. One Health, one medicine: Tackling the challenge of emerging diseases. *Transboundary and Emerging Diseases* 57:1–2.

Angelos, J., A. Arens, H. Johnson, J. Cadriel, and B. Osburn. 2016. One Health in food safety and security education: A curricular framework. *Comparative Immunology, Microbiology and Infectious Diseases* 44:29–33.

Arambulo, P. III. 2011. Veterinary public health in the age of 'One Health'. *Journal of the American Veterinary Medical Association* 239(1):48–9.

Asokan, V., Z. Fedorowicz, and P. Tharyan. 2011. Use of a systems approach and evidence-based One Health for Zoonoses research. *Journal of Evidence-Based Medicine* 4:62–5. doi: 10.1111/j.1756-5391.2011.01124.x.

Asokan, G. V., V. Asokan, and P. Tharyan. 2011. One Health National Programme across species on Zoonoses: A call to the developing world. *Infection Ecology and Epidemiology* 1:8293. doi: 10.3402/iee.v1i0.8293.

Atlas, R. M. and S. Maloy. 2014. The future of One Health. *Microbiology Spectrum* 2(1):1–3. doi: 10.1128/microbiolspec.OH-0018-2012.

Barrett, M. A. and T. A. Bouley. 2015. Need for enhanced enviornmental representation in the implementation of One Health. *EcoHealth* 12:212–19.

Bidaisee, S. and Calum N. L. Macpherson. 2014. Zoonoses and One Health: A review of the literature. *Journal of Parasitology Research*: 874345. doi: 10.1155/2014/874345.

Black, P. F. and C. D. Butler. 2014. One Health in a world with climate change. *Revue Scientifique et Technique-Office International des Epizooties* 33(2):465–73.

Blaha, T. 2012. One world—One Health: The threat of emerging diseases: a European perspective. *Transboundary and Emerging Diseases* 59(Suppl. 1):3–8. doi: 10.1111/j.1865-1682.2011.01310.x.

Bokma, B. H, E. P. J. Gibbs, A. A. Aguirre, and B. Kaplan. 2008. A resolution by the society for tropical veterinary medicine in support of 'One Health'. *Animal Biodiversity and Emerging Diseases: Annals of the New York Academy of Science* 1149:4–8. doi: 10.1196/annals.1428.053.

Buttke, D. E. 2011. Toxicology, environmental health, and the 'One Health' concept. *Journal of Medical Toxicology* 7(August 5):329–332.

Cantas, L. and K. Suer. 2014. Review: The important bacterial Zoonoses in 'One Health' concept. *Frontiers in Public Health* October 14:1–8. doi: 10.3389/fpubh.2014.00144.

Cardona, C., D. A. Travis, K. Berger, G. Coat, S. Kennedy, C. J. Steer, M. P. Murtaugh, and P. Sriramarao. 2015. Advancing One Health policy and implementation through the concept of one medicine one science. *Global Advances in Health and Medicine* 4(5):50–54. doi: 10.7453/gahmj.2015053.

Centers for Disease Control and Prevention. 2015. Multistate Outbreak of Listeriosis Linked to Blue Bell Creameries Products (Final Update). June 10. Atlanta. Accessed May 27, 2016. http://www.cdc.gov/listeria/outbreaks/ice-cream-03-15/index.html

Centers for Disease Control and Prevention. 2016. *List of Selected Multistate Foodborne Outbreak Investigations. May 13.* Atlanta. Accessed May 27, 2016. http://www.cdc.gov/foodsafety/outbreaks/multistate-outbreaks/outbreaks-list.html

Choffnes, E. R., D. A. Relman, L. A. Olsen, R. Hutton, and A. Mack, Rapporteurs. 2012. *Improving Food Safety through a One Health Approach: Workshop Summary.* Institute of Medicine. Washington, DC: The National Academies Press.

Cleaveland, S., M. Borner, and M. Gislason. 2014. Ecology and conservation: Contributions to One Health. *Revue Scientifique et Technique-Office International des Epizooties* 33, (2):615–627.

Coker, R., J. Rushton, S. Mounier-Jack, E. Karimuribo, P. Lutumba, D. Kambarage, D. U. Pfeiffer, K. Stark, and M. Rweyemamu. 2011. Towards a conceptual framework to support One-Health research for policy on emerging zoonoses. *Lancet Infectious Diseases* 11:326–31. doi: 10.1016/S1473-3099(10)70312-1.

Collignon, P. 2013. The importance of a One Health approach to preventing the development and spread of antibiotic resistance. In *One Health: The Human-Animal-Environment Interfaces in Emerging Infectious Diseases.* Current Topics in Microbiology and Immunology, vol. 366, edited by J. S. Mackenzie, M. Jeggo, P. Daszak, and J. A. Richt, pp. 19–36. Heidelberg: Springer.

Conrad, P. A., L. A. Meek, and J. Dumit. 2013. Operationalizing a One Health approach to global health challenges. *Comparative Immunology, Microbiology and Infectious Diseases* 36:211–16.

Corning, S. 2014. World Organisation for Animal Health: Strengthening veterinary services for effective One Health collaboration. *Revue Scientifique et Technique-Office International des Epizooties* 33, (2):639–50.

Courtenay, M., J. Sweeney, P. Zielinska, S. B. Blake, and Roberto La Ragione. 2015. One Health: An opportunity for an interprofessional approach to healthcare. *Journal of Interprofessional Care* 29, (6):641–42. doi: 10.3109/13561820.2015.1041584.

Currier, R. W. and J. H. Steele. 2011. One Health—One Medicine: Unifying human and animal medicine within an evolutionary paradigm. *Annals of the New York Academy of Sciences* 1230:4–11. doi: 10.1111/j.1749-6632.2011.06138.x.

Food and Agriculture Organization of the United Nations. 2016. About FAO. Rome. Accessed May 27, 2016. http://www.fao.org/about/en/

Garcia, A., J. G. Fox, and T. E. Besser. 2010. Zoonotic enterohemorrhagic *Escherichia coli*: A One-Health perspective. *ILAR Journal* 51, (3):221–32.

Glynn, M. K. and N. Brink. 2014. Perspectives on One Health: A survey of National Delegates to the World Organisation for Animal Health, 2012. *Revue Scientifique et Technique-Office International des Epizooties* 33(2):433–41.

Godfroid, J., S. Al Dahouk, G. Pappas, F. Roth, G. Matope, J. Muma, T. Marcotty, D. Pfeiffer, and E. Skjerve. 2013. A 'One Health' surveillance and control of brucellosis in developing countries: Moving away from improvisation. *Comparative Immunology, Microbiology and Infectious Diseases* 36:241–48. doi: 10.1016/j. cimid.2012.09.001.

Golz, G., B. Rosner, D. Hofreuter, C. Josenhans, L. Kreienbrock, A. Lowenstein, A. Schielke, K. Stark, S. Suerbaum, L. H. Wieler, and T. Alter. 2014. Relevance of campylobacter to Public Health—The need for a One Health approach. *International Journal of Medical Microbiology* 304:817–23. doi: 10.1016/j.ijmm.2014.08.015.

Grace, D. 2014. The business case for One Health. *Onderstepoort Journal of Veterinary Research* 81(2):725. doi: 10.4102/ojvr.v81i2.725.

Hasler, B., L. Cornelsen, H. Bennani, and J. Rushton. 2014. A review of the metrics for One Health benefits. *Revue Scientifique et Technique-Office International des Epizooties* 33(2):453–64.

Haxton, E., S. Sinigoj, and A. Riviere-Cinnamond. 2015. The network for evaluation of One Health: Evidence-based added value of One Health. *Infection Ecology and Epidemiology* 5:28164. doi: 10.3402/iee.v5.28164.

Heymann, D. L. and M. Dixon. 2013. The value of the One Health approach: Shifting from emergency response to prevention of zoonotic disease threats at their source. *Microbiology Spectrum* 1(1):OH-0011–2012. doi: 10.1128/microbiolspec. OH-0011-2012.

Hilborn, E. D. and V. R. Beasley. 2015. One Health and cyanobacteria in freshwater systems: Animal illnesses and deaths are sentinel events for human health risks. *Toxins* 7:1374–1395. doi: 10.3390/toxins7041374.

Hope, J. 2013. Bovine spongiform encephalopathy: A tipping point in One Health and Food Safety. In *One Health: The Human-Animal-Environment Interfaces in Emerging Infectious Diseases*. Current Topics in Microbiology and Immunology, Volume 366, edited by J. S. Mackenzie, M. Jeggo, P. Daszak, and J. A. Richt, pp. 37–47. Heidelberg: Springer.

Hueston, W., J. Appert, T. Denny, L. King, J. Umber, and L. Valeri. 2013. Assessing global adoption of One Health approaches. *EcoHealth* 10:228–33. doi: 10.1007/ s10393-013-0851-5.

Infectious Diseases Society of America (IDSA). 2016. *Ending Non-Judicious Use of Antibiotics in Agriculture.* 2016. Accessed May 27, 2016. http://www.idsociety.org/Agriculture_Policy/

Jeggo, M. and J. S. Mackenzie. 2014. Defining the future of One Health. *Microbiology Spectrum* 2(1):OH-0007-2012. doi: 10.1128/microbiolspec.OH-0007-2012.

Lammie, S. L. and J. M. Hughes. 2016. Antimicrobial resistance: Food Safety and One Health: The need for convergence. *Annual Review of Food Science and Technology* 7:287–312. doi: 10.1146/annurev-food-041715-033251.

Lapinski, M. K, J. A. Funk, and L. T. Moccia. 2015. Recommendations for the role of social science research in One Health. *Social Science & Medicine* 129:51–60. doi: 10.1016/j.socscimed.2014.09.048.

Lee, K. and Z. L. Brumme. 2013. Operationalizing the One Health approach: The global governance challenges. *Health Policy and Planning* 28:778–785. doi: 10.1093/heapol/czs127.

Leung, Z., D. Middleton, and K. Morrison. 2012. One Health and EcoHealth in Ontario: A qualitative study exploring how holistic and integrative approaches are shaping public health practice in Ontario. *BMC Public Health* 12:358. http://www.biomedcentral.com/1471-2458/12/358.

McMahon, B. J., P. G. Wall, S. Fanning, and A. G. Fahey. 2015. Targets to increase food production: One Health implications. *Infection Ecology and Epidemiology* 5:27708. doi: 10.3402/iee.v5.27708.

Min, B., L. K. Allen-Scott, and B. Buntain. 2013. Transdisciplinary research for complex One Health issues: A scoping review of key concepts. *Preventive Veterinary Medicine* 112: 222–29. doi: 10.1016/j.prevetmed.2013.09.010.

Na Ayudhya, S. N., P. Assavacheep, and R. Thanawongnuwech. 2012. One world—One Health: The threat of emerging swine diseases. An Asian perspective. *Transboundary and Emerging Diseases* 59(Suppl. 1):9–17.

Nakao, J. H. et al. 2015. 'One Health' investigation: Outbreak of *Salmonella* Braenderup infections traced to a Mail-Order Hatchery—United States, 2012–2013. *Epidemiology and Infection* 143:2178–2186. doi: 10.1017/S0950268815000151.

Rubin, C., B. Dunham, and J. Sleeman. 2014. Making One Health a reality—Crossing bureaucratic boundaries. *Microbiology Spectrum* 2:1. doi: 10.1128/microbiolspec.OH-0016-2012.

Shomaker, T. S., E. M. Green, and S. M. Yandow. 2013. Perspective: One Health: A compelling convergence. *Academic Medicine* 88, (1):49–55.

Silva, C., E. Calva, and S. Maloy. 2014. One Health and food-borne disease: *Salmonella* transmission between humans, animals, and plants. *Microbiology Spectrum* 2, 1. doi: 10.1128/microbiolspec.OH-0020-2013.

Transnational Development Clinic, Jerome N. Frank Legal Services Organization, Yale Law School, Global Health Justice Partnership of the Yale Law School and Yale School of Public Health, and Association Haitienne de Droit de L'Environment. 2016. Peacekeeping without Accountability: The United Nations' Responsibility for the Haitian Cholera Epidemic. 2013. Accessed May 27, 2016. https://www.law.yale.edu/system/files/documents/pdf/Clinics/Haiti_TDC_Final_Report.pdf

United Nations. 2016. *UN Projects World Population to Reach 8.5 Billion by 2030, Driven by Growth in Developing Countries.* New York. Accessed May 27, 2016. http://www.un.org/sustainabledevelopment/blog/2015/07/un-projects-world-population-to-reach-8-5-billion-by-2030-driven-by-growth-in-developing-countries/

Wall, P. 2014. One Health and the food chain: Maintaining safety in a globalised industry. *Veterinary Record* February 22:189–192. doi: 10.1136/vr.g1512.

Wielinga, P. R. and J. Schlundt. 2013. Food safety: At the center of a One Health approach for combating zoonoses. In *One Health: The Human-Animal-Environment Interfaces in Emerging Infectious Diseases. Current Topics in Microbiology and Immunology*, vol. 366, edited by J. S. Mackenzie, M. Jeggo, P. Daszak, and J. A. Richt, pp. 3–17. Heidelberg: Springer.

World Health Organization. 2003. *Diet, Nutrition, and the Prevention of Chronic Diseases.* WHO Technical Report Series 916. Report of a Joint WHO/FAO Expert Consultation. Accessed May 27, 2016. http://www.fao.org/docrep/005/ac911e/ac911e05.htm

World Health Organization. 2014. *Advancing Food Safety Initiatives: Strategic Plan for Food Safety Including Foodborne Zoonoses 2013–2022.* Geneva. http://www.who.int/foodsafety/publications/strategic-plan/en/

World Health Organization. 2015. *Launch of the WHO Estimates of the Global Burden of Foodborne Diseases.* Geneva. Accessed May 23, 2016. http://www.who.int/foodsafety/en/

World Health Organization. 2006. *The Control of Neglected Zoonotic Diseases.* Geneva. Accessed May 23, 2016. http://www.who.int/zoonoses/control_neglected_zoonoses/en/

15 Food literacy

What is it and why does it matter?

Georgia Jones

Current knowledge of food

Unfortunately, Western countries have experienced foundational shifts in eating patterns and skills required to provide food for the family. Entire populations exhibit a lack of confidence in basic food preparation knowledge and skills, which causes a dependence on prepared foods. Approximately 10% of adults in the United States and Australia do not know how to prepare home-cooked meals. Many young adults have limited experience in food preparation and may lack the ability to prepare foods by reading and understanding a recipe or following instructions on a food package (Jones et al. 2014).

An entire industry has grown around food television programming and celebrity chefs (Pray 2016). There has been a growth of farmers' market, local foods, and best-selling cookbooks, but many people do not or cannot cook. According to a 2010 Harris Interactive poll of 2503 adults, 14% do not enjoy cooking, 7% do not cook at all, and 41% prepare meals at home five or more times per week. The results of a North Carolina study found that the proportion of women cooking has declined from 92% in 1965–1966 to 68% in 2007–2008. Those who do cook spend less time doing so. The amount of time spent cooking has decreased from 112.8 minutes/day in 1965–1966 to 65.6 minutes/day in 2007–2008 (Palmer 2013).

There is also a growing focus on the relationship between food and health. Some consumers view food as medicine. At the same time, Americans are spending less time planning meals, preparing food, and dining together. While consumers are becoming more interested in food, they are also becoming more disconnected from it (Pray 2016).

Americans have shifted toward eating out more and cooking at home less. The percentage of daily energy consumed from home food sources and time spent in food preparation decreased significantly for all socioeconomic groups between 1965 and 1966 and between 2007 and 2008. The largest decrease occurred between 1965 and 1992. The American diet has shifted toward foods with decreased nutrient density with less than 20% of the population meeting USDA (United States Department of Agriculture) guidelines for a healthy diet, including fruits, vegetables, whole grains, and low-fat dairy (Smith et al. 2013).

The shift from food prepared at home to increased consumption of convenience/easy-to-prepare and away-from-home food may have important nutritional implications. Cross-sectional and longitudinal studies have shown that away from home foods have been associated with increased energy intake and decreased nutritional quality, as well as increased weight gain (Palmer 2013; Smith et al. 2013). In contrast, eating foods prepared from scratch is associated with increased intake of fruits, vegetables, and whole grains. Increased cooking has also been linked to better overall health and a decrease in BMI (body mass index) (Smith et al. 2013).

Food literacy as a method to reduce obesity

Obesity is one of the most serious public health challenges of the twenty-first century. Increasingly, researchers are focusing on factors that influence the establishment of behavioral risk factors for obesity and related chronic diseases, especially health-related behaviors established in adolescence. A diet consisting mainly of fast foods, away-from-home meals, and packaged snacks promotes weight gain and is associated with increased risk of obesity, type 2 diabetes, cardiovascular disease, and some forms of cancer. Therefore, it is essential that public health promotion strategies and interventions focus on promoting healthy dietary intake, especially during adolescence (Vaitkeviciute et al. 2014).

Interventions to reduce obesity are generally successful in increasing nutrition-related knowledge but do not necessarily improve dietary intake. Research suggests that knowledge alone is not sufficient to change individual behavior. Interventions need to move beyond knowledge to concepts like food literacy to positively impact dietary change. It has been suggested that these outcomes have occurred because interventions have failed to connect nutrition-related knowledge, skills, and critical decision-making about dietary intake. Collectively, these concepts are called "food literacy" and could be the key to improving dietary outcomes (Vaitkeviciute et al. 2014).

Food literacy: A tool for developing a healthy relationship with food

The Food Literacy Center defines food literacy as an understanding of the impact of food choices on health, the environment, and your community. Being food literate empowers consumers to make informed food choices (The Food Literacy Center, accessed on September 8, 2015). Food literacy consists of the everyday practicalities associated with navigating and using the food system to ensure a regular food intake consistent with nutrition recommendations.

Food literacy is composed of a collection of interrelated knowledge, skills, and behaviors required to (1) plan and manage, (2) select, (3) prepare, and (4) eat food to meet needs and determine intake (Vidgen and Gallegos 2014). It is unlikely that an individual would demonstrate all components of food literacy simultaneously or all of the time. That is, all components may not be present in every individual, but each is important and strengthens one's relationship with food. When a component is missing, the relationship with food is weaker, and one is less able to respond to change (Vidgen and Gallegos 2014).

Planning and management refers to making time for food and eating, having a plan to ensure this happens, and having skills to construct a feasible plan capable of delivering the expected outcome. Selection refers to the ability to choose foods in grocery stores and restaurants. Preparation refers to the ability to prepare food. Moreover, lastly, eating refers to the ability to understand that food has an impact on personal well-being, a self-awareness of the need to personally balance food intake, and to consume food in a social manner (Vidgen and Gallegos 2014).

Cullen et al. (2015) proposed that the definition of food literacy should include the positive relationship built through social, cultural, and environmental experiences with food preparation, enabling people to make decisions that support health. Cullen et al. (2015) stated that food literacy should be situated at the intersection between community food security and food skills. Food behaviors and skills cannot be separated from their environmental or social context. Increasing the population's food literacy will allow and empower people to engage in society and influence their local food systems (Cullen et al. 2015).

Meckna (2006) defined food literacy as the degree to which individuals have the capacity to obtain, process, and understand basic food and food preparation information for appropriate food decisions. This definition is based on the CDC (Centers for Disease Control and Prevention) definition of health literacy (Selden et al. 2000). When defined in this manner, food literacy is not only nutrition knowledge; it includes skills and behaviors, from knowing where food comes from to the ability to select and prepare foods and consume it in a manner consistent with nutrition guidelines (Vaitkeviciute et al. 2014).

According to Selden et al. (2000), health literacy is the degree to which individuals have the capacity to obtain, process, and understand basic health information and services needed to make appropriate health decisions. In addition to basic literacy skills, health literacy requires the additional knowledge of health topics. People with limited health literacy often lack knowledge or have misinformation about the body as well as the nature and causes of disease. Without this knowledge, they may not understand the relationship between lifestyle factors such as diet and exercise and various health outcomes (Selden et al. 2000).

Nutrition literacy: The ability to access, interpret, and use nutrition information

Nutrition literacy has been conceptualized as a specific health literacy domain that reflects the ability to access, interpret, and use nutrition information. This broad definition could arguably encapsulate a range of knowledge and competencies. Defining health and nutrition literacy is complex. Both terms "can mean different things to different people, such as understanding the politics of food, gauging the sugar content of a soda and buying and preparing a healthy meal" (Velardo 2015). The ability to understand nutrition concepts is perceived to be particularly significant if an individual has a disease with nutritional implications, such as diabetes and hypertension (Velardo 2015).

The competence to use any dietary information is characterized by the acquisition of food preparation knowledge and cooking skills (Pendergast et al. 2011). Practical skills need to be an integral part of the nutrition literacy concept. Nutrition literacy may also include choosing healthier alternatives when selecting convenient and prepared foods. Although food preparation knowledge and cooking skills are extremely important, it is important to acknowledge the ubiquity of a contemporary food environment that is saturated with convenience foods (Velardo 2015).

Culinary nutrition: Application of nutrition and food science principles

Culinary nutrition is the application of nutrition and food science principles displayed through a mastery of culinary skills. Merging nutrition and food science with the culinary arts will help consumers become aware of nutrition and confident to prepare food. Gaining an awareness of nutrition and learning to prepare food will enable consumers to develop healthy eating behaviors (Condrasky and Hegler 2010).

An example of culinary nutrition is the pairing of chefs with nutrition educators, most often seen in community outreach programs. Together, this team bridges the gap between the culinary and nutrition worlds, and individually can meet the demands set by each field. As a team, they set the standard for the meshing of the two fields. Both nutrition and culinary arts must be available to one another to successfully translate nutrition concepts and healthy cooking techniques into sustainable eating practices (Condrasky and Hegler 2010).

Food literacy, nutrition literacy, and culinary nutrition: Enabling personal and community empowerment

The International Federation for Home Economics identified three components of health and food literacy as functional (knowledge), interactive (skills), and critical (transformation and empowerment) (Murimi 2013). Functional literacy focuses on the communication of information while interactive literacy moves to the more complex development of personal skills. The basic level, interactive nutrition, reflects the ability to translate declarative knowledge into positive dietary choices, such as knowing that too much saturated fat is a problem and choosing a product lower in saturated fat. Critical health literacy is the development of capacities to enable personal and community empowerment. A community that lobbies against the establishment of a fast-food restaurant opposite a local school is exhibiting critical health literacy. More recently, the term "food literacy" as a component of health literacy has emerged, adopting the three levels of functional, interactive, and critical (Pendergast et al. 2011).

While nutrition education focuses on food intake and how the body utilizes nutrients for growth, development, and health, food literacy has a wider scope that ranges across food production, procurement, preparation, processing, packaging, and labeling to food choice and consumption (Murimi 2013). When examining the discourse surrounding food literacy, cooking arguably emerges as a fundamental theme. The significance of cooking has gained momentum in light of the demise of food preparation skills and their continual devaluation in Western society (Vidgen and Gallegos 2014).

Food literacy, nutrition literacy, and culinary nutrition are often used interchangeably. There is no consensus regarding the definitions, constituents, or relationship to each other. As currently defined, they are slightly different. However, food is a component of each. Considering the literature to date, empowerment lies at the core of current conceptualizations (Velardo 2015). Factors that contribute to poor dietary practices are complex and require an interdisciplinary approach. Therefore, it is important to continue to refine food and nutrition-related literacy terminology.

The path to food illiteracy

Historically, the path from field to plate to waste was easily identified and widely understood. The current food system is more complex and distant, rooted in global political and economic systems. Food decisions are still made individually, with the choice influenced by personal and external factors (Cullen et al. 2015). In the 1920s, food companies worked to persuade women that it was better to buy prepared food than to cook from scratch. With the 1920s came an increase in the availability and purchase of processed food. Women allowed themselves to lose their cooking skills, partly because no value was placed on cooking. They were told that smart women do not cook (Hall 1992).

Food marketers and researchers say that despite the desire to cook, the cooking skills of Americans have declined (Hall 1992). Cooking has evolved into an optional activity. Supermarkets carry a variety of convenience products, such as rotisserie chicken and fresh prepacked meal kits. Many young adults never learned how to cook, or they simply do not bother, because there are so many other choices, like fast food, takeout, or frozen dishes that can be microwaved. The National Pork Producers Council administered a cooking test to a sample of 735 adults. About 75% of the participants failed. Fifty percent of respondents did not know how to thicken gravy, and only 55% knew there are three teaspoons in a tablespoon (Hall 1992).

The "obesity–hunger paradox" arises not only from a lack of nutritious, affordable alternatives to fast food but also from a lack of knowledge about how to prepare nutritious food at home with inexpensive, basic ingredients. At the other extreme, high-end kitchen appliances now feature "smart" options that allow those with minimal cooking skills to prepare dishes or entire meals with the push of a button (Lichtenstein and Ludwig 2010).

According to Cullen et al. (2015), there are gaps in consumers' knowledge and skills surrounding food, particularly an understanding of how they are connected to the food they consume. The majority of Canadians' food purchases represent "ultra-processed" foods, exceeding the World Health Organization's upper limits for fat, saturated fat, sugars, and sodium with less fiber than recommended (Cullen et al. 2015). Research shows that the combination of insufficient vegetable and fruit consumption, increased frequency of away-from-home meals, poor food preparation skills, and increased portion size have all contributed to the rise in obesity and related chronic diseases (Condrasky and Hegler 2010). According to Condrasky and Hegler (2010), Americans have increased reliance on convenience products and have drastically different cooking and eating practices than previous generations. Changes in dietary patterns, such as increased consumption of processed food and insufficient vegetable and fruit consumption, parallel global shifts associated with rising rates of obesity and onset of chronic diseases (Cullen et al. 2015).

Why does the public need to be food literate?

Since nutrition is known to play a major role in health, food preparation and cooking skills have the potential to affect one's well-being and health (Anonymous 2011). Research shows multiple health benefits of eating home-cooked meals as opposed to eating out or relying on prepared foods. In addition, there is a growing demand for a more culinary-focused approach to health (Krieger 2014). Consumers want food that is good and not just good for them.

Adolescents who dine with their family have increased intake of dark green and orange vegetables. Conversely, consumption of saturated and trans fats, soft drinks, and fried foods is negatively associated with family meals. Overall, people who prepare food in the home are more inclined to eat smaller portions and consume fewer calories and less fat, salt, and sugar, which is more likely to result in healthy weight and chronic disease prevention (Jones et al. 2014).

During the past 30 years, the link between diet and certain chronic diseases, such as heart disease, hypertension, and certain types of cancer, has become well recognized. Chronic disease prevention requires consistency in the selection of appropriate food and long-term maintenance of health habits. The increase in diet-related diseases has been linked to poor eating habits and a perceived diminishing understanding and skill set around food and its use (Vidgen and Gallegos 2014). The ability to prepare food and follow a recipe can have an impact on one's food choices. If a person becomes reliant on foods requiring minimal preparation, or food prepared for them, it puts a constraint on their choice such that consumers will become increasingly disconnected from preparation (Meckna 2006).

Child and adult obesity is a growing concern among affluent nations. Recent studies reveal that a high standard of living is often positively correlated with health-related diseases, including obesity, heart disease, and cancer. The World Health Organization has declared that childhood obesity is one of the most serious public health challenges of the twenty-first century (Pendergast et al. 2011). Nearly one-third of U.S. children aged 2–19 are overweight or obese, according to a 2014 report from the Centers for Disease Control and Prevention. The childhood obesity rate has more than tripled over the past four decades, though rates have leveled off in recent years. While some progress has been made, data show that significant racial/ethnic and socioeconomic disparities persist in obesity prevalence (Kidsdata.org).

According to Cullen et al. (2015), food-related health problems are on the rise in Canada. Attention to our relationship with food may be a step toward addressing these health-related problems (Cullen et al. 2015). The unprecedented increase in diet-related diseases has been linked to poor eating habits and perceived diminishing understanding and skill set around food and its use (Vidgen and Gallegos 2014). Skills in food preparation are considered an essential component of translating nutrition knowledge into dietary practices (Velardo 2015).

Americans spend less time cooking than people in many other countries. Countries, where individuals spend more time preparing foods, have lower obesity rates (Palmer 2013). Although the optimal diet for obesity and chronic disease prevention remains the subject of investigation, broad consensus exists regarding the benefits of home-prepared meals. Research suggests that frequent consumption of restaurant food, take-out food, and prepared snacks lowers dietary quality and promotes weight gain. Food preparation by adolescents and young adults may have the opposite effect by displacing poor choices (Lichtenstein and Ludwig 2010).

How do we increase food literacy?

There is a growing interest in food, cooking, and nutrition due to the increasing number of celebrity chefs, cooking magazines, and cooking-related television shows. Although there is growing curiosity about food, it is not being met with the nutrition knowledge to link food preparation techniques to effectively alter eating behaviors (Condrasky and Hegler 2010).

Owing to an increased reliance on convenience products, Americans possess drastically different cooking and eating practices compared with previous generations (Condrasky and Hegler 2010). In 2014, American consumers spent more money for food in away-from-home establishments than for meals prepared and consumed at home. Spending at away-from-home food establishments accounted for 50.1% of the $1.46 trillion spent on food and beverages (USDA, accessed on May 5, 2016).

Nutrition and culinary arts are needed as one entity working together for a common cause of outreach during this diet-related health crisis. In other words, making vital nutrition information easily accessible is useless without also making it practical (Condrasky and Hegler 2010). Knowledge alone has proven ineffective in altering eating behavior, but offering hands-on cooking and tasting demonstrations appears to be far more beneficial. The transition from knowledge to practice is viewed as a vital component of food literacy. Pairing nutrition and culinary arts is a natural way to further nutrition awareness and knowledge. Cooking education can provide participants with a sense of control over ingredients, preparation style, and portion sizes. Pairing culinary arts with nutrition incorporates food qualities like taste, satiety, and appearance along with nutrition goals. Applying nutrition principles to food preparation transforms learning into a delicious, nutritious experience by allowing people to actually see, feel, and taste what nutrition is all about (Condrasky and Hegler 2010).

To improve eating and cooking habits, the concepts of culinary nutrition must be shared. While nutrition and health intervention programs have traditionally focused on changing knowledge, attitudes, and behaviors, the addition of hands-on cooking activities allows all three focus areas to come together. Nutrition classes lead to increased nutrition knowledge but not necessarily changes in dietary habits; cooking classes improve food preparation abilities but may not translate into healthy cooking. Although cooking skills alone, without other diet-related education, will not completely change eating behaviors, there is a connection between confidence in cooking abilities and healthy eating habits. General knowledge about nutrition, analytical skills for planning and evaluating nutritionally sound meals, technical knowledge, and refined cooking skills are all needed in order to improve eating behavior (Condrasky and Hegler 2010).

One method of implementing culinary nutrition is through hands-on education programs. While there are numerous nutrition education programs and just as many cooking programs, there are very few that pair the two fields together. Although the literature is limited, researchers have begun to evaluate the effects of implementing cooking activities into nutrition education programs. Preliminary evidence shows that an increase in cooking knowledge and skills can help improve eating behaviors (Condrasky et al. 2011). With all sorts of barriers to maintaining a healthy lifestyle, such as frequency of dining out, lack of time or money, taste preferences, and lack of nutrition knowledge and skills, developers of successful nutrition education programs must broaden their scope of implementing nutrition in a quick, easy, affordable, and convenient manner (Condrasky and Hegler 2010).

Potential interventions to increase food literacy

Revive home economics programs

Parents and caregivers cannot be expected or relied upon to teach children how to prepare healthy meals. Since many parents never learned to cook, children rarely experience what a true home-cooked meal tastes like, or what goes into preparing it. Work schedules and child extracurricular activities frequently prevent involving children in food shopping and preparation (Lichtenstein and Ludwig 2010).

Home economics, otherwise known as domestic education, was a fixture in secondary schools through the 1960s. The underlying concept was that future homemakers should be educated in the care and feeding of their families. This idea seems quaint, but in the midst of a pediatric obesity epidemic and concerns about the poor diet quality of adolescents in the United States, instruction in basic food preparation and meal planning skills needs to be part of any long-term solution (Lichtenstein and Ludwig 2010).

According to Dyas (2014), universities started to defund home economics programs during the Cold War era. Also, the increase in convenience foods made-from-scratch cooking seems irrelevant. As college-level courses disappeared, those at the high school level lost their appeal. Home economics became associated with dead-end high school classes for girls (Dyas 2014).

A new home economics curriculum should teach males and females basic principles they will need to feed themselves and their families within the current food environment. Through a combination of instruction, demonstrations, and field trips, this new home economics curriculum would aim to transform meal preparation from an intimidating chore into a manageable and rewarding pursuit. It is important to dispel the myth that cooking takes too much time or skill and that nutritious food cannot be delicious. As youth transition into adulthood, they should be provided with the knowledge to prepare meals that are quick, delicious, and nutritious (Lichtenstein and Ludwig 2010).

The Queensland Government has developed an initiative to improve the food literacy of its youth. The project aims, through the development of food literacy, to change eating habits, particularly those of children, leading to a reduction in overweight and obesity levels in the community. One part of the initiative is running a kitchen that will deliver six cooking classes a day, 6 days a week, and 48 weeks a year for 4 years. Students are exposed to food preparation skills so that they not only gain a theoretical understanding of appropriate nutrition, but also acquire skills to enact this knowledge (Pendergast et al. 2011).

Youth cooking programs

The younger generation has taken an interest in cooking (Stanton 2016). Cooking is frequently a part of afterschool programs. When cooking clubs are offered in after school programs, they are some of the first clubs to reach maximum enrollment. An after school program offered by Jones (2015) teaches basic cooking skills to middle school youth. It is a hands-on program with each child participating in the food preparation process.

Jones (2015) offers a 5-week cooking class to college students. The class easily and quickly fills its 20 slots. Upon completion of the course, students state that they feel more capable of preparing food for themselves. When one student was asked why he took the class, he stated that he would soon be living on his own and did not want to consume only processed foods (Jones 2015).

The National Restaurant Association offers a cooking program, ProStart® for high school students. This program targets those students wanting to pursue a career in the restaurant and food service industry (https://www.chooserestaurants.org/ProStart). Some universities also offer culinary arts camps for high school students (http://4h.unl.edu/big-red-camps).

Food literacy partners program

The Food Literacy Partners Program (FLPP) is a program developed by the University of North Carolina to expand the number of individuals capable of delivering credible nutrition information to the community. It is based on the

Master Gardener model of "learn and serve" (Rawl et al. 2008). The FLPP provides 20 hours of food and nutrition education to volunteers in exchange for 20 hours of community nutrition education service. It focuses on delivering food and nutrition to help individuals make appropriate eating decisions (Rawl et al. 2008).

Grocery store dietitians

In the 1980s, five or six supermarkets had dietitians. The number of supermarket dietitians has been increasing (Schwartz 2016). These dietitians' job responsibilities are wide and varied, from developing brochures to hosting to cooking demonstrations to giving grocery store tours. However, they all have one common goal—to help Americans make better food choices every day. The reason for this trend includes consumer interest in nutrition education and special dietary requirements. Also, people are not cooking the way they used to. They want to know how to put together meals that are quick, easy, and good value (Schwartz 2016).

Food processors/kids in the kitchen

For years the food industry lamented that consumers lacked the ability to cook. They stated that things were better when consumers cooked from scratch. There now may be a resurgence of cooking (Stanton 2016). Food companies, magazines, and cookbook publishers appear to be encouraging this trend. Most food companies now have a food preparation section on their website. Some have a section that targets children. In addition to recipes, websites also give tips for parents of picky eaters and for parents to help children to develop food preparation skills. Uncle Ben's website (Ben's Beginners™) makes this statement about teaching children to cook. "Ben's Beginners is a movement that inspires healthy beginnings by encouraging families to cook together. When parents and kids connect in the kitchen, children make healthier decisions about eating. They also discover that home-cooked meals aren't just better for them, they're also fun to make!" (Uncle Ben's website, n.d.). For the digital natives, websites can be a good place to help develop food preparation skills.

Subscription food services

Subscription food services, such as Plated, Hello Fresh, Peach Dish, and Blue Apron, are gaining in popularity. A subscription service appeals to consumers who want fresh, authentic food, and control over what they are eating. These services promise delicious food and convenience. Each package contains everything an individual needs to cook, including a recipe card and the necessary pre-portioned ingredients. They only ship what you need to make a recipe, so there is less waste. You will not need a pantry of unfamiliar spices that you may never use again. These services offer convenience, a way to cook more, eat healthy, and waste less.

Subscription food services allow consumers to have restaurant quality meals at home for less money than at an actual restaurant. A subscription food service does not eliminate the need to go to the grocery store. Consumers only receive meal kits for a few dinners. Generally, they do not provide sufficient ingredients for leftovers. A subscription service will save shopping time, but may not save preparation time. Ingredients still need to be chopped and measured. Also, if you like to "throw together" something, a service might not be for you (Lazzaro 2016).

Implications for the future

Public excitement over cooking programs is an opportunity for public health professionals to harness this energy and discover the most beneficial approaches to promote long-term dietary changes and subsequent health outcomes. Continued conversation about the direction of cooking initiatives and implementation of these initiatives alongside interrelated measures such as increasing food accessibility and affordability are essential. Owing to the current rates of overweight and obesity in the United States, strong public enthusiasm for cooking classes provides a rare public health opportunity to engage the community while working to affect dietary outcomes, overweight, and obesity, and related health conditions (Reicks et al. 2014).

REFERENCES

Anonymous. 2011. Can cooking skills be the key to health? *Food Today* 11. Accessed April 28, 2016. http://www.eufic.org/en/healthy-living/article/can-cooking-skills-be-the-key-to-health

Condrasky, M. and M. Hegler. 2010. How culinary nutrition can save the health of a nation. *Journal of Extension* 48(2). Accessed April 28, 2016. http://www.joe.org/joe/2010april/comm1.php

Condrasky, M., J. Williams, P. Catalano, and S. Griffin. 2011. Development of psychosocial scales for evaluating the impact of a culinary nutrition education program on cooking and healthful eating. *Journal of Nutrition Education and Behavior* 43:511–516.

Cullen, T., J. Hatch, W. Martin, J. Higgins, and R. Sheppard. 2015. Food literacy: Definition and framework for action. *Canadian Journal of Dietetic Practice Research* 76:140–145.

Dyas, B. 2014. Who killed home Ec? Here's the real story behind its demise. *The Huffington Post* September 29. Accessed August 28, 2016. http://www.huffingtonpost.com/2014/09/29/home-ec-classes_n_5882830.html

Hall, T. 1992. New 'Lost Generation': The Cooking Illiterate. *The New York Times* January 15. Accessed May 10, 2016. http://www.nytimes.com/1992/01/15/garden/new-lost-generation-the-cooking-illiterate.html?pagewanted=all

Jones, G. 2015. Unpublished data.

Jones, S., J. Walter, L. A. Soliah, and J. Phifer. 2014. Perceived motivators to home food preparation: Focus group findings. *Journal of the Academy of Nutrition and Dietetics* 114:1552–1556.

Kidsdata.org. Accessed August 28, 2016. http://www.kidsdata.org/topic

Krieger, E. 2014. 2013 Lenna Frances Cooper Memorial Lecture: Bringing cooking back: Food and culinary expertise as a key to dietitians' future success. *Journal of the Academy of Nutrition and Dietetics* 114:313–319.

Lazzaro, S. 2016. We tried Blue Apron, Hello Fresh and their 4 competitors – One was clearly the best, the observer. Accessed May 15, 2016. http://observer.com/2016/01/we-tried-blue-apron-hello-fresh-and-their-4-competitors-one-was-clearly-the-best/

Lichtenstein, A. and D. Ludwig. 2010. Bring back home economics education. *Journal of the American Medical Association* 303:1857–1858.

Meckna, B. 2006. Assessing the food literacy of college students. *Master's thesis*, University of Nebraska.

Murimi, M. 2013. Health literacy, nutrition education, and food literacy. *Journal of Nutrition Education and Behavior* 45:195.

Palmer, S. 2013. Get clients cooking!. *Today's Dietitian* 15:28–32.

Pendergast, D., S. Garvis, and H. Kanasa. 2011. Insight from the public on home economics and formal food literacy. *Family and Consumer Sciences Research Journal* 39:415–430.

Pray, L. 2016. *Food Literacy: How Do Communications and Marketing Impact Consumer Knowledge, Skills, and Behavior?* Washington, DC: The National Academies Press. doi: 10.17226/21897.

Rawl, R., K. Kolasa, J. Lee, and L. Whetstone. 2008. A learn and serve nutrition program: The food literacy partners program. *Journal of Nutrition Education and Behavior* 40:49–51.

Reicks, M., A. Trofholz, J. Stang, M. Laska. 2014. Impact of cooking and home food preparation interventions among adults outcomes and implications for future programs. *Journal of Nutrition Education and Behavior* 46:259–276.

Schwartz, K. 2016. The Supermarket RDN, Eat Right Pro. Accessed May 15, 2016. http://www.eatrightpro.org/resource/news-center/in-practice/dietetics-in-action/the-supermarket-rdn

Selden, C. R., M. Zorn, S. C. Ratzan, and R. M. Parker. 2000. *National Library of Medicine Current Bibliographies in Medicine: Health Literacy*. NLM Pub. No. CBM 2000-1. Bethesda, MD: National Institutes of Health, U.S. Department of Health and Human Services.

Smith, L., S. Ng, and B. Popkin. 2013. Trends in US home food preparation and consumption: Analysis of national nutrition surveys and time use studies from 1965–1966 to 2007–2008. *Nutrition Journal* 12. Accessed April 28, 2016. doi: 10.1186/1475-2891-12-45.

Stanton, J. 2016. Market view: Kids are discovering cooking. *Food Processing*. Accessed February 18, 2016. http://www.foodprocessing.com/articles/2016/market-view-kids-cooking/

Uncle Ben's. Ben's Beginners. n.d. https://beginners.unclebens.com/ accessed May 17, 2016.

Vaitkeviciute, R., L. Ball, and N. Harris. 2014. The relationship between food literacy and dietary intake in adolescents: A systematic review. *Public Health Nutrition* 18(4):649–658. doi: 10.1017/S1368980014000962.

Velardo, S. 2015. The nuances of health literacy, nutrition literacy, and food literacy. *Journal of Nutrition Education and Behavior* 47:385–389.

Vidgen, H. and D. Gallegos. 2014. Defining food literacy and its components. *Appetite* 76:50–59.

Part VI

Changing food and health policy

16 Toward a just food system

Megan McGuffey and Anthony Starke

When does life begin? Is physician-assisted suicide a viable option for terminally ill patients? What is the proper role of government? All of these questions may seem out of place in a book about the food system; however, in some small way, they are relevant. Each of these questions, as well as many more seemingly unrelated ones, offers some insight into our individually held beliefs about what is right and what is wrong. More importantly, the answers to these questions espouse the values that contribute to the ideologies that shape our worldview. "An ideology is a relatively coherent system of ideas (beliefs, traditions, principles, and myths) about human nature, institutional arrangements, and social processes held by individuals and groups in society" (Abramovitz 2004, p. 19).

In this chapter, we will discuss the concept of justice and its application to food, the food system, and its associated politics. The scope of discussions regarding food justice can be defined as "seeking to transform where, what, and how food is grown, produced, transported, accessed, and eaten" (Gottlieb and Joshi 2010, p. 5). What you will not find in this chapter is a formula, recipe, or prescription for justice, but rather we will present things to be considered when evaluating fairness within the food system. Food is a highly politicized terrain, and this chapter will: review theories of justice, survey policy and program analysis techniques, and present a concise history of food justice literature and initiatives. Since justice is an abstract construct, this chapter will provide readers with the tools to identify what they believe are the attributes of justice and the skills for assessing a system's ability to manifest those characteristics. We will also argue for the importance of including justice as a key consideration for any policy proposal impacting food issues. Finally, we will take our discussion of food justice and public policy and explore a future research agenda that places food issues as a concern for the field of public administration.

Food and the modern political agenda

Across the globe, governments at all levels are attempting to address food issues in new and innovative ways through public policy. A recent court case in Italy found that it may not be a crime to steal small amounts of food if the theft was committed for essential and immediate survival (Pianigiani and Chan 2016). In

2016, the French Senate passed a law making it illegal for grocery stores to throw away or destroy their unsold food, forcing them to donate it instead (Chrisafis 2016). Cities across the United States are changing local laws to allow people to grow and sell food in urban areas (Mukherji and Morales 2010). Food issues are not new to the public policy agenda; nonetheless, this interest is taking on new dimensions.

Food policy has increased in complexity from its beginnings as a relatively technical and narrow policy field. The passage of farm bills now includes an expanded number of policy issues and an increasing number of interest groups are involved in the legislative debates (Lehrer 2010). In 1900, 41% of the work-force was employed in agriculture, but technological advancements and the industrialization of agriculture created the current conditions where just 2% of the population is employed in this industry (Dimitri, Effland, and Conklin 2005). Policy debates on food issues at the federal level are still dominated by commodity agriculture, but recent farm bills and work by the United States Department of Agriculture (USDA) have recognized a trend toward local and regional food systems that are redirecting some resources and attention to the specific policy needs of this area (United States Department of Agriculture [USDA] 2015). Many municipal governments are also prioritizing food issues on their policy agendas (Stockman 2012). Revising land-use laws, creating policies that encourage agriculture as a land use, promoting community and school gardens, and supporting farm-to-school initiatives are just a few of the most popular approaches currently in use.

The United States has a deeply rooted history with agriculture. In early American history, most families grew a large portion of their own food for survival, making agriculture a largely private concern. As our nation grew and urbanized, there was a greater need to specialize industries and exchange goods, including agricultural products. More and more people became disconnected from the sources of their food, gradually creating a regulatory role for government. The Farm Bill is the major legislation influencing federal food policy. The earliest versions of these laws focused on stabilizing the farm economy through policy measures such as price supports and production controls. The first farm bill was passed in 1933 by President Roosevelt during the height of the Great Depression, in order to level out the "booms and busts of agricultural production" (Lehrer 2010, p. 9). While the concerns of food producers have continued to dominate discussions of federal food policy, the needs of consumers have become a substantial component of federal spending in this area.

Beginning with the National School Lunch Act of 1946, social welfare programs have gradually been added to the Farm Bill. While smaller feeding programs had been piloted during previous periods of economic crisis, it was this change in the farm bill that permanently joined the interests of agricultural policy and social welfare policy, as they relate to food. Beyond school feeding programs, additional social welfare programs now include the Supplemental Nutrition Assistance Program (SNAP; also known as food stamps), the Women, Infant, & Children (WIC) nutrition program, food benefits for seniors, and others. These programs now dominate federal spending, accounting for 79% of the Farm Bill budget (Plumer 2013). Other interests now incorporated in modern farm bills include conservation efforts, funding for local and regional food development, and a greater focus on renewable energy (Lehrer 2010). As food moved from the private to the public realm and the impact of policy-making in this area reached larger and larger numbers of citizens, a greater diversity of perspectives need to be considered and the potential for marginalization increased.

Injustice in food policy

Since the scope of food policy has expanded, the gap between political winners and losers has increased, often to the detriment of society's most vulnerable members. We will show that there is a history of food policy adversely affecting the minority and politically weak populations in the United States, which suggests the need for special attention to justice in future food policy discussions. Moreover, different actors in the food arena have different concerns, which may or may not be addressed in food-related policies. For example, food system workers, ranging from farm workers to those employed in food retail, face several occupational safety issues. Many of these jobs are high-risk, and employees often do not receive health insurance or paid sick days, proper safety training or equipment, and only 13.5% receive a living wage (Shannon et al. 2015). These issues are worsened by the fact that agriculture has historically been exempt from many labor laws (Shannon et al. 2015).

Furthermore, policies are often structured in ways that harm different minority populations, which is not always unintended. Large states with influential agricultural industries, such as California, helped push for many of these laws. The Bracero Program that began during WWII and continued well into the 1960s was a migrant labor program for Mexican agricultural workers mostly in California. While it had the potential to improve labor laws and treatment of agriculture workers, policy stakeholders instead managed to use it to preserve low wages and poor standards of living for these workers in violent and racialized ways (Mitchell 2010).

The issues faced by African American farmers, while also understudied, reveal the troubling legacy of injustice in food policy (Green, Green, and Kleiner 2011; Petty and Schultz 2013). Many theoretical and empirical works do not specifically address Black farmers, despite the fact that this group has engaged in U.S. agriculture since the time of slavery (Green, Green, and Kleiner 2011). African American farmers have faced discriminatory practices such as sharecropping and unfair treatment in federal agriculture programs (Green, Green, and Kleiner 2011; Petty and Schultz 2013). With fewer resources and greater institutional barriers, Black farmers have been disproportionately driven out of agriculture by agricultural crises and there has been a huge loss of land and farm ownership in this group (Green, Green, and Kleiner 2011). The USDA has one of the most troubling and persistent histories with discrimination of any federal agency, which has helped create or made these problems worse (Petty and Schultz 2013). While local political control has been popular across policy areas in recent years and particularly touted by food movement activists, a knowledge of agricultural history for African Americans brings forth justice concerns with such approaches. The USDA has a long history with local control of agricultural programs, which allowed White elites to control these programs and harm poor and minority farmers (Petty and Schultz 2013).

There is an overall dearth of data available on rates of food insecurity among Native Americans in the United States (Gunderson 2006; Jernigan et al. 2013; Skinner, Prately, and Burnett 2016). The United States government has a history of poor treatment of Native Americans including, but not limited to, stripping them of their land and property and relocating them to reservations as well as the forced enrollment of Native American children in boarding schools where they were separated from their families and cultures. Part of the legacy of these injustices has been disproportionately low economic prosperity leaving this group vulnerable to food insecurity (Gunderson 2006). While high overall, rates of food insecurity and the specific challenges faced vary based on Native American peoples' environment, whether it be reservations, rural, or urban (Skinner et al. 2016). Compounding these problems, many traditional strategies for food access that could serve Native American families through personal consumption and sales (such as hunting and foraging) may not be included in mainstream food policies (Stroink and Nelson 2013). Nuanced and in-depth examinations of the unique challenges resulting from injustices, policy-related and otherwise, are warranted.

As demonstrated by this brief review, there is a long history of food policy harming the minority and politically weak populations in the United States. This historical perspective should encourage us to put justice at the forefront of any assessment of future food policies. Of note is the de jure and de facto nature of discrimination in food legislation. If we continue to overlook these inequalities and assume neutral and/or positive effects, many people who have been marginalized will continue to be adversely affected.

Understanding justice

Given the historical injustices of food policy, how then are we to avoid these pitfalls in the future? Some might assume that justice-oriented policies are the proper mechanism for overcoming injustice. However, this presumption begs the question, "What is justice?" Perhaps the most well-known justice theorist is political philosopher John Rawls (1971), who argued the two principles of justice: basic freedom and the difference principle. That is (a) human beings have a reasonable expectation of equal basic liberties and (b) inequalities must be to the benefit of the least advantaged. More importantly, Rawls' thought experiment, *The Veil of Ignorance*, compels others to critique their society from a position of imaginary ignorance, in which achievement is the function of fortune rather than merit. Rawls does this by asking his audience to imagine a state of consciousness before birth, wherein the subject has no possible conception of the fortune into which they will be born. How then would they desire the society to be structured? Rawls asserts that therein lies the answer to how we ought to improve our society. In this thought tradition, justice is characterized as fairness. For the purposes of this chapter, we define justice, from an ontological perspective, as a moral assessment of human decision-making. Consequently, justice can be understood as the outcomes of human activities, with social justice emphasizing the distribution of burdens and benefits across groups of individuals. Our individual and collective experiences, as well as past policies, have also shaped the discourse of who is and who is not deserving (Katz 2013; Schneider, Ingram, and deLeon 2014), thus altering our perceptions of right, wrong, and obligation.

Political ideologies are undergirded by assumptions about human nature, each of which has implications for how we desire social arrangements to be. While conservatives contend that many public social policies and programs are ineffective wastes of taxpayer dollars, incentivize laziness, promote dependency, and inhibit enterprise (Chelf 1992), liberals conversely "see social welfare policies as the legitimate function of a government that cares about the welfare of its citizens" (p. 9). Libertarians argue that in a society there is no central distributor but rather the results of a conglomeration of individual decisions, each of which is not unjust (Winfrey 1998). For libertarians, the concept of social justice itself is a fabricated fallacy because there is no single agent, such as government, that consciously and biasedly distributes benefits and burdens. Communitarianism counters the Western emphasis on individualism. This ideology contends that it is "natural to have individual and social needs" and views the nature of society as "cooperative and participatory" (Winfrey 1998, p. 14). Here, we can see that each of these views can lead to very different expectations of societal arrangements. Other examples of the various nuanced ideologies include social conservatism, laissez-faire economic conservatism, pragmatic liberalism, humanistic liberalism, radicalism, Marxism, liberal feminism, cultural feminism, and socialist feminism, to name a few (see Abramovitz 2004). Nevertheless, our individual political ideologies provide different criteria for assessing the justice and fairness of particular policies.

Assessing fair and just public policy

As an enterprise of practice and scholarship, the domain of public administration entails the implementation of public policy and the management of public programs (Denhardt and Denhardt 2009). Some public administration scholars claim that the undergirding philosophy of public administration is "the ideal of science, the absence of poverty, the end of waste and corruption, and the elimination of extreme inequality" (Miller 2012, p. 63). In attempts to live up to this ultimate purpose, public administration scholars and practitioners continually assess and evaluate practices, policies, and programs in hopes of optimizing the principles of economy, efficiency, effectiveness, and/or equity, at no cost to the others (Norman-Major 2011). However, as the discipline has evolved over time, justice and fairness have become concepts emblematic of the public's interest. In public administration, "The first question is whether an existing public program or proposed program is effective or good. The second question is more important. For whom is the program effective or good?" (Frederickson 2005, p. 36). Thus, the concept of *equity* seeks to answer the question "justice for whom?" (Gooden 2015).

"Social equity is used as a descriptor for those administrative activities implemented in pursuit of fairness, justice, and equality" (Frederickson and Henry 1990, p. 78). According to Fredrickson and Henry's Compound Theory of Social Equity, there are six dimensions of equality which provide an analytical framework for assessing equity (Table 16.1).

Norman Johnson and James Svara (2011) have conceptualized four dimensions for the analysis of social equity: procedural fairness, access, quality, and outcome. Taken together, these dimensions are intended to promote and ensure equal protection, appropriate resource allocation, consistent quality of service, and the absence of disparities. Other scholars have applied the concept of Catholic Social Theory to the administration of public goods and services (Abel 2014). In the Catholic conception of justice, the three guiding principles of administration are

Table 16.1 Compound Theory of Social Equity

Equality	Description
Simple individual	"Individual equality consists of one class of equals, and one relationship of equality where intrinsic or extrinsic factors do not constitute a justification for variation."
Segmented	"Segmented equalities call for equal treatment within segments and unequal treatment between them."
Block	"Block equalities call for equality between groups or subclasses. It argues that one block is equal to the other while recognizing considerable variation within each."
Domain of equality	"The domain of equality is the sphere or range where decisions are made about what is to be distributed. Domains of equality constantly shift, aggregate, and disaggregate. There is a domain of allocation based on available resources, and a domain of claims which accounts for what people in blocks or segments wish to have equally distributed."
Equalities of opportunity	"Equalities of opportunity are divided into prospect and means. In the abstract, prospect equality is compelling, the idea being that everyone has equal prospects for achievement. However, because each one of us is different and, in a sense, unequal, means equality comes into play."
Values of equality	"Values of equality can be money, power, prestige, or whatever is divisible. On the surface, the equitable distribution of services or dollars may seem fair, yet fail to recognize the wide variations in need."

Source: Frederickson, H. G. and B. M. Henry. 1990. Social equity for nursing administration and knowledge-development. In *Practice and Inquiry for Nursing Administration: Intradisciplinary and Interdisciplinary Perspectives: Solicited Papers and Proceedings of the Santa Fe Conference*, edited by B. M. Henry, pp. 76–100.

distributism, subsidiarity, and solidarity. In all, the three principles of Catholic Social Theory attempt to (a) minimize disparity by distributing benefits and burdens in their most effective manner, (b) accentuate the empowerment of both the individual and the group, and (c) emphasize the importance of trust among actors.

When multiple actors and/or multiple interests are at play, it is generally the case that decision-making becomes a much more complicated task. Often, "a moral dilemma arises when we must choose between two or more apparently conflicting moral choices" (Winfrey 1998, p. 2). In this instance, it is necessary to determine which ethical dimension you will use to assess the alternatives. Teleological and deontological are two such philosophical approaches. That is, either a consideration of the consequences of actions or the obligation to others, respectively. Teleological approaches evaluate the consequences of actions. Deontological approaches, on the other hand, examine the fairness of the processes. From a policy or program evaluation standpoint, this is akin to an outcomes versus a process evaluation, wherein to evaluate the efficacy of a program or policy intervention, it is first necessary to specify the attributes under investigation (i.e., outcome or process). For example, would you consider a policy just or fair if all affected parties were able to provide input in the policy design process, or would the policy be considered just or fair if all affected parties were better off as a result of the policy? Either approach would be an acceptable method of assessment.

Anne Ingram and Helen Schneider are the architects of Democratic Policy Design theory (Schneider, Ingram, and deLeon 2014). This theory, which emphasizes the social construction of target populations, "incorporates the social construction and power of target populations to understand the development and implications of policy design" (Pierce et al. 2014, p. 1). Democratic Policy Design theory presumes that policy designs reinforce the socially constructed knowledge and perpetuate a socially constructed reality (Pierce et al. 2014; Schneider, Ingram, and deLeon 2014). This is, in fact, an acknowledgment of Theodore Lowi's assertion that policies influence politics (Ingram and Schneider 1997). The five basic propositions of the theory are as follows:

1.   The distribution of benefits and burdens is contingent upon a group's political power and social construction.
2.   Policy designs have effects on the attitudes and political participation of groups.
3.   Social constructions materialize from emotional reactions and value-laden judgments.
4.   Changes in social constructions may often occur as a result of unintended consequences to previous policies.
5.   Policy change is dependent upon the power and social construction of target groups.

Schneider and Ingram's approach reinforces the study of social equity by introducing the concept of deservingness into the study of public policy. Its use of the dual dimensions of social construction and power allows scholars to address what Laswell and Kaplan identified as the longstanding questions of "who gets what, when and how" (Pierce et al. 2014, p. 3), or what social equity scholars refer to as the second question—that is, policy for whom? Other theories are not as readily capable or explicitly committed to addressing such issues. This is not to say that other theories do not have implications for how we are to assess the fairness of public policies. For example, Public Choice Theory, which views constituents as consumers, encourages a market-based approach to public service, wherein citizens are given the power to make decisions about who or what agency provides their publicly funded service. This approach, not unlike libertarianism, believes justice and fairness are present when we allow individuals to make the decision.

What is presented here illustrates that there are multiple ways of defining justice, each of which leads to its own beliefs about what is and what is not just. More importantly, multifaceted issues, such as food, that involve various actors make it much more difficult to develop an all-encompassing and just policy. Therefore, it is imperative that we remain cognizant of how our individual ideologies may conflict with someone else's views regarding justice and fairness.

Approaches to studying and practicing food justice

In studying and working within the food system today, we see many advances as well as increased attention to considerations of food issues, but many complex problems remain. Everybody eats; therefore, issues of food call upon deeply held beliefs and assumptions for any individual. Our cultures and indeed our very identities are intertwined with our food (e.g., what we eat, how it is prepared, and how it is consumed). This results in passionate opinions about any food policy under consideration. There is no universally accepted definition of what activities and scholarship qualify as food justice. Our goal in this chapter is to ensure that justice is a key consideration in any policy discussion related to food. When we engage in discussions of justice in the food system, it becomes especially important to uncover and examine the many assumptions built into our historical understanding of the food system and how those assumptions continue to impact modern assessment and advocacy in this arena.

To quote a public administrator of the Truman Era, Rufus Miles, "where you stand depends on where you sit" (p. 399). Miles's original quote referred to how individuals' perspectives will change based on what organization they work for since our loyalties and perspectives are shaped by our professional associations (Miles 1978). We believe this quote can also be applied to the influence of personal and political ideologies on questions of justice. As citizens, and especially as public administrators, we must be aware of our ideological commitments and how they color our evaluations of public discourse and policy proposals, especially in the evolving arena of food policy.

The modern food movement is a diverse and sometimes internally conflicted social movement. Advocates and grassroots actors operating from a variety of perspectives have identified numerous problems with the existing structures of our industrialized food system. While a plurality of ideas and proposals for change have emerged from diverse perspectives, the dominant narrative appears to have a largely White and middle-class character. This narrative draws on a nostalgia for the past, ignoring the varied histories and experiences of different groups during those times. Consequently, recommended solutions assume that all people have the same needs from the food system and that they have similar resources to reshape it along the lines of these idealized proposals (Hope Alkon and Agyeman 2011).

One symptom of this problem in the dominant food movement narrative is the "local trap" or "...the tendency of food activists and researchers to assume something inherent about the local scale" (Born and Purcell 2006, p. 195). With the negative reaction to the globalized and industrial food system, many people falsely attribute positive traits to local food, without specifying or critically examining what makes local better. Local is a scale, and so it does not inherently assure that broad concerns of the food movement will be prioritized in implementation, including, but not limited to, ecological sustainability, social and economic justice, food quality and human health (Born and Purcell 2006). Hinrichs (2003) discusses the problematic nature of trying to frame globalization and localization as distinct movements on opposite poles, as well as conflating local with "good" and global with "bad" qualities when these are actually related and mutually conditioning concepts. In Europe, scholarship has grown around the idea of "alternative food networks," but scholars acknowledge the difficulties in using this concept, which is often built around different and competing definitions leading them to call for research to clarify these issues (Sonnino and Marsden 2006).

Community food security (CFS) is a concept with roots in antihunger, community development, and sustainable agriculture activism (Palmer, Chen, and Winne 2014). CFS is viewed both as a social movement and as (a) an analytic tool for understanding the issue of food security, (b) a method for developing food-secure communities, and (c) as a goal in and of itself (Palmer et al. 2014). While CFS has been successful in bringing diverse stakeholders together, practitioners and academics in this area have struggled to develop standardized measures of CFS. Furthermore, there are calls for more rigorous research and greater sharing between communities.

The right to food and the right to health were established in the International Bill of Human Rights in 1948 through the United Nations.* Despite this long history, many justice issues remain in our food system. Shannon et al. (2015) have advanced the United Nations' definition by detailing the interconnectedness of health and food and the important dimensions of these two (i.e., availability, accessibility, adaptability). Additionally, they hold that sustainability must also be interlinked with the right to food and the right to health (Shannon et al. 2015).

* http://www.ohchr.org/Documents/Publications/FactSheet2Rev.1en.pdf

The advocacy organization, *Just Food*, defines food justice as follows: "communities exercising their right to grow, sell, and eat healthy food. Healthy food is fresh, nutritious, affordable, culturally-appropriate, and grown locally with care for the well-being of the land, workers, and animals."* While the issues falling under the umbrella of food justice are as old as human civilization, the modern vocabulary for these concerns and the related scholarship has seen rapid growth in attention during the past decade (Gottlieb and Joshi 2010). Individuals across many disciplines are approaching food justice through their unique lenses while we collectively attempt to operationalize these ideas. Gottlieb and Joshi (2010) note that

> In some ways, food justice has become a way to express discontent about the food system and the desire for change, without necessarily providing a clearly defined agenda for how to bring about that change. Even among advocates and groups that have adopted the term *food justice*, there remains contradictions or at least differences in translating understanding to action. (p. xiv)

The historical background of food policies in the United States and discussion of the various definitions and conceptual approaches to food justice provided above are shared in hopes of demonstrating the diversity of this body of scholarship and the enormous potential for further study. We may not have a singular definition or approach to food justice, but this variation is a strength that can allow voices that have been marginalized to be heard and a plurality of disciplines to tackle this worthy topic.

The state of food justice in public administration

Food is an important issue that needs consideration. Within the food system, there are multiple groups of actors, including producers and consumers, each with their own justice concerns. These concerns can clash at times, calling for scholars and practitioners to have coherent understandings of these issues when weighing the consequences—intended and otherwise—of various food policies. Our brief survey of food justice literature serves as a point of departure for considering the design and implementation of food policy. We bring special attention to the issue of food justice, both because it is a fairly new concept to many administrators and because it has such a far-ranging impact on the general public.

As a field of scholarship and practice, the domain of public administration is the implementation of public policy. Since it relates to the topic at hand, the assessment of issues of justice emphasizes action rather than intent. While elected officials are charged with creating our laws and policies, the complexity of implementing even a fairly straightforward law leaves much room for interpretation by public administrators. It is in this process of transforming ideas into actions that

---

* http://justfood.org/advocacy/what-is-food-justice

justice is either achieved or forfeited. For that reason, food justice is an important equity concern which public administrators and scholars should be aware of in their work. As Desmund Tutu once said, "If you are neutral in situations of injustice, you have chosen the side of the oppressor." We believe that public administrators hold positions that vest them with the opportunity to positively affect social justice through their work.

It is our belief that, from a public administration standpoint, an understanding of the lived experience of those within the food system is lacking. As a result, the existing knowledge within the field on topics such as policy evaluation, program design, and program administration, which have the potential to greatly impact the food system, is incapable of achieving their fullest potential within the food arena. Furthermore, public administrators work within silos, often encapsulated in a specific policy arena, and are unaware of how the many decisions in the food arena are shaped by and also shape the broad constellation of public policies that have an effect on people in their everyday lives.

The future of food justice

We contend that any consideration of policy proposals impacting the food system should include a discussion of food justice. Since food issues have gained prominence on governmental agendas at all levels, public administrators and community activists need to decide how they will educate themselves about the policy options available and what criteria they will judge policy options by. The extant literature certainly indicates that there is a need for more research specific to food justice. However, by informing ourselves about the historical injustices that have previously been built into food policies, we can recognize that the impact of any food policy has the potential to reinforce or subvert structural trends in food justice. Public policies, however their champions might frame them, are never neutral in their impacts. We believe policy stakeholders can, at a minimum, actively consider what the impact of any food policy will be on social justice concerns for the diverse citizenship of our society. Such a heightened awareness has the potential to prevent historical injustices from repeating themselves as we envision and reshape the future of food.

Moving forward, researchers and food justice advocates must grapple with questions such as: What is the proper realm of food: is food a public or private issue? Is food a right? Is food property? Who, if anyone, is responsible for preventing hunger and starvation? As citizens, it is imperative that we ask ourselves these questions because, while there is no one correct answer, our individually held interests are informed by them. Each of these questions has implications for how we develop food policy. Moreover, these policies then shape perceptions and attitudes about welfare (i.e., worthiness, the deserving poor), thereby potentially promoting discursive inequalities.

Future scholarship relating to food justice has the potential to fill the gap in this burgeoning nexus between public administration and food policy within our contemporary environment. While planning scholar Catherine Brinkley says that those in the planning discipline were "last to the table" in comprehensively incorporating food systems research as part of their profession, public administration may yet be behind planning in this regard (Brinkley 2013, p. 245). As food policy continues to be elevated on government agendas through the work of disciplines such as planning and advocacy from various community groups promoting their favored food issues, public administration scholars will need to build the academic and professional literature required to educate those working in the public and nonprofit sectors. Much of this scholarship will focus on practical and/or technical concerns. The nuts and bolts of structuring food policy across various disciplines and professions are vital work, but just as crucial will be a critical awareness and assessment of justice concerns within the food system.

With roots in multiple social movements, food systems research can be motivated by activists promoting their desired solutions to the problems they perceive in our existing food system. Future research in public administration and other disciplines concerned with food systems can help critically examine those activist-motivated policy problems and alternatives by giving special weight to food justice criteria. This could be applied in a case where a public administrator is called upon to evaluate a particular food policy proposal in their community; they can assure that food justice is a criterion that is measured and assessed in determining the desirability of that policy. Beyond adding food justice as an evaluative criterion for future food policy work, additional scholarship is needed to critically examine the food justice impacts of historical food policies and other public policies which ultimately had detrimental impacts on the food systems and the aforementioned vulnerable populations (e.g., housing policy and food deserts). What we are suggesting is that the generalist nature of the field of public administration allows for the sort of system-wide examinations food justice issues require.

REFERENCES

Abel, C. F. 2014. Toward a theory of social justice for public administration. *Administrative Theory & Praxis* 36(4):466–488.

Abramovitz, M. 2004. Ideological perspectives and conflicts. In *The Dynamics of Social Welfare Policy*, edited by J. Blau and M. Abramovitz. New York, NY: Oxford University Press, pp. 119–173.

Born, B. and M. Purcell. 2006. Avoiding the local trap. Scale and food systems in planning research. *Journal of Planning Education and Research* 26:195–307.

Brinkley, C. 2013. Avenues into food planning: A review of scholarly food system research. *International Planning Studies* 18(2):243–266.

Chelf, C. P. 1992. *Controversial Issues in Social Welfare Policy: Government and the Pursuit of Happiness*. Newbury Park, CA: SAGE Publications.

Chrisafis, A. 2016. French law forbids food waste by supermarkets. *The Guardian*. February 4. Retrieved from: http://www.theguardian.com/world/2016/feb/04/french-law-forbids-food-waste-by-supermarkets

Denhardt, R. B. and J. V. Denhardt. 2009. *Public Administration: An Action Orientation.* Belmont, CA: Thomson Higher Education.

Dimitri, C., A. Effland, and N. Conklin. 2005. *The 20th Century Transformation of U.S. Agriculture and Farm Policy*, USDA EIB-3. Washington, DC: U.S. Department of Agriculture. Economic Research Service.

Frederickson, H. G. 2005. The state of social equity in American public administration. *National Civic Review* 94(4):31–38.

Frederickson, H. G. and B. M. Henry. 1990. Social equity for nursing administration and knowledge-development. In *Practice and Inquiry for Nursing Administration: Intradisciplinary and Interdisciplinary Perspectives: Solicited Papers and Proceedings of the Santa Fe Conference*, edited by B. M. Henry, pp. 76–100.

Gooden, S. T. 2015. PAR's social equity footprint. *Public Administration Review* 75(3): 372–381.

Gottlieb, R. and A. Joshi. 2010. *Food Justice: Food, Health, and the Environment.* Cambridge, MA: MIT Press.

Green, J. J., E. M. Green, and A. M. Kleiner. 2011. From the past to the present: Agricultural development and black farmers in the American South. In *Cultivating Food Justice: Race, Class, and Sustainability*, edited by A. Hope Alkon and J. Agyeman. Cambridge, MA: The MIT Press, pp. 47–64.

Gunderson, C. 2006. *Measuring the Extent and Depth of Food Insecurity: An Application to American Indians in the United States.* Ames, IA: National Poverty Center Working Paper Series, Iowa State University. Retrieved from: http://www.npc.umich.edu/publications/workingpaper06/paper02/Gundersen.pdf

Hinrichs, C. C. 2003. The practice and politics of food system localization. *Journal of Rural Studies* 19:33–45.

Hope Alkon, A. and J. Agyeman (eds.) 2011. *Cultivating Food Justice: Race, Class, and Sustainability.* Cambridge, MA: The MIT Press.

Ingram, H. and A. Schneider. 1997. Constructing citizenship: The subtle messages of policy design. In *Public Policy for Democracy*, edited by H. Ingram and S. Smith. Washington, DC: The Brookings Institution, pp. 68–94.

Jernigan, V. B. B., E. Garroutte, E. Krantz, and D. Buchwald. 2013. Food insecurity and obesity among American Indians and Alaska Natives and Whites in California. *Journal of Hunger and Environmental Nutrition* 8(4):458–471.

Johnson, N. J. and J. H. Svara. 2011. Social equity in American society and public administration. In *Justice for All: Promoting Social Equity in Public Administration*, edited by N. J. Johnson and J. H. Svara. Armonk, NY: M.E. Sharpe, pp. 3–25.

Katz, M. B. 2013. *The Undeserving Poor: America's Enduring Confrontation with Poverty.* New York, NY: Oxford University Press.

Lehrer, N. 2010. *U.S. Farm Bills and Policy Reforms: Ideological Conflicts over World Trade, Renewable Energy, and Sustainable Agriculture.* Amherst, NY: Cambria Press.

Miles, R. E., Jr. 1978. The origin and meaning of Miles' Law. *Public Administration Review* 38(5):399–403.

Miller, H. 2012. *Governing Narratives: Symbolic Politics and Policy Change.* Tuscaloosa, AL: The University of Alabama Press.

Mitchell, D. 2010. Battle/fields: Braceros, agribusiness, and the violent reproduction of the California agricultural landscape during World War II. *Journal of Historical Geography* 36:143–156.

Mukherji, N. and A. Morales. 2010. Zoning for urban agriculture. *Zoning Practice* 3:1–7. Chicago, IL: American Planning Association.

Norman-Major, K. 2011. Balancing the four Es; or can we achieve equity for social equity in public administration? *Journal of Public Affairs Education* 17(2):233–252.

Palmer, A. M., W.-T. Chen, and M. Winne. 2014. Community food security. In *Introduction to the U.S. Food System: Public Health, Environment, and Equity*, edited by R. Neff's. San Francisco, CA: Jossey-Bass, pp. 135–156.

Petty, A. and M. Schultz. 2013. African-American farmers and the USDA: 150 years of discrimination. *Agricultural History* 87(3):314–367.

Pianigiani, G. and S. Chan. 2016. Can the homeless and hungry steal food? Maybe, an Italian court says. *The New York Times*. Retrieved from: http://www.nytimes.com/2016/05/04/world/europe/food-theft-in-italy-may-not-be-a-crime-court-rules.html?_r=2

Pierce, J. J., S. Siddiki, M. D. Jones, K. Schumacher, A. Pattison, and H. Peterson. 2014. Social construction and policy design: A review of past applications. *Policy Studies Journal* 42(1):1–21.

Plumer, B. 2013. The Senate is voting on a $955 billion farm bill. Here's what's in it. *Washington Post*. Retrieved from: https://www.washingtonpost.com/news/wonk/wp/2013/06/10/the-senate-is-voting-on-a-955-billion-farm-bill-heres-whats-in-it/

Rawls, J. 1971. *A Theory of Justice*. Cambridge, MA: BelkPress of Harvard University Press.

Schneider, A., H. Ingram, and P. deLeon. 2014. Democratic policy design: Social construction of target populations. In *Theories of the Policy Process*, edited by P. Sabatier and C. Wieble. Boulder, CO: Westview Press, pp. 105–150.

Shannon, K. L., B. F. Kim, S. E. McKenzie, and R. S. Lawrence. 2015. Food system policy, public health, and human rights in the United States. *Public Health* 36:151–173.

Skinner, K., E. Pratley, and K. Burnett. 2016. Eating in the city: A review of the literature on food insecurity and indigenous people living in urban spaces. *Societies* 6:7.

Sonnino, R. and T. Marsden. 2006. Beyond the divide: Rethinking relationships between alternative and conventional food networks in Europe. *Journal of Economic Geography* 6:181–199.

Stockman, D. P. 2012. The new food agenda: Municipal food policy and planning for the 21st century. Doctoral dissertation, University of Michigan.

Stroink, M. L. and C. H. Nelson. 2013. Complexity and food hubs: five case studies from Northern Ontario. *Local Environment* 18(5):620–635.

United States Department of Agriculture (USDA). (2015). Local and regional food systems. Retrieved from: http://www.usda.gov/wps/portal/usda/usdahome?contentid=usda-results-local.html

Winfrey, J. C. 1998. *Social Issues: The Ethics and Economics of Taxes and Public Programs*. New York, NY: Oxford University Press.

17 School lunch reform and the problem with obesity

Jennifer Geist Rutledge

Introduction

In December of 2010 Congress passed the Child Nutrition Act, reauthorizing spending on a variety of food and nutrition programs, including the national school lunch and school breakfast programs, and upgrading the nutritional standards for these meals. While in many ways a mundane spending reauthorization bill, in fact this act represents the first significant change to the nutritional standards of these meals in 15 years and the first significant change to the financing for these meals in 30 years. These changes affect 31 million school children that eat school meals on a daily basis, 21 million of whom eat free or reduced-price lunch.* There are the many vested interests in maintaining school food as it was, including the USDA, agribusiness companies, and schools. What then explains this policy change after so many years of stasis?

I argue that the changes to the school meal program in 2010 reflect the emergence of obesity as a public health problem. While school meals became increasingly unhealthy beginning in the 1970s as schools privatized their meal programs, unhealthy meals consumed primarily by poor people were not seen as a problem. It was not until a concern with obesity became an overriding issue in the political system that policy change was possible. This concern is reflected in the bill's focus on the consumption of vegetables, low-fat milk, and calorie maximums for each meal, all of which differ significantly from previous incarnations of the program which focused on encouraging consumption of often unhealthy commodity agricultural products.

Obesity emerged as a policy problem to be solved due to the efforts of child and public health advocates to construct obesity as a public health epidemic. As such, this case exemplifies problem definition in the policy process. Using insights from multiple streams analysis, which focuses on the merging of the separate problem, policy, and politics streams to explain how certain issues arrive on the policy agenda, I focus on problem definition as an inherently political act. Through this case study of school meal reform in 2010, I demonstrate that the

---

* This is out of a school age child population of approximately 49.5 million; 62% of children in the United States eat these meals.

three streams should not be regarded as separate and independent but instead are interrelated. In particular, precisely because problem definition is political it can rightly be understood as being in both the problem and politics stream. As such, I demonstrate that when obesity, rather than unhealthy food, became the problem to be solved, this act of problem definition had an effect on the politics stream such that change was necessary.

Using primary sources, including newspaper articles, legislation, committee reports, and articles in the Congressional Record, this paper presents a narrative account of this policy change. I first briefly discuss multiple streams analysis and position my argument within that body of literature. I next review the history of the national school lunch program, before turning to a discussion of problems with school meals, largely represented by poor quality and corporate control over the food itself. I then outline the changes to the meal programs created by the 2010 Child Nutrition Act and 2012 USDA Nutrition Standards, which highlights the significance of this policy change. Next I analyze the emergence of obesity as a public health problem and particularly the way in which it began to motivate legislative changes in the early 2000s. Following this I investigate the particular legislative moment in which the 2010 Act was created, which was affected by both the Great Recession and debates around the Affordable Care Act; these two events focused legislative attention on the twin concerns of health and economy, making obesity a particularly relevant problem during the discussions about the school meal program.

Multiple streams model

In this chapter I use insights from multiple streams analysis, first developed by John Kingdon (2003) to explain how policies rise onto the agenda. In particular, Kingdon focuses on three streams—the politics, policy, and problem stream. The problem stream refers to any issue that could require government action, while the policy stream refers to the potential solutions to that problem. The politics stream refers to aspects of public opinion, general political attitudes of the moment, and changes in the administration. Kingdon argues that these three streams primarily exist independently from one another and that when they merge, this merging can be regarded as a policy window that creates the possibility of a new policy being placed on the legislative agenda. Streams merge when there are changes in how the problem is understood, when critical events occur that bring attention to a problem, or when there are routine changes to the politics stream, such as a new administration.

The streams metaphor points our attention to the way in which policy change occurred only after the problem of unhealthy lunches in schools became defined as the public health problem of obesity, and once indicators, or statistics, about obesity had risen to an alarming level. However, the streams metaphor, which keeps the streams separate for analytic purposes, tends to obscure the messy nature of policy change (Sabatier 1999; Robinson and Eller 2010). In this case the obesity statistics rose for a number of different reasons, but the Centers for Disease Control popularized a narrative that saw obesity as a result of a lack of exercise and overconsumption of food which had the effect of shutting out those who argued that obesity should be understood as a result of systemic forces in the American food, agricultural, and welfare systems. As such, the advocates for this particular understanding of the problem affected the politics stream by altering the national mood, while at the same time being themselves created by a politics stream that seeks incremental change and individualistic solutions to problems. This process, the contentious process of problem definition, points our attention to the way the streams overlap and are interrelated as the problem and politics streams are in fact mutually constituted.

The problem: Agriculture commodities for lunch

In order to understand the magnitude of the changes put in place by the 2010 Act, I review the history of school lunches briefly in order to situate the issues that motivated school food reform. Although local efforts to feed hungry children began in the late 1800s, with Philadelphia creating the first citywide school lunch program in 1894, federal interventions into school meals did not begin until the Great Depression, when national concern with both hungry children and farmers created Public Law 320, allowing the Secretary of Agriculture to remove surplus foods from the market in order to not interfere with normal sales. These surplus commodities were sent to schoolchildren in order to dampen consumer anger over the Corn-Hog program that had simply destroyed surpluses (White 2014). The Federal Surplus Commodities Corporation began distributing surplus foods to schools in 1933; this organization worked specifically with state and local authorities, Parent Teacher Associations (PTAs), and other voluntary organizations to ensure the expansion of school lunch programs. Funding for this program continued even as the Depression lessened in intensity, due to pressure from agricultural producers.

While funding for school meals wavered during World War II, as commodities were funneled into the war effort, a variety of actors began to argue for a national school meal program, both for the benefit to school children, as well as the benefit to agricultural producers once the war was over. In fact, the bill creating the National School Lunch Act, passed in 1946, makes clear that supporting domestic agricultural production was an essential part of the school lunch program by stating, in its opening measures:

> As a measure of national security, to safeguard the health and well-being of the Nation's children and to encourage the domestic consumption of nutritious agricultural commodities and other food, by assisting the States, through grants-in aid and other means, in providing an adequate supply of food and other facilities for the establishment, maintenance, operation and expansion of nonprofit school lunch programs.
>
> (House of Representatives 1946)

The legislation clearly specifies that the primary concern of the program is to further the interests of agricultural producers. Indeed, for the first 30 years of its existence, the program ran largely as a commodity distribution program which was conceived of as an insurance policy against market-distorting agricultural surpluses (Levine 2010, p. 93). The Secretary of Agriculture determined each year which products were considered to be in surplus and thus eligible for subsidies for the school lunch program. As such, the foods for meals tended to be inconsistent, dependent on the lobbying power of different commodity groups. While schools were assured a steady supply of dried milk, lard, flour, rice, and cornmeal, the other foods waxed and waned from year to year (Levine 2010, p. 94). This inconsistency made any nutrition goals the program might also claim difficult to achieve.

In addition to being held captive to the commodity markets, school meal programs have become increasingly privatized and outsourced to food service companies such as Aramark or Sodexo. These companies work with food manufacturers to process the raw materials provided by the federal commodity programs and raise the cost to schools. For instance, food processers contract with schools to turn free raw chicken into chicken nuggets, which costs the school two to three times the price of the raw commodities. This processed food is usually higher in fats and sugars, leading to lower quality meals. The argument behind the rise in private contracting is that schools will save on labor costs as they no longer have to pay for on-site cooks, yet studies have found that savings were minimal as schools paid higher rates in fees and supplies (Komisar 2011).

Corporations first worked their way into the lunchrooms in the late 1960s. The 1966 Child Nutrition Act created the School Breakfast Program as a pilot program specifically for poor children and appropriated funds for the first time for free lunches for poor children. This shift to focus the meals on poor children grew out of the War on Poverty and had important demographic and financial implications for the lunch program. In particular, although the federal government increased the funds for free meals, this funding still did not pay for a full meal. Therefore, local governments and school boards raised the cost of the meal to students paying full price in order to make up the difference, with the rather predictable consequence that many of those students stopped buying meals, leaving the meal programs chronically underfunded. In addition, as more poor students took advantage of the free meals, the meal program as a whole began to be associated with poverty, further driving full-paying students away (Levine 2010, p. 154). Thus, local school boards, who needed to meet their federal obligations of providing free meals, began to look for cost-cutting measures, which were offered by food corporations.

By the late 1970s most school meal programs were run as public/private partnerships in which corporations both supplied the food and in many cases also ran the meal programs (Levine 2010, p. 152). Driven therefore by profit motives, these corporations began to look at ways to cut costs, which often involved the introduction of fast foods into the cafeteria. Not only were these types of food more efficient to produce, but they had the added benefit of drawing full-paying students back to the cafeteria. At the same time the Department of Agriculture began to loosen its nutrition standards and its regulations for reimbursement with the result that less nutritious offerings were available. For instance, a new rule in 1979 "stipulated that if the 'food' supplied more than 5% of the RDA of just one basic nutrient in a 100 calorie serving, the item could be served for lunch. If the nutrition value fell below that already low bar, the sale of the product was restricted to after lunch hours" (Levine 2010, p. 164). While nutrition had never been the main goal of the school lunch program, all of these changes made any hope of nutritional value from the meals increasingly unlikely.

While children's advocates argued for improving the nutrition of these meals, the meals programs have long been unable to shake the commodity agricultural agenda that motivated the program. For instance, by the late 1990s, the federal government bought up more than $800 million worth of farm products every year and turned them over to schools (Yeoman 2003). This was despite a USDA report in 1992 that highlighted the poor quality of school lunches as containing too much fat, too much salt, not enough carbohydrates, and clearly not meeting nutritional standards of the time (Burros 1993), and which had spurred the Clinton administration to pass changes to the school meal program requiring adherence to the National Dietary Standards of the time by 1996. The focus at the time was on reducing the fat and cholesterol in meals (Krauss et al. 1996), but there was little enforcement or incentives for schools to meet these standards. For instance, "in 2003 USDA spent $939.5 million dollars buying surplus commodities for School Lunch. Two-thirds of that bought meat and dairy, with little more than one-quarter going to vegetables that were mostly frozen" (Parker-Pope 2009). With these inputs, many of the menus focused on meat and cheese entrees with few fresh vegetables; the only available fruits were those that travel and store well such as apples or oranges. As such, schools were likely to violate existing government standards for fats in school meals, largely due to the types of foods made available to the schools by the government. Even those schools that sought to work within government guidelines have historically only focused on reaching a minimum calorie limit, which has meant that individual schools can apportion the calories as they see fit, by, for instance, tossing on an extra slice of bread to bring up the calorie count (Alderman 2010). For many children, and parents, the resulting meals are unappealing and unhealthy.

The policy: 2010 Child Nutrition Act and 2012 Nutrition Standards

In December 2010, Congress approved the Healthy, Hunger-Free Kids Act of 2010, which was a reauthorization bill that covered federal school meal and child nutrition programs. While the school meal program, for instance, does not expire, it is required to be periodically reviewed and the funding reauthorized. The bill included a number of changes to the federal meal programs, the most significant of which are that the USDA now has the authority to set nutritional standards for all food sold in schools, including vending machines as well as the cafeteria, and additional funding for schools that meet the new nutritional standards. In other words, the bill creates a performance incentive for schools to improve the quality of their meals. The bill does a number of other important things, such as requiring access to drinking water, providing assistance for schools to establish farm-to-school networks to encourage the use of local foods, and creating better school wellness policies. In addition to these provisions that focus on improving nutrition, the bill also increases access to meal programs by, for instance, using census data to determine school eligibility for free meals rather than requiring individual applications, as well as increasing program monitoring. All of these provisions taken together represent a significant change to the federal school meal programs.

The 2010 Act authorized the USDA to set new nutritional standards for school lunches, updating these standards for the first time since 1995. The standards are based on the work of the Institute for Medicine, which was asked by the USDA to provide recommendations for revising the nutrition standards for both the school lunch and school breakfast programs in 2009 (Institute of Medicine 2009). Following the passage of the 2010 Act the USDA began, based on the Institute of Medicine's recommendations, to mold their own standards and revealed their final rule, *Nutrition Standards in the National School Lunch and School Breakfast Program* on January 12, 2012 which began to be applied in the 2012–2013 school year. Basically, the rules require a doubling of the amount of fruits and vegetables, as well as a greater diversity of vegetables,* to be served per day, the use of whole grains in foods, whereas before the use of whole grains was encouraged but not required, a requirement to offer only fat-free or low-fat milk, and a requirement to offer meat alternatives. In addition, schools must reduce the use of sodium and eliminate trans-fats, which previously was unregulated. Further, whereas the meal program had for years had minimum calorie require-ments, but no maximums, the meals are now bound by calorie minimums and maximums. These new standards have generally been well received by nutrition and food advocates, while food industry representatives have given the standards cautious approval (Nixon 2012).

The politics: Obesity, recession, and the ACA

In multiple streams analysis, the politics stream refers to the public mood, national ideology, the composition of Congress, and changes in the administra-tion (Kingdon 2003, p. 145). Clearly, part of the responsibility for the passage of the 2010 Act with this emphasis on sound nutrition lies with the fact that there were both a Democratic majority in Congress, and a Democratic President. But what multiple streams analysis best explains is how certain items rise to the agenda and thus the question remains, why did a concern with obesity and school meals rise to the agenda for this Democratic leadership to address? I argue that there had been a concrete shift in the national mood such that there was a pre-vailing public concern with obesity. This concern with obesity reflects the con-struction of obesity as a public health epidemic, which is exemplified in Michelle

* There is now a weekly requirement for dark green, red/orange vegetables and beans/peas.

Obama's Let's Move Campaign which itself served as an important source of political attention on the problem of obesity as hearings for the 2010 Act began.

Obesity is understood as a public health problem; and public health problems necessitate certain kinds of government interactions. Obesity as a public health problem is not without merit; recent studies indicate that at least one-third of all Americans qualify as obese (Ogden et al. 2014), based on a body mass index (BMI) between 25 and 29.9 being considered overweight and those with a BMI over 30 being considered obese. Indeed, obesity leads to a number of health complications, including diabetes, heart disease, strokes, cancer, sleep apnea, and other chronic diseases, which were estimated to have cost $147 billion in 2008 (Kuchler and Ballenger 2002; Hammond and Levine 2010). In addition to the direct medical costs of obesity, further economic costs arise from lost productivity when workers are either absent or do their work more slowly, increased transportation costs as heavier people use more fuel and require larger vehicles, and in some cases costs on human capital accumulation as heavier people are absent from school more often and are less likely to complete higher grades (Hammond and Levine 2010). If these indirect costs of obesity are added to the direct medical costs, the literature suggests annual economic costs of roughly $215 billion. These costs alone are enough to suggest a public health crisis and require government intervention.

And yet, obesity did not necessarily have to be understood as a public health problem. Instead, obesity could be understood as the result of U.S. agricultural policy or the construction of the suburbs or endocrine disrupting chemicals in the environment and in food, all of which probably help to explain the rise in obesity (Guthman 2011; Ludwig and Pollack 2009). Indeed, there is a strong critical understanding of obesity as being due to the built environment which presents us with far too much cheap and fattening food as well as a lack of opportunity for physical exercise. However, the dominant way in which obesity has been constructed is as the energy imbalance model: In this construction, obesity is caused by personal choices to consume too many calories and exercise too little (Guthman 2011).

This particular construction of obesity, which focuses on the overconsumption of unhealthy foods, clearly assigns blame at the individual level first and at the community level second. The solutions proposed by this understanding of the obesity problem are clear—more physical exercise, access to healthy foods, and education (Guthman 2011, p. 20). Thus, all the government needs to do is offer access to healthy foods and encourage children to eat it, rather than attempt any sort of structural reforms to agricultural or economic policy. Further, by placing responsibility primarily on the individual, food corporations are either left free from responsibility, or can position themselves as part of the solution, as they did during the Child Nutrition Act hearings. This clearly reflects the work of numerous actors, most prominently the CDC, to construct obesity as a public health problem. Public health professionals worked over the years to construct obesity as a public health epidemic, while simultaneously a variety of other actors, concerned with issues as diverse as family farms and national security, worked to construct school lunches as one of the necessary sites at which to challenge this epidemic. The framing of obesity as a public health problem has certain implications: Problems that are construed in a public health frame are constituted as both curable and preventable. These problems then are curable by the techniques and rationalizations of science, instead of fundamental change in the social order.

The act of defining problems is in many ways the beginning of the policy process, as various parties seek to define their problem as the one deserving attention and action (Rochefort and Cobb 1993). Certainly there are many problems, but only a few of them receive attention or end up on the agenda. In order to receive attention, these issues must be perceived as problems, rather than conditions about which nothing can be done (Kingdon 2003, p. 109). For instance, in this case, nutritional deficiencies in the meals, corporate influence in the cafeterias, or the large number of poor children and children of color who rely on the meals could have been seen as problems. However, these factors were never successfully defined as problems. Instead, obesity became defined as a problem serious enough for government action and is the main justification behind the most recent changes to the Child Nutrition Act.

Defining something as a problem is most likely to happen when "participants perceive the discrepancy between (a problem) and some ideal state or social goal" (McDonnell and Weatherford 2013). This discrepancy is most likely to happen when those issues violate important values or are defined in such a way that it forces action (Kingdon 2003). However, it is necessary for policy entrepreneurs to make the case for their particular construction of the problem. Further, they often have to wait until there are changes in indicators, focusing events, a crisis of some sort, or feedback effects from existing policies in order for any particular problem to make it onto the policy agenda (Kingdon 2003). In this case the indicators, the statistics, about obesity pointed to a steep rise in obesity amongst children, which helped put changes to school meals onto the policy agenda.

In the 1980s, roughly 8% of children in the United States could be considered obese, while by 2009 that number was 17% (Schanzenbach 2009). For adults in 1990, only 15% could be considered obese, while that number rose to 30% in 2010 (Ogden et al. 2014). Based on these numbers, obesity has been declared a public health epidemic (Hill and Peters 1998; Mokdad et al. 1999), but up until the mid-1990s obesity had remained only on the radar of public health professionals. However, in 1996, the National Center for Health Statistics (a division of the CDC) reported that overweight people outnumbered other Americans. At this point, the issue took off in the media, garnering a 50% increase in coverage in the *New York Times* from the previous year, and increasing in all news outlets each following year (Lawrence 2004).

Following this coverage and the public's increasing concern with the issue, obesity began to appear with some regularity in the legislative records in the early 2000s. A search of the legislative record reveals that the first time obesity was mentioned in Congress was in 1979 in a bill discussing diet programs and was mentioned again in the early 1980s in two separate bills seeking to regulate diet pills; both bills died in committee. While obesity began to appear occasionally,

Table 17.1 Obesity in Congressional Literature

Congressional Session (Years in Parentheses)	Legislation that Mentions Obesity
96 (79/80)	1
97 (81/82)	0
98 (83/84)	1
99 (85/86)	1
100 (87/88)	0
101 (89/90)	4
102 (91/92)	8
103 (93/94)	8
104 (95/96)	5
105 (97/98)	9
106 (99/00)	15
107 (01/02)	30
108 (03/04)	83
109 (05/06)	86
110 (07/08)	132
111 (09/10)	171

the legislative record indicates a rapid upswing of discussion around obesity during the 108th Congress, in 2003/2004, and demonstrates that a concern with obesity began to compel government action. Table 17.1 shows this large increase in legislation that explicitly discusses obesity and clearly demonstrates that obesity had become an entrenched part of the congressional discussion by the time of the 2010 Child Nutrition Act.

In particular, people began to link school lunches and obesity; public health professionals had long linked the quality of school meals, composed largely of fatty and salty foods to childhood obesity, and the public began to as well. For instance, a study in 2005 utilized panel data from the Early Childhood Longitudinal Survey to demonstrate that children who eat school lunches are more likely to be obese than their counterparts who bring their lunches to school, and in particular, that those who are eligible for the free or reduced school lunches are likely to weigh more and be obese (Schanzenbach 2009). In addition, a 2008 study demonstrated a causal link between the consumption of school lunches and an increase in obesity, while simultaneously demonstrating a beneficial link between the School Breakfast Program and the reduction of obesity (Millimet et al. 2010). Further, a study in 2010 of schoolchildren in Michigan found a link between school lunch and childhood obesity, finding that those who ate school lunch were 29% more likely to be obese (Eagle et al. 2010).

Obesity appeared in school meal legislation for the first time in 2004 in the 2004 Child Nutrition Reauthorization Act, the act directly preceding the 2010 act under discussion here. In this act, in addition to reauthorizing the meal programs, schools were required to create wellness policies that would include "goals for nutrition education, physical activity (and) nutrition guidelines... with the objective of improving student health and reducing childhood obesity" (Section 204 of Public Law 108-264, June 30, 2004). Further, obesity is mentioned 18 times throughout the text of the bill, including a Miscellaneous section that specifically explores the "Sense of Congress Regarding Efforts to Prevent and Reduce Childhood Obesity" (Public Law 105-336, June 30, 2004). This is the first time that obesity is mentioned in legislation related to school meals: Obesity is not mentioned at all in the text of the 1998 William Golding Child Nutrition Reauthorization Act.

However, it was not the first time obesity was connected to school meals in committee discussions and legislative debates. The first time obesity was connected to the school lunch program was actually in 1991, when Senator Lugar introduced a bill to eliminate the requirement that whole milk be served in school lunches, in favor of allowing schools to serve 2% milk if they chose. In his statement about his bill Sen. Lugar connected obesity rates to high-fat milk (Congressional Record 1991). After that obesity was not connected to school meals again until the 107th Congress in 2001/2002. For instance, in 1995/1996 there were 1038 congressional statements about school lunches and eight pieces of legislation about obesity, but no connections between obesity and school lunches. Concern with obesity had not yet become dominant and no one was making the connection between obesity and school meal reform.

This changed rapidly in the early 2000s. Table 17.2 shows the rapid increase, beginning in 2003/2004, between obesity and school lunches in statements from Congress, either in the form of legislation, Committee Reports, or articles in the Congressional Record. While school lunches were regularly discussed in Congress, we can clearly see that by 2004 obesity as a public health problem had

Table 17.2 School Meals in Congressional Literature

Congressional Session (Years in Parentheses)	School Lunches Discussed in Legislation, Committee Reports, or Congressional Record	Connection Made between Obesity and Improving School Lunches in Legislation, Committee Reports, or Congressional Record
101 (89/90)	204	0
102 (91/92)	258	1
103 (93/94)	257	0
104 (95/96)	1038	0
105 (97/98)	331	0
106 (99/00)	318	0
107 (01/02)	272	6
108 (03/04)	418	48
109 (05/06)	287	11
110 (07/08)	386	31
111 (09/10)	423	54

rapidly emerged into the national dialogue as an idea able to compel action on changing school lunches. The link between school meals and obesity was well established by the time of the 2010 Act.

The process of problem definition can be understood as the strategic representation of situations (Stone 2002) and as such is explicitly political (Allison 1971; Baumgartner and Jones 1993; Schneider and Ingram 1993). Relatedly, problem definition is also interpretive; it requires the construction of a causal story, which in turn allows us to assign responsibility for problems (Stone 2002). While there can be accidental, inadvertent, and mechanical causes, it is the intentional causes that are most powerful as it casts blame directly at someone for willfully and knowingly causing harm. In the case of school meals, it could easily be argued that the poor nutrition in the meals was caused by a confusing mix of inadvertent and mechanical causes, including agricultural subsidy formulas first developed in the 1940s and the creation of public–private partnerships designed to make the meal programs sustainable. Sorting out the causal arrow for poor nutrition in this case would be difficult, if not impossible, and it would be hard to argue that any one particular entity was to blame. Thus, it was hard to create a compelling causal story around the school meal programs and therefore difficult to compel action to improve the meals. However, with the construction of obesity as a public health problem in the mid-1990s (Hill and Peters 1998; Mokdad et al. 1999), it became easy to link obesity to school meals and therefore a variety of actors were able to frame changes to school meals as one of the most important solutions to childhood obesity.

These constructions, this definition of the problem, changed the risk calculations for legislators who could no longer vote for obesity by refusing changes to school lunches. In other words, the link between obesity and school lunches was so strong that legislators had to vote for changes, despite the costs and objections by food corporations, as to vote against these changes was a vote to condemn children to a lifetime of obesity with its attendant economic and health costs. Likewise, food corporations who had arguably contributed to the problem in the first place found it necessary to reframe themselves as interested in solving the obesity problem that they had created. One of the first hearings on the reauthorization bill in March of 2009 included representatives from a dairy company, Mars Snackfood and the American Beverage Association, as well as prepared statements from ConAgra Foods, the American Frozen Food Institute, the Potato Industry Child Nutrition Working Group, the National Dairy Council, and the Schwan Food Company. Most of these prepared statements mention the health of schoolchildren as one of the company's motivations and the people who spoke at the hearing, in front of the Senate Committee on Agriculture, Nutrition and Forestry, all discuss obesity and weight and focus on how their products—milk, snack foods, and beverages—can contribute to lowering obesity rates (United States Senate Hearing, March 31, 2009). Food corporations recognize that they are operating in a changed social environment that requires them to market themselves as antiobesity and in favor of changed school lunches, despite their previous vested interest in maintaining the status quo.

Thus, one important element in the politics stream was the inherently political act of problem definition, where the problem became not the unhealthy food supplied by corporations in cafeterias but instead obesity. Another important element in the politics stream was the Obama administration, and in particular Michelle Obama as she came to the White House with a particular focus on childhood obesity. Michelle Obama created the Let's Move Campaign in February, 2010, while legislative hearings were ongoing for the School Meals Act. This campaign is dedicated to eradicating childhood obesity within a generation and focuses its efforts on "empowering parents and caregivers, providing healthy foods in schools, improving access to healthy, affordable foods (and) increasing physical activity" (Boyle and Holben 2012, p. 442). While the very title of the campaign emphasizes the physical activity component of the campaign, a review of press coverage reveals that the press focused almost entirely on the diet elements, and particularly the suggested changes to school meals.* This move likely reflects the general national understanding that tied obesity directly to food consumption without a more holistic look into the causes of obesity. Despite this, we can understand that the Let's Move Campaign, and Michelle Obama's high profile position helped keep school meal reform, and a focus on obesity, high on the legislative agenda.

However, it is not enough to simply define an issue as a problem in order to ensure policy change or have high profile advocates. In addition, there must be an opportunity for change to occur, most commonly through the opening of a policy window. Policy windows present opportunities for action on a given agenda item, and open both frequently, as in the case of reauthorization bills, and infrequently, as in the case of unexpected election results, which might allow one party more votes than expected (Kingdon 2003, p. 166). In this case, the 2010 reauthorization bill was an expected policy window in which child advocates, nutritionists, parents, teachers, and food corporations would be able to push their agenda. However, the 2010 policy window was different from an expected policy window; the combination of the Great Recession and the health-care debate created not just a policy window, but a window of opportunity.

Following the onset of the Great Recession in 2008, policymakers became more concerned with both the cost of government programs, and the effects of rising poverty in the country. The Subcommittee on Children and Families of the Senate Committee on Health, Education, and Labor ran a series of hearings on the State of the American Child in the summer of 2010 that looked specifically at the impact of the recession on the health and well-being of children. These hearings were concerned with the long-term impacts for children living in poverty on their education, health, social connectedness, and empathy, just to list a few (United States Senate Hearing November 18, 2010). This series of hearings demonstrates the openness of policymakers to ideas that might improve these factors at this particular time. In fact, the Senate legislation authorizing the 2010 CNA

---

* "Michelle Obama's Let's Move is Losing Its Footing" http://healthaffairs.org/blog/2011/06/28/michelle-obamas-lets-move-is-losing-its-footing/. Accessed in April 2016.

specifically mentions the recession as a driving factor in the changes to the school meals programs contained in the act (Senate Report, May 5, 2010).

In addition to a heightened concern with child poverty starting in 2009, the debates around the new health-care law highlighted for policymakers the costs of health care and particularly the long-term costs of malnutrition and obesity. In three separate Senate hearings on Obesity, the Farm-to-School program, and Federal nutrition programs, testimony included discussion of these specific issues, tying improved nutrition for children into a reduction in long-term health-care costs (United States Senate Hearing March 31, 2009; May 15, 2009; March 4, 2010). The health-care debate was another opportunity for those concerned with reforming the school food program as it focused governmental and public attention on the cost of health care and possible interventions to reduce those costs over the long term.

These two prior legislative moments focused attention on the costs of government programs, as well as the cost of health care, and meant that during the hearings on the Child Nutrition Act, which began in 2009, lawmakers were particularly attuned to arguments that focused on health-care costs and a concern with childhood poverty. Thus, during the Child Nutrition Act hearings lawmakers were both expecting and particularly receptive to arguments that focused on reducing obesity-related health-care costs, due to the heightened level of concerns with these issues at this particular time period. Federal lawmakers were particularly open to claims not only about obesity, but also poverty and health-care costs, due to the Recession and the debates around the health-care bill. These events, considered along with the pervasiveness of the concern with obesity, created a changed social environment such that lawmakers and food corporations had to support programs that worked to reduce obesity.

Conclusion

This chapter analyzed the way in which the construction of obesity as a public health problem changed the risk calculations for both legislators and agri-food corporations, thus necessitating changes to the school meal program. Further, by focusing on the passage of the Healthy, Hunger-Free Kids Act of 2010, this chapter seeks to critically evaluate the way in which problem definition is explicitly political, and as such can be understood as part of both the problem and politics stream in multiple streams analysis. The construction of obesity as a public health problem also foreclosed other potential solutions to both obesity and unhealthy school meals. As such, this chapter implicitly considers the inadvertent consequences of problem definition.

However, in the case of school meals, perhaps one of the original goals of school meal reformers is being addressed after all. While legislators and even agribusiness approved of the 2010 Child Nutrition Act and the 2012 Nutrition Standards, some students have been less excited. A wave of publicity in the fall of 2012 highlighted student complaints that the new meals were too small and too healthy. For instance, students have staged boycotts and some schools have experienced a drop-off in the number of students buying the lunches (Yee 2012). However, in schools that have large populations of students that receive free or reduced-price lunches, the criticism has been more muted and many of these schools have embraced the changes as a critical component in improving the lives of children of color (Diaz 2013). Only 28% of white students receive free or reduced-price lunches, while 74% of black students and 77% of Latino students are eligible for the meals (National Center for Education Statistics 2016). In this way, the prevailing public concern with obesity, which closed off the opportunity to think more critically about the causes of obesity, might in fact be working to achieve the underlying goal of the initial advocates for reform: social justice.

REFERENCES

Alderman, L. 2010. Putting nutrition at the head of the lunch line. *New York Times*, November 5.

Allison, G. T. 1971. *Essence of Decision: Explaining the Cuban Missile Crisis*. Boston: Little Brown.

Baumgartner, F. R. and B. D. Jones. 1993. *Agendas and Instability in American Politics*. Chicago: University of Chicago Press.

Burros, M. 1993. Eating well. *New York Times*, March 17.

Congressional Record. Statements on Introduced Bills and Joint Resolutions (Senate— February 26, 1991).

Diaz, V. 2013. Whatever Happened to Michelle Obama's Lunch Program? Retrieved from: http://civileats.com/2013/10/08/what-ever-happened-to-michelle-obamas-school-lunch-program. Accessed on January 10, 2014.

Eagle, T., R. Gurm, and C. S. Goldberg. 2010. Health status and behavior among middle-school children in a midwest community: What are the underpinnings of childhood obesity? *American Heart Journal* 160:1185–1189.

Guthman, J. 2011. *Weighing In: Obesity, Food Justice, and the Limits of Capitalism*. Berkeley: University of California Press.

Hammond, R. A. and R. Levine. 2010. The economic impact of obesity in the United States. *Diabetes, Metabolic Syndrome and Obesity: Targets and Therapy* 3:285.

Hill, J. O. and J. C. Peters. 1998. Environmental contributions to the obesity epidemic. *Science* 280(5368):1371–1374.

Institute of Medicine. 2009. Report Brief. School Meals: Building Blocks for Healthy Children.

Kingdon, J. 2003. *Agendas, Alternatives, and Public Policies*, Second Edition. New York: Longman.

Komisar, L. 2011. How the food industry eats your kid's lunch. *New York Times*, December 3.

Krauss, R. M. et al. 1996. Dietary guidelines for healthy American adults: A statement for health professionals from the nutrition committee, American Heart Association. *Circulation* 94(7):1795–1800.

Kuchler, F. and N. Ballenger. 2002. Societal costs of obesity: How can we assess when federal interventions will pay? *Food Review* 25(3):33–37.

Lawrence, R. G. 2004. Framing obesity the evolution of news discourse on a public health issue. *Harvard International Journal of Press/Politics* 9(3):56–75.

Levine, S. 2010. *School Lunch Politics: The Surprising History of America's Favorite Welfare Program*. Princeton: Princeton University Press.

Ludwig, D. S. and H. A. Pollack. 2009. Obesity and the economy: from crisis to opportunity. *JAMA* 301(5):533–535.

McDonnell, L. M. and M. S. Weatherford. 2013. Evidence use and the Common Core State Standards movement: From problem definition to policy adoption. *American Journal of Education* 120(1):1–25.

Millimet, D. L., R. Tchernis, and M. Husain. 2010. School nutrition programs and the incidence of childhood obesity. *Journal of Human Resources* 45(3):640–654.

Mokdad, A. H. et al. 1999. The spread of the obesity epidemic in the United States, 1991–1998. *JAMA* 282(16):1519–1522.

National Center for Education Statistics. www.nces.ed.gov. Accessed on February 4, 2016.

Nixon, R. 2012. New rules for school meals aim at reducing obesity. *New York Times*, January 25.

Ogden, C. L., M. D. Carroll, B. K. Kit, and K. M. Flegal. 2014. Prevalence of childhood and adult obesity in the United States, 2011–2012. *JAMA* 311(8):806–814.

Parker-Pope, T. 2009. Obama's new chef skewers school lunches. *New York Times*, January 29.

Robinson, S. E. and W. S. Eller. 2010. Participation in policy streams: Testing the separation of problems and solutions in subnational policy systems. *Policy Studies Journal* 38(2):199–216.

Rochefort, D. A. and R. W. Cobb. 1993. Problem definition, agenda access, and policy choice. *Policy Studies Journal* 21(1):56–71.

Sabatier, P. 1999. *Theories of the Policy Process*. Boulder, CO: Westview Press.

Schanzenbach, D. W. 2009. Do school lunches contribute to childhood obesity? *Journal of Human Resources* 44:684–709.

Schneider, A. and H. Ingram. 1993. Social construction of target populations: Implications for politics and policy. *American Political Science Review* 87(2):334–347.

Stone, D. 2002. *Policy Paradox: The Art of Political Decision Making*. New York: Norton.

United States House of Representatives. Report No. 2080, May 20, 1946.

United States Senate Hearing 111-242, Beyond Federal School Meal Programs: Reforming Nutrition for Kids in Schools. March 31, 2009.

United States Senate Hearing 111-245, Benefits of Farm-to-School Projects: Healthy Eating and Physical Activity for School Children. May 15, 2009.

United States Senate Hearing 111-1130, Childhood Obesity: Beginning the Dialogue on Reversing the Epidemic, March 4, 2010.

United States Senate Hearing 111-1142, The State of the American Child. June 8, 2010.

United States Senate Hearing 111-1163, The State of the American Child. November 18, 2010.

United States Senate Report 111-178, May 5, 2010.

White, A. F. 2014. *Plowed Under: Food Policy Protests and Performance in New Deal America*. Bloomington: Indiana University Press.

Yee, V. 2012. No appetite for good-for-you school lunches. *New York Times*, October 5.

Yeoman, B. 2003. Unhappy meals. *Mother Jones* 28(1): 40–45, 81.

18 Leadership, partnerships, and civic engagement

A case study of school food reform in California

Helena C. Lyson

Introduction

Childhood obesity has become one of the greatest public health crises of our time. As of 2014, approximately 17.2% of U.S. children and adolescents aged 2–19 years, or 12.7 million youth, were classified as obese, compared to only 5% of children and adolescents in the early 1980s (CDC 2011, 2015). This tripling of the childhood obesity rate since the 1980s has helped fuel mounting public concern about the health and well-being of the nation's children and has landed childhood obesity as a major focus of public health initiatives throughout the country. The nation's federal school meal programs, in particular, have been hurtled to the forefront of efforts to improve children's diets—and for good reason. Together, the national school lunch program (NSLP) and school breakfast program (SBP) are two of the nation's largest food and nutrition assistance public welfare programs (Morgan 2015). They play an important role in the diets of hundreds of thousands of children, including many low-income and minority youth who have been disproportionately affected by obesity (CDC 2011). National data has shown that foods eaten at school comprise anywhere from one fifth to one half of children's total daily energy intake (Stallings and Yaktine 2007, p. 103). Federal school food programs are critical in the battle against childhood obesity, as they can provide youth with critical access to healthy food groups including fruits, vegetables, and calcium-rich dairy beverages (Ralston and Newman 2015).

As a result of the increased emphasis on school food as a solution to addressing childhood obesity concerns throughout the country, the school lunchroom has become a site for reform efforts targeted at improving the nature and quality of school food. In particular, school food reformers have launched a growing, grassroots farm to school (FTS) movement around the country that promotes the local procurement of foods for school meals from small-scale, sustainable farms; agriculture or nutrition-based educational activities in the classroom; field trips to farms or farmers' markets; educational sessions for parents and the community; and tending to school gardens (USDA 2016). FTS programs have had documented success in increasing student access to, and consumption of, locally sourced fruits and vegetables, as well as improved student attitudes toward trying and eating fresh fruits and vegetables (Bontrager Yoder et al. 2014; Nicholson et al. 2014). FTS programs, moreover, have grown rapidly in recent years, from fewer than 10 programs in 1998, to programs in approximately 42% of school districts nationwide in 2015 (Joshi et al. 2008, p. 230; USDA 2015).

This chapter explores how groundbreaking school food reform efforts unfolded in a large, urban school district in California to address childhood obesity concerns and institutionalize farm to school programming. My research reveals that school food reform efforts transpired in the district through three interrelated processes: (1) the sustained involvement of civically engaged parent-activists advocating for substantial changes to the district's school meals program; (2) the passion and leadership capacity of the district's school food service director to champion farm to school efforts and facilitate key partnerships to envision and oversee reform efforts; and (3) widespread community support to fund and implement the proposed reforms. I draw from Lyson's (2004, 2005) theory of civic agriculture, as well as social movement and organizational theories on leadership (Aldon and Staggenborg 2004), institutional entrepreneurship (DiMaggio 1988; Fligstein 1997, 2001), and partnerships and alliances (Van Dyke and McCammon 2010) to structure an explanation of the interrelated processes of social change in the district. This chapter illuminates the dynamic relationship between food and public health by exploring how social change efforts coalesced in a case study school district to transform existing public school food program arrangements, so as to implement widespread reforms to benefit the health and well-being of youth in the community.

Theory

Civic agriculture

Lyson's (2004, 2005) theory of civic agriculture provides a useful framework for examining the dynamics of food system social change efforts that are embedded within the structure of local communities. Blending social science theories of civic engagement with the sociology of food and agriculture, the concept of civic agriculture provides a way to understand what Lyson identified as the trend toward locally based agriculture and food production that is tightly linked to a region's social and economic development. Representing a community-oriented, sustainable alternative to the market-based model of large-scale, industrial agriculture, civic agriculture "embodies a commitment to developing and strengthening an economically, environmentally, and socially sustainable system of agriculture and food production that relies on local resources and serves local markets and consumers" (Lyson 2005, p. 94). The organizational manifestations of civic agriculture include farmers' markets, neighborhood and school gardens, community supported agriculture operations and kitchens, and roadside fruit and vegetable stands (Lyson 2004).

Central to the concept of civic agriculture is civic participation and the notion of community problem-solving: "The locally based organizational, associational, and institutional component of the agriculture and food system is at the heart of civic agriculture," Lyson (2004, p. 63) writes. Lyson (2005, pp. 97–98) saw increasing civic engagement with the food system through the presence of organizations established to promote a flourishing localized agriculture as evidence of local problem-solving activities that are central to the functioning of civic agriculture in local communities. Expanding on Lyson's (2005) initial formulation of problem-solving and civic agriculture, Bagdonis, Hinrichs, and Schafft (2009, p. 109) contend that Lyson's use of the concept of civic engagement in the context of civic agriculture emphasizes the orientation of citizen efforts toward the needs and concerns of their wider community, and involvement that is thoughtful, deliberate, and reasoned.

Bagdonis et al. (2009, p. 109), however, argue that Lyson provides limited empirical findings on the practices and social interactions within communities that might foster civic agriculture beyond just the presence of associations and initiatives, and that we still know little about the texture and evolution of civic practices related to localized food and agriculture projects. Drawing on social movement theories of framing, Bagdonis et al. (2009) attempt to fill this lacuna in the literature by illuminating how activists with two FTS initiatives in Pennsylvania construct meaning and possible solutions to particular problems in order to shed light on how civic engagement ensues on the ground in relation to local agriculture projects. In the same vein, I build on the efforts by Bagdonis et al. (2009) to provide empirical evidence detailing the evolution and dynamics of civic practices associated with local food and agriculture social change efforts to contribute to the growing literature on civic agriculture and food system activism. In particular, I attend closely to the role of civically minded parent-activists in mounting school food reform efforts in the district and the ultimate widespread community buy-in for the proposed FTS initiatives in the case study school district.

Social movement leadership and institutional entrepreneurship

In exploring the key role of the district's food service director in bringing about school food reform, I draw from theories of action and leadership at the nexus of social movement and organizational theory. Traditionally, social movement scholars have been slow to theorize the role of movement leaders for fear of overemphasizing human agency at the expense of structural conditions that give rise to collective action. However, scholars have increasingly begun to recognize that leaders are critical to social movement success as "they inspire commitment, mobilize resources, create, and recognize opportunities, devise strategies, frame demands, and influence outcomes" (Aldon and Staggenborg 2004, p. 171). Importantly, social movement scholars have noted that leaders generate social change as strategic decision-makers who inspire and organize others, formulate ideologies, synthesize information, dialogue with stakeholders, network, and build coalitions (Aldon and Staggenborg 2004, p. 175).

The recent cross-pollination between social movement theory and organizational theory has offered yet more perspectives on agency and action in institutional settings that shed light on the role that key actors play in social change efforts. In particular, neoinstitutionalist theories of institutional entrepreneurs seek to account for action-oriented institutional change despite pressures toward stasis by emphasizing how actors leverage resources to create new, or transform existing, institutional arrangements (DiMaggio 1988, 1991; Fligstein 1997, 2001). Echoing social movement theories of leadership, organizational scholars emphasize how institutional entrepreneurs engage in key actions including agenda setting, framing action, aggregating interests, and networking and coalition building to motivate change in an institutional setting (Fligstein 1997). Institutional entrepreneurs, moreover, are change agents who initiate divergent actions that challenge existing institutional logics, or established ways of doing things, and actively participate in the implementation of these changes (Battilana, Leca, and Boxenbaum 2009). Drawing from these theories of leadership and agency in social change processes, I explore how the district's nutrition services director played a key role in school food reform efforts.

Social movement alliances, partnerships, and coalitions

Key external partnerships were also crucial in bringing about change in the district under study. Social movement theories on alliances, partnerships, and coalitions are helpful in exploring this phenomenon. Drawing from social movement and organizational scholars' identification of the important role that institutional entrepreneurs and movement leaders play in terms of networking and alliance building to enact institutional change agendas, scholars of social movements have delved deeper into how strategic partnerships, alliances, and coalitions function to achieve social change. Transcending notions of social movements as homogenous social entities, the notion of social movement coalitions allows researchers "to grasp more fully the varied constituencies, ideological perspectives, identities, and tactical preferences different groups bring to movement activism" (Van Dyke and McCammon 2010, p. xii). Diani and Bison (2004, p. 283), for example, note that inherent to social movement processes is the presence of "dense informal interorganizational networks" in which "both individual and organized actors, while keeping their autonomy and independence, engage in sustained exchanges of resources in pursuit of common goals." Moreover, Staggenborg (2010, p. 316) writes that coalitions have become a central focus of social movement scholars and contends that "by combining resources and coordinating strategies, movements, and their allies are bound to be more effective in achieving goals and creating social changes in culture, institutions, and public policy."

Coalition work in social movement activism ranges from loosely coupled activities aimed at similar goals to formal coalitions of organizations that bring together different types of actors to focus on particular social change campaigns or efforts (Staggenborg 2010, p. 317). Research on movement coalitions and partnerships indicates that these alliances generally emerge out of the identification of shared interests and identities, as well as preexisting networks and a history of cooperation (Staggenborg 2010). And as indicated above, institutional entrepreneurs and movement leaders often play a key role in establishing these crucial partnerships. Informed by the literature on social movement coalitions and partnerships, I explore the extent to which school food reform efforts in the case study school district relied on key partnerships between school officials and external groups, including a local nonprofit organization, to facilitate change to the school meals program.

Research site and context

Out of the nearly 15,000 school districts in the United States today, the largest districts have a disproportionate share of low-income students who rely on school food as a crucial source of nutrition. In the context of childhood obesity and school food reform efforts, it is these largest school districts that require the most attention, as their school food programs are critical in the battle against childhood obesity (Poppendieck 2010). As a state commanding one of the most significant portions of the federal school food program budget and serving meals to the second largest number of students in the country behind Texas, California is an ideal state to study school food programs (USDA FNS 2016). According to 2012 U.S. Department of Education statistics, 30 of the 200 largest school districts by enrollment size in the nation are in California. As such, qualitative research for this chapter was conducted in one of these 30 school districts in California—hereafter referred to as Pacific City School District (PCSD),* to explore how school food reform efforts have unfolded in a large, diverse, urban school district that plays an important role in the fight against childhood obesity.

As outlined in Table 18.1, district facts indicate that students in PCSD are primarily Black and Hispanic, with these two racial/ethnic groups comprising nearly 70% of the student population. Moreover, almost 75% of students qualify for free or reduced-price lunches in the district. Out of the 86 total schools in the district, the school nutrition program operates cooking kitchens at 25 of them, where meals are produced on-site. Two of these cooking kitchens serve as central kitchens, preparing the majority, nearly three-quarters, of food for the district. Sixty-four out of the 86 schools in the district receive meals from these central kitchens and are known as "satellite" school sites, which do no on-site cooking. Although food prepared at the central kitchens is scratch-cooked as much as possible, the extent of scratch cooking that is feasible is limited by old and nonfunctional existing equipment.† Moreover, the current

---

* Names of all organizations referenced and individuals interviewed have been changed to protect confidentiality.
† Scratch cooking is not a reality for many school districts across the country today, as most lost skilled workers and the infrastructure needed to prepare fresh meals throughout the 1970s during the transition to serving highly processed, frozen heat-and-serve foods. According to a 2012 survey, 88% of school nutrition officials surveyed nationwide said their district lacks the appropriate infrastructure needed to prepare items from scratch including knives, refrigerators, and other equipment (The Pew Charitable Trusts and the Robert Wood Johnson Foundation 2013). Although PCSD's two central kitchens incorporate scratch cooking as much as possible into meal preparation, the district is similar to others nationwide in that the poor condition of the existing equipment in the central kitchens limits the extent of scratch cooking that is possible.

Table 18.1 Pacific City School District Facts, 2014–2015

Total enrollment	37,147
Total number of schools	86
Student racial/ethnic composition	
White	11.8%
Black	29.7%
Hispanic	39.3%
Asian	13.9%
Other	5.2%
Free and reduced price lunch eligible students	73.4%
Average number of breakfasts served daily	7491
Average number of lunches served daily	20,705

Source: Adapted from Pacific City School District, internal data, 2015.

Notes: Deidentified source material available upon request.

kitchen system requires that the food service staff prepare most meals several days in advance of service, and then pack these meals in plastic to be sent to the school sites and then reheated. Finally, nutrition services for PCSD is entirely self-operated, meaning the district employs school food service staff to run the program, rather than contracting out the operating of the program to a private food service management company (FSMC). Although the number of school districts that contract out their meal services to a FSCM has steadily increased in recent decades to around 17% of districts nationwide (The Pew Charitable Trusts 2014), the majority of school districts still manage their own meal services like PCSD.

In the district, overall school meal program improvement was an on-going process, beginning in the 2009–2010 school year when a group of concerned parents began advocating for widespread changes. This parent activism, combined with the leadership of the food service director, led to the formation of a crucial partnership with an external nonprofit organization the following school year to initiate and execute a detailed study on the feasibility of large-scale school food reforms in the district. The study recommended the building of a state-of-the-art central kitchen and educational farm to drastically improve meal offerings. The central kitchen would be the hub of a new kitchen system in the district that would eliminate nearly all prepackaged food and allow students to eat meals freshly prepared at their school sites, the same day. In addition, the educational farm would allow for increased local sourcing of food for school meals, and a unique opportunity for students to engage in hands-on learning in the areas of agriculture and nutrition. School food reform efforts in the district ultimately culminated in the passage of a community-backed bond measure in 2012 to fund the building of the central kitchen and educational farm.

Research questions and design

Questions

This study examines the following research questions: (1) what were the processes that facilitated groundbreaking school food reform efforts in a large, urban school district to address growing childhood obesity concerns and (2) how were these processes affected by the local community context of the school district.

Methods

Data for this chapter come from 8 months of qualitative fieldwork throughout 2015 in the case study district including semi-structured interviews with 46 school food stakeholders, participant observation at school cafeterias, kitchens, and food service and school board meetings, and archival document analysis of key school documents including official reports, press releases, and media coverage. All audio recordings of the interviews were transcribed, and I used NVivo 11 for Mac to analyze the transcripts, field notes, and archival documents—employing a combination of inductive and deductive methods to develop analytical categories and themes based first on the qualitative data collected, and second on broader analytical concepts derived from the theoretical literature relevant to the research. The findings presented here should be regarded as exploratory, as the research focuses on the dynamics of school food reform efforts in one case study school district in California. Moreover, because of the uniqueness of the case study district as large, diverse, urban, and with a significant number of students that participate in the school meals program, the findings from the study may not necessarily be generalizable to other school districts across the country. Nevertheless, the research provides a useful framework for understanding the challenges and successes of school food reform efforts beyond the case study district based on key community-level factors that will likely resonate with any school district in the United States, regardless of size, location, or demographic composition.

Results and discussion

My research demonstrates that school food reform efforts in PCSD were facilitated in large part by three interrelated processes:

1. The sustained involvement of civically engaged parent-activists advocating for change.
2. The passion and leadership capacity of the district's school food service director as a champion for reform.
3. Widespread community support to fund and implement reforms.

In what follows, I detail the complexities of each of the three processes and find support for previous research emphasizing that school food reform efforts like farm to school projects rely on the dedication and coordination of a variety of actors from a diversity of sectors working together to reorient school meal programs toward local, sustainable, and healthy alternatives (e.g., Trainor 2006; Bagdonis et al. 2009; Conner et al. 2011; Buckley et al. 2013).

Parent-activists

Concerned parents who identified the need for reform in their community and organized themselves into an association committed to improving school food were the early initiators of improvement efforts in PCSD. One parent activist I interviewed, Lily, described to me in detail the early stages of her involvement in seeking to bring about healthy change to the district's school meals. After noticing that the quality of school lunches was not what it should be at her child's elementary school, she was inspired to promote change. Through involvement in the school's parent–teacher association, she took on the responsibility of contacting NourishYouth, a new Pacific City-based organization that had been started by two local business school graduates and was committed to serving healthy, freshly prepared meals to students in local schools, to see what it would take to get them into her child's school. As she describes it:

> …it seemed like a really exciting company, and the thought of having organic food and some of it locally sourced seemed like a really great opportunity for the school. And I was a new parent. I had no idea at all what was involved. I had just thought, 'This is a school, and they can have lunch with whoever they want, and we'll get [NourishYouth] to write up a contract with us.' And then, all of a sudden, 400 students are getting fresh, organic meals…And to me, at the time, I thought, 'Wow, if I could get organic food on 400 plates for lunch, that has an impact.' It felt like a huge impact to me to alter that. And I had no idea like, what was really possible at that time. But that seemed like a really great step. So, I decided to take this on. So, I reached out to [NourishYouth] (Interview, April 17, 2015).

Through her contact with this organization, Lily discovered that they were not able to contract with individual schools and would, instead, have to contract with the district's entire school meals program. She also learned that a number of other parents had also recently independently contacted NourishYouth to look into getting them into the PCSD. As Lily remarked, "They were [Pacific City] parents who were doing the same thing at the same time—like, picking up the phone—actually, before me—picking up the phone and saying, 'We want [NourishYouth].' " Motivated by their mutual interest in getting better food into the district, the concerned parents decided to work together on this issue and formed the Pacific City Cafeteria Collaboration—a volunteer group eager to improve food quality in the district.

They pursued getting NourishYouth into the entire district by meeting with Cindy, the district's nutrition services director, to see what was possible.

The parents quickly found out, however, that although Cindy indicated she was open to ways to improve the food quality in the district, the meal program was already tied to other contracts with food service vendors and would not easily be able to begin contracting with NourishYouth. "There was the contract issues with the vendors. There was the labor contract issues. Layers and layers of complexity," Lily described, "And I sort of sat back, and I was like, 'Well, you know, this is just classic bureaucracy, right?'" Lily remarked that district budget cuts contributed to evaporating the dream to get NourishYouth in the district and that:

> ...fairly quickly it became clear that there wasn't enough money for us to engage with [NourishYouth]. And at that point in time, the [parent] group was starting to solidify and decided that we wanted to move forward with our own reform...what became clear was...the way to real systemic change would be to change the system itself. So, we decided to take that on at that point (Interview, April 17, 2015).

With that, the parent activist group ramped up their engagement with the school district and the community. Lily described that the Collaboration's bimonthly meetings gathered as many as 200 people, with participants ranging from parents and teachers to other interested community members. Nonetheless, a core group of around 12–15 people were the main leaders of the group. As Lily's recounting of the formation of the Cafeteria Collaboration reveals, concerned parents who were committed to working for change in the district were a crucial component to beginning school food reform efforts in the district. These civically oriented parent-activists, who were passionate about food and agriculture system reform in their community, brings to mind Lyson's (2004, 2005) melding of civic engagement and food system transformation. These parents' early efforts to seek out local solutions in the form of a partnership with a local food and agriculture organization to begin sourcing fresh, local, and healthy food for students in the district to solve a problem they collectively identified demonstrates the problem-solving capacity of local communities that was so central to Lyson's (2004, 2005) concept of civic agriculture and the move toward a healthier, more sustainable, and locally embedded food system. Although Lily and the other parents' initial concern regarding school food began with observations from their own children's schools, they quickly realized that reform in the entire district was a critical need for the wider community, and they were deliberate and reasoned in their decision to take on problem-solving the issue of poor school meal quality for the entire district through their formation of the Cafeteria Collaboration.

School food service director leadership

When Lily and the other parents first approached Cindy, the school food service director, about potentially contracting with NourishYouth, Lily recalled that the meeting was somewhat adversarial. Cindy laid out all the reasons why that route to improvement was not going to be possible, mainly pointing to the current contracts the district was already in and budget issues. Importantly, however, Lily recalled that Cindy was not opposed to school food reform, and in fact, said she was willing to engage with the parents and work with them, but that they would need to find another way. Cindy's openness to pursuing reforms with the parents would prove to be crucial to the ultimate success of the efforts. School food service directors are charged with overseeing all aspects of a district's food service program including procurement, menu planning, food preparation, financial management, and personnel management. With such significant control over a district's program, food service directors can often make or break reform efforts targeted at overall meal improvements.

Mark, a nonprofit activist who works on school garden programming at the state level, remarked on the general importance of school food service directors in making FTS programs happen in districts:

> ...the interesting thing about farm to school, there's no cookie cutter approach to it, it is not institutionalized, everybody has to figure it out on their own and where we see great strides being made is when you have a proactive, supportive school food service director. They're kind of the gatekeeper for farm to school to happen, in my opinion... I believe that districts, based on whether it's the school board or parent pressure, are going to be looking to replace their food service directors with more farm to school or nutrition-minded food service directors and I think 'cause they're the kind of champions that can make or break it (Interview, January 22, 2015).

Kristen, a school food service director in a southern California school district, reinforced this idea of school food service directors as gatekeepers for instituting progressive reforms to school food programs, when she discussed how school food service directors are the ones who have full control over deciding what kind of food sourcing and distribution the district will use and the difficulties in moving away from the established ways of doing things:

> The challenge is, I think, getting food service directors to be willing to venture away from the typical distribution setup. I know it's a lot of work, but if you really want to do farm to school, you have to look at alternative distribution so that you can get food from [local] farms...You're taking on one more huge task, without any help. It's daunting, to say the least. And especially if you don't have the passion for it. Like, if you don't get why it's important for kids to eat local, sustainably produced foods, you're not going to put a ton of extra work into that (Interview, March 6, 2015).

In addition, Maggie, a nonprofit staff member who partners with school districts throughout California to promote farm to school programming, told me that activists like her can do as much as they want in terms of facilitating farm to school efforts, but "you just have to have really motivated food service directors that are really sold on the idea [of farm to school]" because "they're the ones, in the end, that make the buying decisions and do the purchasing. All I can do is just the groundwork."

In the case of PCSD, Cindy ultimately emerged as a champion of school food reform efforts, and many people I spoke with attributed the district's success in terms of school food reform efforts directly to her passion and motivation. For example, Julia, a strategic planner who worked closely on school food reform efforts in the district, talked about how Cindy was at the vanguard of the district's efforts to improve school food in the early stages:

> Cindy, she's really an amazing woman…She was always two steps ahead…I couldn't believe how she was doing what she was even doing with the budget she had…it was really remarkable. She was already going to the farmers markets and gardens and all the things that the [Cafeteria Collaboration] really wanted (Interview, May 19, 2015).

Importantly, Cindy had the passion and the interest to start serving healthier foods to PCSD students. As Drew, a nonprofit activist, remarked about Cindy's early desire for change:

> Cindy wanted to serve more local food, fresh food, healthier food. This was seen as a positive health intervention in [Pacific City], and if you look at that disparity and life expectancy in different parts of [Pacific City] and a lot of it is tied to food and food security and all these things, [Pacific City] is a really interesting place to create those changes. And there was this willingness (Interview, May 28, 2015).

The narrative of change in Pacific City is woven around Cindy and her motivation to do things differently for PCSD's students. As Mark said reflecting on the progress Pacific City has made, "Like you look at [PCSD] and Cindy, and she's behind it, and great things are happening all over the place." In the same vein, Ana, a school food service director for another local school district commented, "I do have a ton of admiration for what [Pacific City] is doing, and what Cindy is doing." These comments reveal how Cindy's name goes hand in hand with discussions of school food reform efforts in Pacific City and emphasize the important role she has had in spearheading reform efforts to improve the quality of school food in the district.

In particular, Cindy's initial openness and subsequent ongoing commitment to school food reform enabled her to mobilize a broad base of support for school meal improvement efforts in the district through key actions, including networking and dialoguing with stakeholders in the community. As a skilled leader, or institutional entrepreneur, Cindy was able to interface with both the parent-activist group and a local nonprofit organization focused on youth education for sustainable living, the Institute for Green Education, that happened to be searching for a school district to partner with at around the same time. As Lily described it to me:

> So, [the Institute for Green Education] had feelers out and they were looking for a district....And they were interested in [another local school district], and obviously, that would have been a great district to take on, but what they found was that there were not—the players were not aligned and ready to go....And when they came to [Pacific City], what they found is they had a really active parent group, they had a nutrition services director who was on board (Interview, April 17, 2015).

As a result of Cindy's interfacing with both groups, the Institute for Green Education joined forces with the parents and district to help realize school food change. With the support of grant funding, the Institute helped produce a feasibility study that provided a concrete path forward for bringing about the changes that the district wanted, including ways to fund these changes. Central to this plan was a $40 million building project to create modern kitchens throughout the district, as well as a new, state-of-the-art central kitchen and educational farm. All of these changes would allow for more on-site preparation of healthy meals throughout the district instead of serving reheated frozen meals; increased local sourcing of food directly from the educational farm; and an opportunity for students to learn about where their food comes from through classes at the educational farm.

Cindy's leadership, then, was the second major element responsible for facilitating the transition to healthier school meals in the district. This finding supports previous research demonstrating that supportive school food service directors are central to improving school food programs on the ground (Bagdonis et al. 2009; Buckley et al. 2013). Bagdonis et al. (2009, p. 111), in particular, found that FTS "champions" can play a pivotal role in linking other stakeholders and maintaining the energy, enthusiasm, and forward momentum of local FTS efforts. In PCSD, Cindy's passion and openness to help facilitate reform efforts in the district enabled her to use her integral position as the director of the program to become an internal champion for change and interface with stakeholders. My findings also coincide with previous research on the important role of movement leaders and institutional entrepreneurs in facilitating social change efforts by actions including aggregating interests, networking, and coalition building, as detailed in the social movement and organizational theory literature.

In addition, by combining resources and coordinating strategies, the partnership between the parent-activists, the district, and the Institute for Green Education allowed the reform efforts to be more successful than they would have been if any single group had been acting on its own. Cindy or the parent-activists, for example, would likely not have had the time or expertise to come up with such a grandiose plan for school food reform in the district on their own. The partnership with experts at the nonprofit organization, who had expertise in the arena of large-scale school food reform, enabled the reform efforts that had been discussed to become a reality. This finding, thus, reinforces previous research on the benefits of social movement coalitions in effecting change. Research on food system social change efforts, in particular, has similarly found that key partnerships with outside nongovernmental organizations are crucial in developing and spearheading change initiatives. Studies conducted by Bagdonis et al. (2009) and Trainor (2006), for example, concluded that nonprofit partnerships with school districts play a key role in the success of FTS programs.

Local community support

Finally, widespread support from the local community was the last factor facilitating school food reform in PCSD. The proposal developed by the Institute for Green Education for the central kitchen and educational farm stipulated that funding was not going to come from private donors, but would, instead, require widespread community buy-in and support. In this way, a citywide bond measure became the focal point of funding the path forward for school food reform efforts in PCSD. The bond would provide for district access to $475 million in facilities upgrade funds, with roughly $44 million to be designated for revamping school kitchens and the construction of a central kitchen in Pacific City, including a 1.5-acre educational farm that would eventually supply some of the district's fresh produce needs. The bond required a 55% supermajority vote for approval. Many of the parent-activists were involved in canvassing the community in support of the bond measure and in November 2012, just over 84% of Pacific City voters approved the bond.

Many people I interviewed about school food reform efforts in PCSD emphasized the various bases of community support Cindy and the district relied on in their efforts to mount change. Mark, for instance, remarked that in addition to Cindy's leadership, "it's the team that makes that [change] happen. She has staff under her, nonprofit support, they got the bond measure, and once again, there's no cookie-cutter way to do it, but if there's a will, there's a way, and there's usually organizations that'll help support it." Rachel, a farm to school nonprofit activist in California, also was careful to characterize change efforts in Pacific City as a community project: "And then, like, PCSD, you know, has been, like, this crazy linchpin, like community change around school food and they've made, like, huge progress...They got, you know, a $475 million bond passed to fund all this stuff." Kristen, too, remarked on the importance of various forms of community backing for Pacific City's success: "I think Cindy's support from her community enabled her to make that change—the bond, the [Institute for Green Education]. That was amazing for Cindy because her task was exceedingly daunting, given the challenges that you face in [Pacific City]." In this way, the widespread community backing for the ultimate passage of the bond measure to fund the new central kitchen and educational farm that will pave the way for institutionalizing farm to school practices in the district reveals a profound prioritizing of local food and agriculture to benefit the health and well-being of the community's youth, and the immense problem-solving capacity of the Pacific

City community that is in line with Lyson's (2004, 2005) vision for civic agriculture projects across the country.

Conclusions

While many challenges limit the ability of school districts to provide healthy and nutritious food environments for students in the face of childhood obesity concerns, this analysis of school food reform efforts in a large, diverse, urban school district reveals the potential of coordinated social change initiatives to bring about large-scale improvements to federal school food programs. In this way, these research findings hold important implications for discussions at the intersection of food and public health, especially in relation to childhood obesity. Moreover, although the research was conducted in a large, urban school district, the lessons generated from the results are nevertheless useful for any school district across the country operating federal school meal programs. All school districts, regardless of their size, demographic composition, or geographic location, operate within a specific community context, and it is this local context that we must be attuned to when mounting school food reform efforts.

In particular, results from this research speak to the importance of locally embedded reform efforts that realize success through their harnessing of the varied assets and resources of the local community to enact change. Importantly, school districts require support from both civically engaged parent-activists and the local community to realize school food reform. The established ways of operating federal school food programs are deeply engrained and require significant motivation, passion, and resources to be changed. Community problem-solving efforts that bring together individuals and organizations from a variety of sectors are integral for challenging the status quo and, in this case, working to institutionalize farm to school practices that will benefit students by both providing them with healthier and fresher foods, and educating them on the importance of local, sustainable agriculture. Facilitating the creation of a vibrant nonprofit sector and active parent-teacher associations is especially crucial then for small, rural, or economically disadvantaged school districts throughout the country to ensure a supportive community context for school food reform.

Reflecting back on PCSD's success at working toward changing the nature and quality of school food in the district, Lily remarked, "It was really an alignment of people and social factors that facilitated this. Because you think about—in another place or another time, this just could have been dead in the water." My research demonstrates that it was, indeed, the confluence of a variety of factors, including the motivation of civically engaged parent-activists; the passion and leadership of a school food service director; the resources and facilitation of a local nonprofit organization; and the far-reaching support of the local community that put PCSD on the path to success to realize genuine school food reform. Hence, this study has contributed to deepening our understanding of the factors that are crucial to enacting school food reform efforts that are at the heart of addressing public health concerns surrounding childhood obesity.

Acknowledgment

Research for this chapter was supported in part by a Doctoral Dissertation Research Improvement grant from the National Science Foundation.

REFERENCES

Aldon, M. D. and S. Staggenborg. 2004. Leadership in social movements. In *The Blackwell Companion to Social Movements*, edited by D. A. Snow, S. A. Soule, and H. Kriesi. 171–196. Malden, MA: Blackwell Publishing.

Bagdonis, J. M., C. C. Hinrichs, and K. A. Schafft. 2009. The emergence and framing of farm-to-school initiatives: Civic engagement, health and local agriculture. *Agriculture and Human Values* 26:107–119.

Battilana, J., B. Leca, and E. Boxenbaum. 2009. How actors change institutions: Towards a theory of institutional entrepreneurship. *Academy of Management Annals* 3(1): 65–107.

Bontrager Yoder, A. B., J. L. Liebhart, D. J. McCarty, A. Meinen, D. Schoeller, C. Vargas, and T. LaRowe. 2014. Farm to elementary school programming increases access to fruits and vegetables and increases their consumption among those with low intake. *Journal of Nutrition Education and Behavior* 46(5):341–349.

Buckley, J., D. S. Conner, C. Matts, and M. W. Hamm. 2013. Social relationships and farm-to-institution initiatives: Complexity and scale in local food systems. *Journal of Hunger & Environmental Nutrition* 8:397–412.

Centers for Disease Control and Prevention. 2011. CDC grand rounds: Childhood obesity in the United States. *Morbidity and Morality Weekly Report* 60(20):42–46. Retrieved from: http://www.cdc.gov/mmwr/preview/mmwrhtml/mm6002a2.htm#fig1. Accessed on April 22, 2015.

Center for Disease Control and Prevention. 2015. *Childhood Obesity Facts*. Retrieved from: http://www.cdc.gov/obesity/data/childhood.html. Accessed on March 9, 2016.

Conner, D. S., B. King, C. Koliba, J. Kolodinsky, and A. Trubek. 2011. Mapping farm-to-school networks implications for research and practice. *Journal of Hunger & Environmental Nutrition* 62(2):133–152.

Diani, M. and I. Bison. 2004. Organizations, coalitions, and movements. *Theory and Society* 33:281–309.

DiMaggio, P. 1988. Interest and agency in institutional theory. In *Institutional Patterns and Organizations*, edited by L. Zucker. 3–22. Cambridge, MA: Ballinger.

DiMaggio, P. 1991. Constructing an organizational field as a professional project: US Art Museums, 1920–1940. In *The New Institutionalism in Organizational Analysis*, edited by W. Powell and P. DiMaggio. 267–292. Chicago, IL: The University of Chicago Press.

Fligstein, N. 1997. Social skill and institutional theory. *American Behavioral Scientist* 40(4):397–405.

Fligstein, N. 2001. Social skill and the theory of fields. *Sociological Theory* 19(2):105–125.

Joshi, A., A. M. Azuma, and G. Feenstra. 2008. Do farm-to-school programs make a difference? Findings and future research needs. *Journal of Hunger & Environmental Nutrition* 3(2–3): 229–246.

Lyson, T. A. 2004. *Civic Agriculture: Reconnecting Farm, Food and Community*. Medford, MA: Tufts University Press.

Lyson, T. A. 2005. Civic agriculture and community problem solving. *Culture and Agriculture* 27(2):92–98.

Morgan, R. B. 2015. U.S. Domestic Food Assistance Programs. *National Council of State Legislatures*. Retrieved from: http://www.ncsl.org/research/human-services/u-s-domestic-food-assistance-programs.aspx. Accessed on April 28, 2016.

Nicholson, L., L. Turner, L. Schneider, J. Chriqui, and F. Chaloupka. 2014. State farm-to-school laws influence the availability of fruits and vegetables in school lunches at US public elementary schools. *Journal of School Health* 84(5):310–216.

Poppendieck, J. 2010. *Free for All: Fixing School Food in America*. Berkeley: University of California Press.

Ralston, K. and C. Newman. 2015. School meals in transition. United States Department of Agriculture (USDA): Economic Information Bulletin Number 143. Retrieved from: https://permanent.access.gpo.gov/gpo61191/Full%20report/eib143.pdf. Accessed on June 1, 2017.

Staggenborg, S. 2010. Conclusion: Research on social movement coalitions. In *Strategic Alliances: Coalition Building and Social Movements*, edited by N. V. Dyke and H. J. McCammon. 316–329. Minneapolis, MN: University of Minnesota Press.

Stallings, V. A. and A. L. Yaktine. 2007. *Nutrition Standards for Foods in Schools: Leading the Way toward Healthier Youth*. Washington, DC: The National Academies Press.

The Pew Charitable Trusts. 2014. *Serving Healthy School Meals in California: The Tools Needed to do the Job*. Philadelphia, PA: The Pew Charitable Trusts. Retrieved from: http://www.pewtrusts.org/~/media/assets/2014/11/kitscaliforniareport111214final.pdf. Accessed on June 1, 2017.

The Pew Charitable Trusts and the Robert Wood Johnson Foundation. 2013. *Serving Healthy School Meals: U.S. Schools Need Updated Kitchen Equipment*. Philadelphia, PA: The Pew Charitable Trusts and Princeton, NJ: Robert Wood Johnson Foundation. Retrieved from: http://www.pewtrusts.org/~/media/assets/2013/12/kits_equipment_report.pdf. Accessed on August 31, 2016.

Trainor, J. K. 2006. Stakeholder roles and perceptions in the creation and success of farm to school programs. *Appetite* 47(3):401.

U.S. Department of Agriculture. 2015. *The Farm to School Census*. Retrieved from: https://farmtoschoolcensus.fns.usda.gov/home. Accessed on April 19, 2016.

U.S. Department of Agriculture. 2016. *The Farm to School Program, 2012–2015: Four years in review*. Retrieved from: https://origin.drupal.fns.usda.gov/sites/default/files/f2s/Farm-to-School-at-USDA--4-Years-in-Review.pdf. Accessed on April 19, 2016.

U.S. Department of Agriculture, Food and Nutrition Service. 2016. Child Nutrition Tables. Retrieved from: http://www.fns.usda.gov/pd/child-nutrition-tables. Accessed on April 27, 2016.

Van Dyke, N. and H. J. McCammon. 2010. *Strategic Alliances: Coalition Building and Social Movements*. Minneapolis, MN: University of Minnesota Press.

19 School food services privatization

Carol Ebdon and Can Chen

Introduction

Since the vast majority of U.S. children consume a significant portion of their daily food intake at school, the school food environment has a vital role in improving public health. Historically, childhood malnutrition was a major reason that schools began to provide meals for children, and for the adoption of the National School Lunch Program (NSLP) in 1946 (Nestle 2002; Levine 2010). By 2012, over 31 million low-cost or free lunches were being provided annually to children (USDA 2013). Beginning in 1970, the federal government allowed school districts to contract with private companies to operate their lunchrooms. This change was due to a recognition that an estimated 9 million children were in schools without lunch facilities (Levine 2010). Since then, the number of districts contracting with food service management companies (FSMCs) has steadily increased, especially since the late 1980s (Nestle 2002). The most current nationwide survey found that about 13% of school districts contract out for food services, but with wide variations across states, ranging from 86% in Rhode Island to six states (e.g., Kentucky) that had no districts with contracts (LaFaive 2007).

Districts are considered as having contracted out services if they use a private vendor for any part of their regular and routine food service operation. Given the critical role of school food services for public health, it is important to examine the impact of the privatization of school food services on school food cost and quality.* While there is a large literature on contracting for other government services, little empirical work exists on the results of contracting for school food services. To fill this void, we conducted interviews with key school district and food service company managers in Nebraska and Florida to explore the rationale for, as well as the benefits and challenges of, contracting versus internal school food service provision. Our results improve our understanding of school food service operations and provide valuable insights for theory and practice in this area.

---

* Privatization and contracting out are used interchangeably in this chapter.

Literature review

Privatization is a topic that concerns many scholars, government practitioners, and citizens. There is a voluminous literature on this subject. In general, privatization research can be categorized into two lines of inquiry. One line of research empirically investigates the motivations and determinants of privatization decisions in different kinds of public services (e.g., Ferris 1986; Brooks 1996; Savas 2000; LaFaive 2007; Curry 2010; Levine 2010). A second line of research examines the effects of privatization on public service delivery (e.g., McGuire and Van Cott 1984; Brooks 1996; Levin and McEwan 2002). A brief summary of each area of research is necessary.

Determinants of privatization

Generally, the literature has found that contracting is done primarily to save money and improve the quality of public services (LaFaive 2007; Curry 2010; Levine 2010). Researchers have also identified several specific factors influencing public agencies' utilization of privatization for the implementation of programs and services. For example, Ferris (1986) examines the determinants of privatization decisions in U.S. municipalities. He finds that large and urban cities are more likely to privatize than small and rural cities. In addition, cities are less likely to privatize when they have a strong labor union and sound fiscal health. Brooks et al. (1994) examine why some cities contract out solid waste collection while others maintain internal operations. They find that municipalities are more likely to turn to privatization when the local tax burden increases, multiple alternative service producers exist, and citizen demand for service increases. Hart et al. (1997) and Boyne (1996) find that public agencies are moving away from internal operation and favoring privatization, due to a growing sentiment that government is too large, less efficient, and untrustworthy.

Effects of privatization

In theory, privatization of government services is assumed to achieve cost savings because of competitive pressures and economies of scale in the private production process. In addition, the incentive structure in the private sector is more conducive to efficient production than its counterpart in the public bureaucracy (Spann 1977). However, studies have found mixed evidence on cost savings. On the positive side, Savas (1977) and Brooks (1996) find that in the case of municipal solid waste service, contracted private sector collection is less costly than public sector collection when the population exceeds 50,000. Similarly, in the area of school bus transportation service, McGuire and Van Cott (1984) assert that substantial savings could result from privatizing. In one of the few empirical studies of school food service contracting, the Mackinac Center in Michigan (2011) found that officials reported saving an average of $34 per pupil on food service contracts.

However, many studies also document negative cost effects of contracting. Harding (1990) and Alspaugh (1996) found that in-house provision is more efficient than the private operation of school bus transportation. Callan and Thomas (2001) found there is no difference between public and private production of municipal solid waste service in Massachusetts. Recently, Bel, Fageda, and Warner (2010) conducted a meta-regression analysis of 27 econometric studies examining privatization of water distribution and found no systematic support for lower costs with private production in municipal solid waste and water services. The U.S. GAO (2009) contends that an estimated $860 million (8.6%) in the school year 2005–2006 was paid improperly to food service contractors because of errors in the number of meals provided. One point emphasized by scholars is that the role of competition is critical for cost savings; if there is little competition among private vendors, there is little incentive for companies to provide low-cost bids (Savas 2000; Curry 2010; Kassel 2010).

Aside from the purported cost effects, the literature on school food services is very limited. It is primarily based on normative criticisms of privatization, including lack of public accountability and transparency, dependency, restricted flexibility, a loss of control, and lower quality (e.g., LeBruto and Farsad 1993; Levin and McEwan 2002; Nestle 2002; VanderSchee 2005; Mathis and Jimerson 2008). Beyond this speculation, we know little about the actual experiences and results of contracting for school food services.

Methodology

This research is exploratory in nature, due to the sparse extant empirical evidence related to school food service privatization. Our intention is to enhance our understanding of the factors that affect contracting and its perceived effects. We focus on school districts in two states: Florida and Nebraska. This selection was partially due to convenience, but the states are quite different in population and school district size, so similarities across these two states may be more generalizable than looking at states that are more alike.

Our primary data collection method was in-depth interviews, but we also reviewed written documents such as school lunch fund financial statements, procurement policies, and contracts. Interviewees included a combination of food service directors and school business managers. We emailed individuals in 18 districts in Nebraska and 20 districts in Florida to seek their participation. Follow-up emails were sent to those who did not respond. The districts were selected based on a combination of factors. In Nebraska, the largest ten districts were selected, then additional districts were added based on the snowball method when interviewees mentioned other districts that had experience with contracting. In Florida, five districts in Florida have privatized their food services, but one of the five declined to be interviewed. Self-operating districts in Florida were selected to represent a balance of diverse geographic locations and district sizes.

A total of eighteen interviews were conducted, eight in Nebraska and ten in Florida. Individuals were from fifteen separate districts, seven in Nebraska and eight in Florida (in some districts both the food service director and business manager were interviewed, while in others only one or the other participated). Eight of the districts provide the service internally (four in Nebraska and four in Florida), while the other seven contract (three in Nebraska and four in Florida). It should be noted that several of the participants had previous experience in other districts, as a contractor and/or a school official, so they had a broad perspective beyond their current district.

In order to obtain candid responses to our questions, interviewees were guaranteed anonymity, so neither the school districts nor the individuals are identified by name. We employed content analysis to distil themes and other insights provided by interviewees. One of us conducted the Florida interviews and the other the Nebraska interviews. We used the same questions and jointly reviewed the notes and discussed the results in depth throughout the analysis.

We asked a series of questions of the interviewees and the questions varied slightly depending on whether the district provides food service internally or contracts for the service. The questions related to the way in which major decisions are made, district procurement policies, perceived advantages and disadvantages of contracting versus internal provision, their opinions of the effects of privatization on costs and food quality, recent efforts made by the district to improve nutrition, and whether the district has recently considered changes in the method of food service. Interviewees from districts that contract were also asked about the history of contracting in the district, terms of the contract, why the decision was made to contract, and how the contract is monitored.

There are limitations to this study. With a small sample size, we may have missed a perspective that is different from the individuals we interviewed. In addition, our work reflects only the experiences in two states and may not be generalizable to other states. However, we found commonalities with responses from interviewees across districts and across states, despite the wide variety of size and circumstances, which mitigates our concerns about these limitations. Overall, we believe that our results can be useful to both scholars and practitioners and help to build our knowledge of school food service operations.

Analysis

The demographics of these two states vary substantially. Florida has a population of 20.3 million, of which 20% are under the age of 18. The land area is 53,625 square miles (U.S. Census Bureau 2015). Florida has 67 school districts, one district per county. There are 3255 schools, with a 2015–2016 membership of 2,646,100. The free and reduced lunch rate is about 46% (Florida School Nutrition Association 2016). Nebraska, on the other hand, is small in population, at 1.9 million (25% under 18), but the state is larger geographically than Florida, at 76,824 square miles (U.S. Census Bureau 2015). This has resulted in a large number of small school districts. There are 245 public school districts in Nebraska, with a 2015–2016 membership of 315,542. The free and reduced lunch rate is about 44% (Nebraska Department of Education 2015).

Our interviews resulted in four primary areas of focus: reasons for contracting, contracting versus internal operations, contracting process and terms, and effects of contracting. We will discuss each of these in turn. Throughout the analysis, we will review similarities and differences within and across states.

Reasons for contracting

The interviewees believed that school districts are increasingly turning to contracting for food service operations. "It's exploding in Nebraska; many districts are going to contracts now." A number of reasons were mentioned for this (Table 19.1).

In Nebraska, one major rationale appears to be the difficulty of finding qualified staff to manage this service, especially in smaller rural school districts. Six of the eight Nebraska interviewees noted that a number of districts have moved to contracting when their long-time directors retired because of the inability to replace the director. "Our food service director was retiring. The next person in line was also retiring. The supervisor at the middle school moved outside the area. So I lost my top three people all in one year. We put an ad in the paper to try to find people, but we just couldn't find anyone. People are not that interested in coming out here to this area. So we said, we have to look at outsourcing." In Florida, an interviewee from a small, rural district with a high poverty rate highlighted the difficulty to get qualified experts. "The reason why we looked at this option was being in a small rural district; we weren't sure that we could acquire the expertise…So, we turned to outsourcing toward a management company. This makes them [experts] palatable to come here as opposed to [for us] getting the talent that we couldn't afford."

A second reason for contracting relates to financial issues and resources. Some districts in both states have had difficulty breaking even on their food operations, or they prefer the national resources that a contractor can bring to the table. For example, interviewees in Nebraska say "There are changes when…the food

Table 19.1 Reasons for Contracting

State	Reasons for Contracting
Nebraska	• Inability to replace the food service director (6)
	• Financial issues and resources (2)
	• Educational philosophy (4)
	• New federal regulations (4)
	• Manage staff better and cut costs (2)
	• Create a one-stop shop by packaging outsourced services (1)
	• Unhappy with food (1)
Florida	• Financial deficit in their operation of food services (3)
	• Educational philosophy (3)
	• New federal regulations (2)
	• Cut employee cost because union is out of control (2)
	• Difficult to get qualified experts (1)
	• Food waste and unhappy with food (1)

service is not doing financially well. That's when they look into it." In Florida, five interviewees from the three privatized districts noted that they had difficulty breaking even on their food service programs. "We lose money in our food service operation. We were in the hole about a million and a half dollars." "The school district was looking at outsourcing to help erase a deficit in food service operation."

The complexity and challenges of the new federal regulations on school food are another reason for districts opting to contract. Four in Nebraska stated that the regulations were a leading factor in privatizing. "This is not the lunch lady land it used to be. There are so many more special diets and special nutritional regulations on the menus. A lot of the old-time veterans are not being able to keep up with all the changes and challenges." In Florida, two interviewees from privatized districts agree. "As long as you have to follow what the government says about the food; I do not see you will be able to improve the food program as much as you think you will be able to do that. That is the biggest problem of new federal regulations." "With new federal guidelines, we became a restaurant. But in a small district, it is very hard to follow the new changes and rules."

Somewhat related to this is the idea that the mission of a school district is to provide an education, not to be a food service provider. This was mentioned as a reason for contracting by several interviewees in both states. For example, one Nebraska interviewee stated, "The district administrators went to school to be teachers—little of their schooling was focused on facilities management and food service. They made a conscious decision to outsource so they could focus on education." And as one Florida interviewee put it, "School districts are in the education business. They are not in the restaurant business."

Several other reasons for contracting were raised by one or two individuals. These include the idea of creating a "one-stop" shop by packaging deals to outsource several operations to one company, such as food and custodial services. Another noted that contractors may be able to manage staff better and make cuts as necessary, particularly in small towns where everyone knows everyone else. One interviewee in Florida points out that private contractors are brought in when the union is out of control. "The union is dictating to the school district, and the school district is paying larger benefit packages and larger salaries to employees. That put the school district out of the business." In some districts, parents and students are not happy with the food, and/or there is food waste and low rates of lunch participation: "We had significant amounts of students not even purchasing the food and significant amounts of food that is actually not consumed...When the food waste exceeded 50%, there is an issue. That needs to be looked at. That was the intent of contracting."

Contracting versus internal operations

Pros and cons of contracting

A variety of opinions were expressed about the advantages of contracting versus providing the service internally (Table 19.2). The perceived benefits of contracting can be grouped into three areas. First, the contractor takes responsibility for

Table 19.2 Contracting versus Internal Operation

State	Main Advantages of Contracting	Main Advantages of Internal Operation
Nebraska	• Contractor takes responsibility for everything, including meeting regulations (7)	• Greater internal control (3)
	• Financial efficiencies (5)	• History and experience (2)
	• Contractor has greater resources (expertise and professional management) (3)	• Longer-term focus (2)
		• Food service is part of the administration team (2)
Florida	• Financial efficiencies (6)	• Keep the connection of between food and student learning (3)
	• Contractor has greater resources (expertise and professional management) (5)	• Greater internal control (2)
	• Cut the employee costs and better manage staff (4)	• A better fit in the educational setting (2)
	• Contractor takes responsibility for day-to-day management (3)	• Provide more personalized service (2)

all aspects of the food service operation (except for collecting funds from parents, processing free and reduced applications, and federal/state reporting). This was cited as a benefit by seven Nebraska and three Florida interviewees. Some districts, perhaps small districts, in particular, prefer to hire firms that are better able to keep up with the regulations. "It relieves the client from dealing with government regulations. We're taking on all his food safety risks, his menu-setting, government meal standards. We take all the risks; that's why he pays me to do that, so he can sleep at night and not have to worry about the challenges." "We do not have to employ inputs and resources. We do not have to worry about complying with new federal regulations. We do not worry about managing food service. We now have a company doing that."

Financial efficiencies were also mentioned as a potential advantage of contracting by five Nebraska and six Florida interviewees. These efficiencies often stem from the large-scale buying power of the firms, which can result in lower purchasing costs, particularly for small districts that do not buy in sufficient quantities to receive volume discounts. For example, one Florida interviewee mentioned "xxx company has a nationwide contractor. Just based on the economy of scale, they have the opportunity to have much lower pricing than the district with 27,000 kids." One individual from Nebraska also mentioned that some districts have purchasing policies that give preference to buying locally, which can result in higher costs, so contracting for this service with regional or national companies, who are not restricted in their food sourcing, can save money.

The ability of contractors to access greater resources was mentioned by three of the Nebraska interviewees and five of the Florida interviewees. These

resources can be useful for meal planning and advice regarding federal regulations. For example, one individual from Florida mentioned "They [private con-
tractors] have the ability to hire people with an appropriate education level and
training experience, such as nutritionists and dietitians at the corporate level or
regional level...They have the ability to design meals at a lower cost than we will
provide because they have the nutritionists and dietitians to serve multiple school
districts and create menus."

On the flip side, three individuals from Nebraska mentioned potential down-
sides specific to contracting. One noted that hiring a regional or national company can hurt local vendors who previously supplied goods to the district. Two
others mentioned that contractors do not always keep their promises; if that happens, it takes time and effort and potentially additional costs to go through the
contracting process again or transition back to internal operation. "If you get
a vendor in place that doesn't deliver on promises, then all of a sudden, you're
forced to rebid every year or every so often if not meeting the expectations from
the bid. We have some districts that are struggling with that part."

Four Florida interviewees mentioned three different disadvantages specific to
contracting. One disadvantage is the complicated contracting process and the
difficulty in the transition period. "It [Contracting] was very intense and a complicated process during the transition time. It was done in a very short period of
time. The level of bureaucracy existed in the transition process..." There can also
be conflicts when working with private contractors: "In our district, we had some
disagreements with the private company. We need to resolve the disagreements
to move forward..." Others pointed out the misalignment between goals: "The
ultimate goal for any business is profit. The ultimate goal for education is to have
student achievement. I do not think they are mutually exclusive, but I do think
when everybody's goal is aligned, you do have the better synergy."

Pros and cons of internal operations

There was more variation both within and across the states regarding the potential advantages of operating food services internally. In addition, the advantages
were largely noted by individuals in districts that provide food services internally.
The first advantage, mentioned by three Nebraska and two Florida interviewees,
is the ability to have greater control over the operation. For example, "We create
our own marketing materials and do our own menu-setting. No company sets the
menu. ...Everything is under control with us."

A number of the internal food service directors have been in their position for
an extensive period of time. Some directors "have worked 15–20 years, so they
have the background of what's happened in the districts. I think you have the
experience and the advantages of a director that's consistent and knows the history." They can provide more personalized services: "Everything is individualized with us. It fits us better because we know what works for us."

Internal operations may also enhance the ability to have a longer-term focus,
and to maintain the focus on the educational goals and student needs. Contractors

are focused on making a profit for this year, or satisfying the terms of the 5-year contract, whereas internal directors are "making decisions that aren't just for 6 months or a year, you're doing them for 5–10 years. I'm buying something that will last a long time." Internal directors are usually part of the administrative team, involved in priority-setting for the district. "We invest in our employees and our cafeterias. Everybody works for the same goal, everybody works for the same person, everybody works in the same place, this creates a clear and very straightforward communication line when it is in-house."

Finally, self-operation is perceived by one individual as very important to keep the connection between food and student learning. "Children absolutely need connection to the earth. Everything cannot be packaged and brought in because they are really kids and they really do not know... Improving that connection is extremely important for kids' learning. This is the key advantage of in-house food service operation."

Contract process and terms

Table 19.3 displays key points about the contracts for the three Nebraska and four Florida districts that are privatized. In both states, the number of years the service has been contracted out ranges from 1 year to more than 20 years.

Table 19.3 Contract Process and Terms

State	Contract Type	Contract Years	Evaluation Criteria	Contract Monitoring
Nebraska	Fixed-price contract (1)	More than 20 years (1)	Most important on income guarantee (1)	CFO (3)
	Cost-reimbursement (2)	5–10 years (1)	Emphasis on other criteria (2)	Contractor administrator (0)
		Under 5 years (1)		Designated food service manager/ director (0)
				Shared responsibility (0)
Florida	Fixed-price Contract (4)	More than 20 years (1)	Most important on income guarantee (3)	CFO (0)
	Cost-reimbursement (0)	5–10 years (2)	Emphasis on other criteria (1)	Contractor administrator (1)
		Under 5 years (1)		Designated food service manager/ director (2)
				Shared responsibility (1)

There are two main types of contracts: fixed price (the district pays a specific price per meal served) or cost reimbursement (the district reimburses for specific contractor costs). Both methods commonly include a guarantee of a certain amount of income to the district. Interviewees noted that the federal government is encouraging the use of fixed price contracts. In Florida, all four districts utilize a fixed-price contract. In Nebraska, one district uses a fixed price contract, and two use cost reimbursement. Of the latter two, one includes an income guarantee, while the other one has a guarantee instead based on the company's volume discount allowance rather than on the district's bottom line budget. The reason for this was based on an experience with a previous contractor where "...every time there was a snow day or field trip the company was going back to xxx to renegotiate – xxx was frustrated with that." The fixed price method is viewed as simpler and less financially risky for the districts: "If the company has guaranteed a certain profit, then there's not a real question as far as how the district will do, the burden will be on the company to meet the bottom line rather than the district." But one CFO for a district with a cost reimbursement contract prefers this because "it's what gives us the opportunity to give kids different things; xxx district went to fixed price; my daughter goes there, and she stopped eating...."

Contracts are on a 1-year basis, with options to renew for up to four additional years. While there are a number of regional and national companies that provide this service, the degree of competition in individual districts appears to be fairly low, especially when the district has a history of contracting. In Florida, the number of received bids ranges from two to five contractors, while the districts that contract in Nebraska have had from one to four bids for the most recent contracts. In one case, about five companies participated in the initial informational meeting, but then only two bids were received. "Sometimes you get a smaller company that comes in and they can see there's not much of a chance of switching... sometimes it might be stealing ideas, they can see what everyone else is doing and go back and put it in their accounts."

Districts noted that they use a point based system to select a contractor, based on a USDA template. The income guarantee is mentioned as being the most important factor in most of these districts, although other considerations were also mentioned, such as capital purchases included in the bid, a la carte sales, snacks, reference letters, staffing, community relationships, and buying from local farmers. On the other hand, the CFO from a Nebraska district has other concerns: "We were most interested in keeping kids on campus...We weren't just focused on the dollars...We're about an hour from the state line, and with Colorado legalizing marijuana, we've had a lot of problems. [We] are seeing more incidents. All the fast foods are on the same street as the high school. If we can incent kids with good food to stay on campus, it's a win."

Contract monitoring varies between the two states. In Nebraska, contracts are typically monitored by the district's chief financial officer. Regular meetings are held between the food service company and the CFO, ranging from every 2 weeks to monthly. Conversely, in Florida, monitoring depends on the managerial structure of each school district. Two Florida districts have designated the internal position of a food service manager or director to monitor the contract. For example: "The food service manager is required every 2 weeks to visit each of the schools to ensure the cafeteria workers are caring for the district's food capital equipment, make sure things and equipment are appropriately used. He also is the chair of the committee of three district administrators and three XXX company employees. They meet on a monthly basis to discuss ways to improve the program and to ensure that the standards are being met as proposed in the contract." Another Florida district relies on the director of purchasing and contracting administration (with the assistance of a full-time food service compliance officer), while the final district shares the responsibility among various administrators.

Effects of contracting on school food cost and quality

We asked specifically about whether contracting has any effects on cost and quality, and received mixed responses within and across states (Table 19.4). Three interviewees in Nebraska and six in Florida felt that contracting can decrease costs for the district. In Nebraska, this was noted mostly as an issue for smaller districts: "It costs more to deliver to smaller schools and they don't buy as much. A small school doing their own isn't getting as good a price." The interviewees from the privatized Florida districts believe that contracting can save money because of economies of scale, larger purchasing power, better expertise, and professional management. In addition, contractors are better able to cut labor costs by paying lower wages and reducing fringe benefits.

However, one Nebraska and three Florida interviewees, all from districts with internal operations, contend that contracting increases the cost because of the management fees paid to the contractors. "If you have a good director, it is much more economical to not pay a contract manager to put a director into your school district." "You might as well keep the revenue in your school district when you outsource you're not doing that." Five other interviewees were of the opinion that contracting has no effect on district costs (surprisingly, most of these were from districts that contract).

There was also significant variation between states regarding the effect on service quality. Five interviewees from Florida, but only one from Nebraska, felt that quality has improved since contracting. For example: "Previously, we had a lot of food that was purchased precooked and flash-frozen. Essentially, our

Table 19.4 Effects of Contracting on Food Cost and Quality

State	Effects on Cost	Effects on Quality
Nebraska	Increase (1)	Increase (1)
	Decrease (3)	Decrease (0)
	No effect (4)	No effect (7)
Florida	Increase (3)	Increase (5)
	Decrease (6)	Decrease (2)
	No effect (1)	No effect (3)

district just warmed it up. Now, XXX brings a lot of fresh fruits and vegetables. They make things from scratch... I have yet to have a student tell me that they don't like the food"; "Oh, absolutely, private contractors improve food quality. If they do not sell the meals, they do not make anything. They have to make food palatable to the kids, otherwise the kids will bring their lunch or parents go to McDonald's to bring in a happy meal." In a district that recently began contracting, the former internal director "...still did all her own baking, but kids want what they get at home, which is store-bought. XXX knows that the majority of the kids get fast food, not homemade buns. So usership is starting to go up now."

Two Florida interviewees from two different internal operation districts argue that contracting will decrease the quality of food service. According to one interviewee, "Outsourcing companies may cut food cost and tend to buy low-quality food. We feel that we are consistent with the school district...For example, we had peaches from Florida this year. They are pretty expensive, but we purchased them because we want kids to get the peaches from Florida. I do not think private food service companies will make that decision." Another interviewee argues that "I do not have to pay a management fee, so I have more money to spend, and therefore, I can buy better quality of food."

Almost all of the Nebraska interviewees were of the opinion that contracting generally does not have any effect on quality. One who has worked for both private companies and school districts said: "I expect quality here like I expected it where I was before." There were some caveats to this, though. One noted that contractors do provide more food choice ("the food choices that the students receive is better than in-house," but another (who works for a contractor) had the perspective that national firms "... are trying to manage things and make a profit, so they have national menus. Some of our creative freedoms may be limited based on corporate standards, where a local school district wouldn't have that." A third mentioned that "XXX brought a lot of southwest food into XXX district, but it wasn't a good fit for Nebraska." So the degree to which contractors are able to tailor their operation to local needs is a question.

Conclusion

There are over 50 million children in K–12 schools in the United States (National Center for Education Statistics 2015). Their nutrition is important for learning as well as for their physical health, and a significant portion of their daily food intake occurs during the school day. The performance of school food service operations is, therefore, vital for public health. This study explored the use of privatization of this function in public school districts in Florida and Nebraska. We found a variety of similarities, as well as some differences, within and across these states.

The general literature on government contracting has found that its primary purpose is to save money and improve public services. While reducing costs and service issues were mentioned as a factor in our interviews, they were not the primary drivers for privatization. Rather, the reasons frequently related to other issues, such as the inability to find experienced internal staff, the increasing complexity of federal regulations, and district administrators preferring to focus on their core mission of education.

While cost was not the main reason for choosing to contract, it is perceived as a benefit, particularly in terms of managing staff and economies of scale in purchasing food and supplies. Cost is also important in selecting a contractor. Florida districts are more likely to focus primarily on the income guarantee as for the deciding factor in this process. The two Nebraska districts that use cost-reimbursement contracts noted that other factors are also very important, such as serving food that is more likely to keep students in school at lunch time.

Having a contractor take over responsibility for this function is also viewed as a relief for districts, especially with the new regulations. There was less agreement about the benefits of internal operations, but these center around maintaining internal control and using experience with the district to better personalize the service, the ability to plan for the long-term, and maintaining a connection between student learning and food.

The biggest disparity between states was seen in the perceived effects on cost and quality. Florida interviewees were most likely to believe that costs go down with contracting, while the Nebraskans were more likely to perceive no effect on costs. Several individuals in districts without contracts think that costs actually increase with contracting. A larger gap between responses was seen in the effects on service. Almost all of the Nebraska interviewees see no effect on quality, while one-half of the Floridians believe that contracting increases quality.

Overall, cost and quality do not appear to be major factors in the decision to contract, and mixed results are seen as to the extent to which contracting results in lower or higher costs and quality. This was not expected, based on the contracting literature. This could be due to distinctions between this service and other government functions that have been studied. It may also relate to differences between different school districts. Interviewees noted, for example, that it is more difficult for smaller districts in rural areas to hire qualified food service directors and to achieve financial savings through volume price discounts. It may be that contracting has greater advantages for these districts than for larger and urban districts.

Another important finding relates to competition. The contracting literature is clear that competition is a key factor in achieving good results with contracting, especially in cost savings. Simply replacing a government monopoly with a private company monopoly generally does not result in efficiency, especially in the long-run. Competition during the bidding process is, therefore, crucial. In our cases, though, the degree of competition does not appear to be high. In one district, the same vendor has had the contract for about 20 years, and no other companies bid the last time the contract was renewed. This again may explain our mixed findings about cost effects of contracting.

There are limitations to this research. We had a small sample of districts in two states, so must be careful about generalizing our results. In addition, we focused on individual perceptions that may not be shared by others (although in some cases we spoke to multiple individuals in the same district and found consistency in responses). For the most part, though, we saw similarities across the cases. With the very limited literature on this topic, this exploratory approach helps to build our understanding of contracting for school food service operations.

There are a number of areas that would be fruitful for future research. First, it would be useful to use these results to design a survey that could be administered on a larger scale, to determine the extent to which these views are shared more broadly. Second, a more in-depth study of how school food service finances changed after contracting would be beneficial. This could be done by focusing on several districts that began contracting in the recent past. Third, given the limited competition in bidding that we found, it would be helpful to look more closely at the companies that are in this business and their decision processes for bidding on these contracts.

Finally, the most important factor is ultimately the ability to get school children to eat healthy foods. All of our interviewees discussed the challenges of finding things that students will eat under the new federal regulations that strictly limit sodium, calories, fats, etc. All districts appear to be struggling with this, whether or not they contract, and are experimenting with a variety of methods, such as self-service. There were significant differences in the opinion in our study as to whether contracting has any effect on quality and service. Future research should focus on better identifying the circumstances in which contracting affects participation rates and other measures of service quality. This would assist in identifying best practices for practitioners as well as expanding contract theory.

REFERENCES

Alspaugh, J. W. 1996. The effects of geographic and management factors on the cost of pupil transportation. *Journal of Education Finance* 22(3):180–194.

Bel, G., X. Fageda, and M. E. Warner. 2010. Is private production of public services cheaper than public production? A meta-regression analysis of solid waste and water services. *Journal of Policy Analysis and Management* 29(3):553–577.

Brooks, R. C. 1996. An analysis of residential sanitation collection pricing under alternative delivery arrangements. *Journal of Public Budgeting, Accounting & Financial Management* 7(4):493.

Brooks, R. C., B. Apostolou, and N. G. Apostolou 1994. Alternative methods of residential sanitation collection. *Research in Government and Nonprofit Accounting* 8:277–290.

Boyne, G. A. 1996. Competition and local government: A public choice perspective. *Urban Studies* 33:703–721.

Callan, S. J. and J. M. Thomas, 2001. Economies of scale and scope: A cost analysis of municipal solid waste services. *Land Economics* 77(4):548–560.

Curry, W. S. 2010. *Government Contracting: Promises and Perils.* Boca Raton, FL: CRC Press.

Ferris, J. M. 1986. The decision to contract out: An empirical analysis. *Urban Affairs Review* 22(2):289–311.

Florida School Nutrition Association. 2016. Florida Fact Sheet Regarding School Breakfast and Lunch Participation. Retrieved from: http://www.floridaschoolnutrition.org/. Access date June 1, 2017.

Harding, R. W. 1990. Contracting out the bussing of school children: An industrial organization approach. *Unpublished Doctoral Dissertation*, University of California, Los Angeles.

Hart, O., A. S. Shleifer, and R. W. Vishny. 1997. The proper scope of government: Theory and application to prisons. *Quarterly Journal of Economics* 112:1127–1161.

Kassel, D. S. 2010. *Managing Public Sector Projects*. Boca Raton, FL: CRC Press.

LaFaive, M. D. 2007. *A School Privatization Primer for Michigan School Officials, Media and Residents*. Mackinac Center for Public Policy. Retrieved from: https://www.mackinac.org/archives/2007/s2007-07.pdf. Access date June 1, 2017.

LeBruto, S. M. and B. Farsad. 1993. Contracted school food service: Advantages, disadvantages, and political concerns. *Hospitality Review* 11(1):57–67.

Levin, H. M. and P. J. McEwan. 2002. Cost-effectiveness and educational policy. In H. M. Lewin and P. J. McEwan (Eds.), *Cost-Effectiveness and Educational Policy*. New York: Routledge.

Levine, S. 2010. *School Lunch Politics: The Surprising History of America's Favorite Welfare Program*. Princeton, NJ: Princeton University Press.

Mackinac Center. 2011. *Michigan School Privatization Survey 2011*. Midland, Michigan: Hohman, J. M. and Kollmeyer, J. M.

Mathis, W. J. and L. Jimerson. 2008. A guide to contracting out school support services: good for the school? Good for the community? *Education and the Public Interest and Education Policy Research Unit (2008)*. Retrieved from: http://greatlakescenter.org/docs/Policy_Briefs/Mathis_ContractingOut.pdf. Access date June 1, 2017.

McGuire, R. A. and T. N. Van Cott. 1984. Public versus private economic activity: A new look at school bus transportation. *Public Choice* 43(1):25–43.

National Center for Education Statistics. 2015. *Digest of Education Statistics*. Retrieved from: http://nces.ed.gov/programs/digest/d15/tables/dt15_205.10.asp. Access date June 1, 2017.

Nebraska Department of Education. 2015. *2015–16 Student Characteristics*. http://drs.education.ne.gov/quickfacts/Pages/StudentCharacteristics.aspx. Access date June 1, 2017.

Nestle, M. 2002. *Food Politics*. Berkeley, CA: University of California Press.

Savas, E. S. 1977. Policy analysis for local government: Public vs. private refuse collection. *Policy Analysis* 3:49–74.

Savas, E. S. 2000. *Privatization and Public–Private Partnerships*. New York: Chatham House.

Spann, R. M. 1977. Public versus private production of governmental services. In *Budgets and Bureaucrats: The Sources of Governmental Growth*, edited by T. E. Borcherding, 71–89. Durham, NC: Duke University Press.

U.S. Census Bureau. 2015. *American Fact Finder*. Retrieved from: http://factfinder.census.gov/faces/nav/jsf/pages/community_facts.xhtml. Access date June 1, 2017.

U.S. Department of Agriculture. 2013. *National School Lunch Program Fact Sheet*. Retrieved from: https://www.fns.usda.gov/sites/default/files/NSLPFactSheet.pdf. Access date June 1, 2017.

U.S. GAO. (2009). *Meal Counting and Claiming by Food Service Management Companies in the School Meal Programs*. Retrieved from: http://www.gao.gov/products/GAO-09-156R. Access date June 1, 2017.

VanderSchee, C. 2005. The privatization of food services in schools: Undermining children's health, social equity, and democratic education. In *Schools or Markets? Commercialism, Privatization, and School-Business Partnerships*, edited by D. R. Boyles, 1–30. Mahwah, NJ: Lawrence Erlbaum Associates.

20 Thinking beyond food and fiber

Public dialogue and group discussion in the New Deal Department of Agriculture

Timothy J. Shaffer

Introduction

In *Food Politics: What Everyone Needs to Know*, Robert Paarlberg writes, "Since biblical times, the policies of governments have shaped food and farming... The food and farming sectors of all states, ancient and modern, foster considerable political activity" (Paarlberg 2013, p. 1). In U.S. history, one of the richest moments in agricultural policy that continues to shape food policy comes from the 1930s and what is popularly known as the "New Deal."

For this volume, the relevance of this chapter is that questions about agriculture and food production were situated within broader framings that went beyond a narrow definition of how some viewed the United States Department of Agriculture's role in society. We cannot think about food policy without thinking about agricultural issues broadly defined. As Luna (2004) has noted, "Food demand and consumption are closely linked to the nation's agricultural agenda... From the New Deal to the contemporary period, the agricultural agenda has not only exerted control over the nation's food supply but also dictated the type of products, the manner, and distribution in which the food supply is made available to consumers" (p. 214). What follows is an introduction to an often overlooked chapter of American history when the federal government, in partnership with state and local organizations, established educational programs that attended to both the challenges to agricultural policy from an economic standpoint as well as a cultural one. Specifically, this chapter will focus on a discussion-based adult education program designed by USDA administrators, implemented by Cooperative Extension agents, and how it was developed in order to help rural Americans understand agricultural policy as a complex issue interwoven with economic, political, and social issues.

Through the use of group discussion, government leaders looked to shape agricultural policy by cultivating opportunities for rural citizens to discuss and understand national and local policy about food production, social and cultural issues, and fundamental issues about the vitality of public life and democracy. But to make sense of the discussion efforts shaped by USDA administrators, it is important to ground it within the context and setting to make sense of how dramatic the idea of democracy as discussion really was. This chapter will explore five ways in which the federal government redefined, briefly, the role of ordinary citizens in relationship to agricultural policy. First, the change in dynamics between the federal government and citizens will be addressed. Second, the implementation of the Agricultural Adjustment Act and the key role of the Cooperative Extension Service will be highlighted as a foundational element of the USDA's efforts to save agriculture. Third, the roots of democratic participation through land-use planning helped to prepare rural communities for more robust forms of engagement. Fourth, we will look at the ways in which, again through Extension, the USDA grounded its work in practices that committed to citizens engaging in dialogue and discussion with one another about the complex challenges they faced. These ranged from the ability to produce agricultural good to more philosophical discussions about the social, cultural, and political changes taking place across the United States and elsewhere. Finally, this chapter will touch on the central theme driving group discussion through Extension but also more broadly—that problems are complex and we must attend to them accordingly.

Redefining the relationship between government and citizens

The Great Depression was, according to one author, "Unforeseen and unexpected, inexplicable and inexorable," impacting the United States well beyond the fateful Black Tuesday of October 29, 1929 (Himmelberg 2001, p. 3). What some first viewed as possibly just a misstep for Wall Street became a catastrophe affecting all aspects of American life. But others saw social, cultural, economic, and political changes brewing for decades (Rauchway 2008, p. 2). This very dramatic event was simply the breaking point. Regardless of whether the economic collapse came as a surprise or was confirmation of common sense, the impact was real. Nearly one in four workers had no employment. Unable to pay mortgages, many Americans lost their homes and savings.

Rural Americans were not immune. The unprecedented economic crisis struck first and hardest at the farm sector. Net income of farm operators in 1932 was less than one-third of what it had been in 1929. Farm prices fell more than 50% while the prices for goods and services necessary for farmers fell 32% (Rasmussen and Baker 1969, p. 69). Low crop yields, notably in 1931, 1934, and 1935, created a need for, "feed and seed loans, emergency forage crops, and information on economic feed use." During the 1930s, farm prices dropped far below the 1910–1914 "parity" level for five of the ten years (McIntyre 1962, p. 122).* The crash brought devastation to every corner of the country. Franklin D. Roosevelt was swept into office on the

---

* This time period in the 1910s was known as the golden age of American agriculture because of the relative prosperity farmers found. Between 1900 and 1920, gross farm income doubled with real farm income increasing 40%. The value of the average farm—smaller than 150 acres throughout this period—tripled during this period. "Midwestern farmers, especially, were making more money and living better than before," wrote historian Eric Mogren. But this prosperity would not last. Starting in 1921 and lasting well into Franklin D. Roosevelt's administration, farmers would face a prolonged depression. New Deal administrators would look back to this period (particularly 1909 to 1914) when shaping agricultural policies for parity: the relative purchasing power of farmers. See Danbom (1995, p. 162), Mogren (2005, p. 25), Libecap (1998, p. 190), and Campbell (1962, p. 4).

platform of a New Deal for the United States, ushering in what one historian called the "Third American Revolution" impacting all sectors and aspects of life (Degler 1959, pp. 379–416). One of the first and most dramatic settings in which the federal government played a crucial role in responding to desperate need was agriculture.

In the midst of widespread and intense efforts by the Roosevelt administration, the USDA implemented policy responding to the needs of farmers, associated industries, and consumers who were increasingly challenged with access to healthy food—or food at all. As one scholar put it, the U.S. government "attempted to resolve two pressing social and political problems... great masses of people in unemployment-induced poverty... and the great bounty of American agriculture that was available at the time but unaffordable and allowed to rot or intentionally destroyed" (Nestle 2014, p. ix). There were inherent challenges to propping up agricultural prices that benefited farmers while responding to the needs of hungry Americans. White (2014) noted that citizens and the federal government "negotiated the tensions between food as a biological necessity and as a vital commercial product" (p. 3). After initiating a response to the economic collapse facing farmers, the USDA developed processes for citizens to understand and address topics such as land-use planning and how the management and future use of land impacted incomes and communities. The idea of government intervention, more so than previously experienced, was to redefine and reshape the relationship between government and citizens, especially when thinking about the intersection of food policy, economic vitality, and civic life. As Henry A. Wallace would write in *America Must Choose*, "Much as we all dislike them, the new types of social control that we have now in operation are here to stay, and to grow on a world or national scale" (Wallace 1934b, p. 1).

Extending federal agricultural policy

On May 12, 1933, the Agricultural Adjustment Administration (AAA) was created within the USDA through the passage of the Agricultural Adjustment Act, the first "Farm Bill." The AAA was the most important agency established during the First Hundred Days of Roosevelt's administration according to one author (Hurt [1940] 1986, p. 18). Through this action, the "new Department of Agriculture" was born and the "picture" of the New Deal became clearer, offering benefits to organized labor and farmers (Baker et al. 1963, p. 245; Roth 2009, p. 131). Working with Extension agents in rural counties, the AAA made payments to farmers in return for reduced crops. In short, it was a production control measure. It benefited most farmers, but it was especially beneficial to those who were commercially successful. For farm workers, sharecroppers, and tenants, the reduction program had adverse effects (Gilbert 2003, p. 132).* The AAA was part of the core of what has been referred to as the "first New Deal," representing its basic plans through

---

* Charles M. Hardin noted that Congress attempted to favor tenants and small farmers in the law, but the AAA obligation to bolstering farm prices meant that the program would have to favor commercial farmers. See Hardin (1952, p. 132) and Harrington (1986, pp. 190–191).

the "retrogressive idea of recovery through scarcity" (Hofstadter 1948, p. 328). There was great hope for farmers and for those who were invested in agriculture. There needed to be. Things had seemingly reached the cliff, and now there was help to pull American agriculture back from the abyss with clear leadership from the executive branch and a more than willing Congress to enact, almost word for word, what President Roosevelt and his advisors saw as the path forward.[*]

President Roosevelt appointed Henry A. Wallace to serve as Secretary of Agriculture, a position Wallace's father held during the Harding and Coolidge administrations starting in 1921. In turn, Wallace would reach out to Milburn Lincoln Wilson—known widely as "M. L."—to help shape the USDA in a way that would embody its commitment to both solving agricultural problems and having the department base its work on democratic ideas. These two, more than any others in the department, saw democratic practices both within the USDA as well as in rural communities across the country as being central not only to their mission but to that of the entire federal government if it was fundamentally concerned with the continuation of America's democratic experiment.[†]

Because the AAA was such a different approach to dealing with agricultural production issues, those in administrative positions realized the necessity for "very far-reaching propagandic campaigns to familiarize farmers with the need for such a program, and the underlying economic facts upon which it was based" (Umberger 1935, p. 106). While the AAA was being set up, Edward A. O'Neal of the American Farm Bureau Federation attended a cabinet conference at the White House regarding the administration of the Act and "vigorously opposed a plan to set up a highly centralized bureaucracy" (Kile 1948, p. 203). He insisted that the existing national Cooperative Extension Service be utilized rather than the creation of an entirely new administrative structure. Secretary Wallace's view aligned with O'Neal's idea for Extension as the means for engaging rural citizens.

Created in 1914 with the passage of the Smith–Lever Act, the Cooperative Extension Service (or "Extension" for short) was established as a cooperative approach to community-based education with the USDA, land-grant universities, and local communities sharing funding responsibilities. The passage of the Act codified what had been taking place for decades, particularly in the South.[‡] The Act states in two places how Extension educators will approach their work: first, Extension agents will "aid in diffusing among the people of the United States useful and practical information on subjects relating to agriculture and home economics, and to encourage the application of the same......." Second, the Act states that Extension work is to "consist of the giving of instruction and practical demonstrations in agriculture and home economics to persons not attending or resident in [land-grant] colleges in the several communities, and imparting to such persons information on said subjects through field demonstrations,

---

[*] Katznelson 2013, p. 123.

[†] The most thorough study of democratic planning and the commitment to USDA administrators is Gilbert (2015).

[‡] On the lead up to the establishment of Extension, see Scott (1970).

publications, and otherwise......" (True 1928, p. 195). The diffusion and transmission of knowledge and information has only been part of Extension's work, especially when considering its civic role.

In addition to the transfer of technical knowledge, Extension's work has gone beyond the application of research-based information to include important community work and leadership development. In Louisiana, Mary W. Mims, who would be involved with the discussion project described in greater detail below, had the official title of "Community Organizer" as an Extension educator with Louisiana State University (McGinty 1978, p. v). Organizing discussion groups, folk schools, and other programs, Mims embodied this larger framing for Extension's work. M. L. Wilson noted how the rise of scientific knowledge led many people to turn major problems over to experts, but "We [are] in danger of forgetting that the democratic process requires participation of all in the decisions of the group; that decisions imposed from above, even though accepted, are not the democratic way" (Wilson 1940b, p. 3). The primary job of the Extension educator, in Wilson's view, was to "help the community analyze its problems in the light of all available information and so to organize itself that the necessary action can be taken" (Wilson 1940b, p. 4). Extension, from its origins, has been comprised of sometimes competing and sometimes complementary approaches to its desire to inform and engage citizens.

Because Extension agents were found in nearly every county and were familiar with agricultural practices and community engagement, Wallace turned to the Extension Service of the land-grant colleges and universities.* Extension had trained field personnel who were "charged with bringing the farmers information on improved agricultural techniques. The county agents knew the local problems; they had the confidence of the local people. Would this not be the ideal field staff for AAA?" Wilson proposed that the State Extension Directors be made the AAA administrators in their states. This approach was because of his "passion for grass-roots participation" (Schlesinger 1958, p. 60). The Extension system was an institution deeply embedded in rural communities, but this approach to agricultural policy was not universally welcomed.

Rexford Tugwell, an agricultural economist from Columbia University at the center of animating Roosevelt's vision for the country, challenged this approach to rely on Extension out of concern that the Extension Service was too closely aligned with commercial farming and the Farm Bureau itself.† The Farm Bureau's

---

* For an account of the tensions within the land-grant and cooperative extension system in relation to the creation of the AAA and the utilization of county extension agents, see Evans (1938).

† This theme has been picked up by Gilbert: "In the 1930s, the Farm Bureau/Extension relationship precluded the development of alternative structures for implementing the Agricultural Adjustment Act—structures that might have been more responsive to popular demands.... In summary, the USDA/land-grant complex developed in a way that increased the class-capacity of the dominant farm classes, subverted that of oppositional groups, and structurally privileged the former within the state" (Gilbert and Howell 1991, 208). On the parallel development of the Extension service and Farm Bureau, see Block (1960, pp. 4–21). In his dissertation on adult education in the 1930s, Ronald J. Hilton wrote about Tugwell's resistance to Extension because of its relationship with big farming and how this issue was "never mentioned in most histories of adult education" (Hilton 1981, pp. 152–153).

interest in large, successful farming marginalized tenant farmers and people of color, not challenging the economic and political barriers that protected certain farmers while further marginalizing others. While this view was true in many ways, the need for swift action helped Wallace make the decision to endorse Wilson's plan to use Extension as the fieldworkers of the AAA in rural communities (Davis 1935; Schlesinger 1958, p. 60).* To quote Russell Lord, "Wilson was strong for using the extension services. Quietly and firmly he worked against an impatient impulse in Washington to set up a hasty new field adjustment force on the side. Tugwell had no firsthand knowledge of county agents and little faith in the extension mechanism" (1939, p. 161).

If Tugwell had more experience with Extension, he might have been able to see beyond the Extension/Farm Bureau relationship. But from his point of view, he saw an educational organization too closely aligned with private interests to accomplish the AAA's work. Van L. Perkins' assessment was more practical: turning to the Extension Service was the only possibility (Perkins 1969, p. 97). More recently, Loss (2012) has shed more light on this episode noting how, "By activating local interests and minimizing the visible presence of the federal government, Wallace, and the AAA achieved administrative capacity and a critical mass of built-in rural support while expending minimal political capital" (p. 62). Each of these perspectives points to one reality: on multiple fronts, Extension was the best choice for implementing the AAA, even if it was not ideal to critics.

Wallace approached C. W. Warburton, director of Extension, about the idea of utilizing Extension as the vehicle for implementing the AAA's program. Warburton was more than willing to participate, but state Extension systems were reluctant to go along unless they could control the program (Perkins 1969, p. 97). Additionally, there was a feeling among county agents that a reduction program could not function effectively because it contradicted "all their previous training and teachings" geared toward increased production and efficiency (Evans 1938, p. 41). Later that year, Wallace spoke to the annual convention of the Association of Land-Grant Colleges and Universities. He challenged the administrators of these institutions by saying how they must, "be prepared to go beyond technical agriculture and engineering and even economics into a new realm which none of us yet fully senses" (Wallace 1934a, p. 42). Land-grant universities and Extension were going to need to adjust to the needs of the country, moving beyond their domain of providing technical knowledge to a new role in coordinating a completely new program. They became the "front line forces" of the AAA (Loss 2013, p. 296).

The country faced a dire situation with the Great Depression and Extension was utilized to assist or, in some situations, to almost take over the administration of the AAA since they were familiar with farmers and the rural community in which they lived. As the Agricultural Adjustment Act had stated, the Secretary of Agriculture had the discretion to choose from a number of alternative policies.

---

* A result of this decision was increased influence and strength for the Farm Bureau. Cf. McConnell (1953, p. 77).

Aside from entering into agreements with farmers and to pay them to reduce their acreage, Wallace was able to also negotiate marketing agreements by which producers would pay farmers a minimum price for their produce in addition to other steps. All of this was done to raise farm income to what was called "parity." That is, "to establish the same relationship between the prices farmers paid and the prices they received as existed in the so-called golden age of American agriculture between 1909 and 1914" (Badger 1989, p. 152). But the path to achieving parity was fraught with undesirable decisions.

One of the lasting impressions on the American mind about the severe instability of the period was the plowing up of cotton and the slaughter of millions of pigs. Despite efforts to push the farm bill through Congress, it reached President Roosevelt's desk "well after spring planting had begun. Seeds had already sprouted in thousands of cotton patches throughout the South and in the rolling wheatfields of the West. Millions of pigs had farrowed in bloodsheds and barnyards across the corn belt" (Kennedy 1999, p. 204). The price for pork was so low that Wallace called it "absolutely ruinous" and thus the USDA took steps to help the market (Reminiscences 1977, p. 263). While drought saved the need to address an overabundance of wheat, cotton plow-up and "pig infanticide" became lasting images of the AAA for many Americans (Kennedy 1999, p. 205). In the summer of 1933, 25% of all cotton planted was destroyed (Poppendieck 2014, p. 109). But whether one was thinking about pigs or cotton, the idea of destroying food during a time when so many lacked adequate nourishment was difficult to accept. People reacted strongly and condemned the actions taken by the government as immoral. In light of this and other perceived missteps taken by the USDA, *Newsweek* caricatured Wallace as the Big Bad Wolf (White 2014, p. 145). Government officials were in the unenviable position of making decisions that impacted people's lives intimately. Wallace would later write, "to have to destroy a growing crop is a shocking commentary on our civilization. I could tolerate it only as a cleaning up of the wreckage from the old days of unbalanced production. Certainly, none of us ever want to go through a plow-up campaign again, no matter how successful a price-raising method it proved to be" (Wallace 1934c, pp. 174–175). The AAA was established as an emergency agency responding to an immediate need. Wallace's reflection suggests how some of the actions taken during this early period of the New Deal showed the extreme steps taken to address agricultural issues through whatever means possible at the time.

The government found itself in the unfortunate position to balance questions about economic health for farmers and the entire farm sector as well as citizens in every community struggling to feed their families and to put clothing on their backs. But while these measures were implemented, there were other aspects that were more positive for rural communities.

Roots of democratic participation

Extension, as a partner with the AAA, utilized its network of county agents to work with farmers to help them meet the requirements for participation in USDA programs. But the AAA efforts also provided an opportunity to bring farm men and women together around issues of local and national importance and to encourage them to view themselves not only as producers but also as civic actors. Chester C. Davis, administrator of the AAA, wrote in 1934 a publication titled "The Farmers Run Their Show" about the ways farmers had gathered together in their communities, especially in response to the severe drought many across the country were experiencing, and to make sense of what was occurring. He wrote: "The question is: Can the old-fashioned democratic processes be successfully used by the farmers to bring order out of economic chaos? The outcome of this experiment, if successful, may give part of the answer to the twentieth century riddle—how to preserve democracy in the machine age" (Davis 1934, p. 1).

The AAA was an experiment that confronted the belief that farmers typically only focused on their own individual concerns. Davis continued: "Unquestionably, millions of farmers, accustomed to going their own way and disregarding their fellows, are giving up their old-style individualism. They are learning the central truth of the New Deal philosophy—that the welfare of the individual is dependent on the welfare of the group." Not only were they learning this philosophy, but they also were putting it into practice. Such a shift did not go unnoticed for those within the AAA who viewed it as something, "significant and of permanent social value" (Davis 1934, p. 2). Farmers, in Davis' view, were not as aware of this simply because they had their backs "to the wall and [were] fighting desperately for the simple right to make a livelihood from the soil" (Davis 1934, p. 3). Even in this challenging and stressful environment, by working together and "organizing along democratic lines, they [could] bring law and order into the economic realm" (Davis 1934, p. 3). Evoking President Abraham Lincoln's famous address at Gettysburg, Davis wrote about farmers working together as being, "For the Farmers, By the Farmers, and Of the Farmers" (Davis 1934, p. 3).

In an article about an Institute of Rural Economics in New Jersey organized by Rutgers University and the American Association for Adult Education with the endorsement of Wallace, Elsie Gray Cambridge referenced Wallace's belief that citizens needed to come together to envision their future and, quoting Wallace, noted how the outlines of long-term planning "can not fully appear until there has been a much more extended debate in the community forums of the cities, the schoolhouses, meetings of the country, the radio, and the press." Wallace hoped that discussion and debate would, "rage with great intensity" that winter of 1934; it would, in fact, in some places (Cambridge 1934, p. 181).

Wallace would later argue that the welfare of the individual was intimately connected with the general welfare and that it was one of the central elements of what he called the "democratic body of faith" (Wallace 1944, p. 141). This shift away from individualism toward greater collaboration was a strong rebuke to one of the central meta-narratives about the American experience. Wilson expressed similar sentiments. In the American Country Life Association's publication *Rural America*, he wrote that any planning in the field of agriculture must be done, "by and through the democratic participation of the millions of farm families throughout the United States." He continued by noting how individual farm families needed to do their own thinking but engage others through various, "avenues for collective expression" (Wilson 1934, p. 3). Men and women were encouraged to come together to learn from and with one another so they could take action to ameliorate the challenges facing rural America.

In many counties, participation in the AAA's domestic allotment plan was more than 90%. Those in the remaining 10% often were tenant farmers, farmers on poor land who were barely subsisting, farmers who would like to participate but were unable to do so, and those who viewed such government intervention as something they objected to because of the restrictions placed on them. A major criticism of the AAA, and the USDA more broadly was the focus on large-scale agriculture and commercial ventures.* As pointed out by Chester C. Davis, that 10% included "tenant farmers whose landlords refuse to sign the contract; farmers on poor land whose production is so small they are virtually on a subsistence basis; farmers who would like to participate but who are prevented by some special complication; and farmers who are suspicious of the Government and object to being restricted in any way" (Davis 1934, p. 8). Overall, however, the adjustment programs helped to restore the "old spirit of neighborliness" (Davis 1934, p. 10). They aided farmers in becoming more aware of the larger social problems at the national and international levels which had repercussions for them at the local level. The county-level production control associations of the AAA, according to Davis, connected deeply to American traditions. He wrote, "in the long view of history, [these associations may] be comparable to the democratic institutions set up by the early American colonists" (Davis 1934, p. 13).

The AAA's Program Planning Division, with encouragement and support from Wallace and Wilson, established the Program Study and Discussion (PSD) Section as part of the USDA's "long-time, more permanent plan for American agriculture" (Gilbert 2015, p. 105). It was in this spirit of what Davis referred to as "democratic institutions" that adult education and group discussion came to be viewed as one of the major pillars of agricultural policy alongside more traditional elements of concern for agriculture such as farm credit, land tenure, foreign trade, and soil conservation (Gilbert 2015, p. 146). Beyond the attempts to control production for the sake of farmers and the establishment of social welfare programs to ensure that people had adequate nutrition (Poppendieck 2014), the USDA embarked upon a democratic experiment that would test the limits of what an agricultural agency could—or *should*—do.

Group discussion at the heart of democracy

One of the most important—and largely overlooked—outcomes of the USDA's work during the 1930s dealt more with how citizens understood agricultural issues as also being deeply social, economic, political, and philosophical issues that required them to engage in thoughtful discussion and deliberation with neighbors and broader community members (Wilson 1940a). As part of what

* On this point, see Wood (2006), Roberts (2015), and Gilbert (2015).

Gilbert (2015) has referred to as the "intended New Deal," the existence of a discussion-based adult education program designed by USDA administrators and implemented by Cooperative Extension agents can help us better under how rural Americans came to understand agricultural policy in its complexity.

While a dominant narrative about the New Deal period is that experts largely shaped the federal government's efforts to respond to a diverse range of public problems,* it diminishes the serious commitment that individuals such as Henry A. Wallace and M. L. Wilson had with respect to creating space for rural men and women to understand and determine their fate (Shaffer 2013, p. 145). Alongside planning programs within the AAA, USDA officials saw an opportunity to think about long-term questions for agriculture and not only immediate or short-term goals. The growth and development of two, complementary educational approaches—adult education and group discussion methods—opened up the possibility that Extension could facilitate community-based discussions. The forum movement offered a model for Extension to apply in rural communities, drawing on the experience of others in urban settings (Coleman 1915; Sheffield 1922; Studebaker 1935; Overstreet and Overstreet 1938; Keith 2007). As Gilbert (2015) puts it: "Probably the most unusual innovation in the New Deal USDA aimed to advance democracy through adult or continuing education" (p. 142).

This "pillar" of the USDA was rooted in the knowledge and experience of citizens. Expert knowledge was important, but it was not to overshadow the opportunity for people to engage in thoughtful discussion about wide-ranging issues. The USDA's interest in this effort was to have people discussion public issues. The government's interest was in guaranteeing that the "facts [were] set forth correctly" (Wilson 1941b, p. 8). The role of the USDA in this setting was to prepare discussion guides and outlines. While the USDA would produce such documents and disseminate them widely, "the handling of the discussion programs [was] entirely up to the States," meaning that Extension agents were critical to its success (Wilson 1935b, p. 33). Wilson was emphatic that the USDA would not advocate for anything other than the opportunity for citizens to learn about the issues facing them during this time of transformation. The agency's leaders "counted themselves among a 'great democratic movement' that had education at its core" (Gilbert 2015, p. 143), as Wilson believed that "free and full discussion is the archstone of democracy" (Wilson 1935a). Drawing on John Dewey's view that democracy and education went hand-in-hand, Wilson sought to ground the USDA's work with Extension in communities as an opportunity to foster democracy as a lived reality rather than an idea to be studied or as only something politicians did in legislatures.†

Because they were based in counties across the country, Extension agents had a close relationship with those they served. They encouraged men and women, young and old, to gather in small groups to discuss topics dealing with issues of economy, agriculture, taxes, urban and rural differences, trade, and so on.

---

* See Badger (1989, p. 6) and Kirkendall (1962, p. 456).
† On the influence of Dewey and pragmatist philosophy, see Gilkeson (2010, p. 62) and Reminiscences (1956, p. 1018).

People gathered in living rooms and grange halls. They were encouraged to be exploratory in their discussions and to consider the tensions and trade offs of different paths forward. In a period when people were discussing the future of democracy against the rise of authoritarian leaders in Europe, the encouragement of diverse views meant that "democracy is safe," in the words of one of the leaders in the discussion and forum movement (Overstreet and Overstreet 1938, p. 216). Alongside the more explicit land-use planning project within the USDA, citizen discussion groups served as an opportunity for citizens to be both informed about what actions the government was taking in regard to a number of issues, but also to make sense of how they might more explicitly be involved in decision-making and informing decisions all the way to the department's leadership (Gaus, Wolcott, and Lewis 1940, p. 469; Kirkendall 1966, p. 161).[*]

For roughly a decade, discussion-based adult education opportunities for men and women blossomed into two interrelated programs, both part of the PSD unit, first housed in the AAA and later in the Bureau of Agricultural Economics: first, discussion groups that were organized and facilitated by local Cooperative Extension agents from land-grant universities with rural men and women; and second, multiday professional development/continuing education opportunities known as Schools of Philosophy that were organized by Extension and facilitated by USDA staff and distinguished scholars (Taeusch 1941; Jewett 2013; Shaffer 2013, 2014; Gilbert 2015; Shaffer 2016).

The PSD prepared and distributed millions of copies of topic-based discussion guides. Participation figures, as complete as possible, suggest that more than 3 million rural men and women participated in discussion groups, 60,000 discussion leaders received training and tens of thousands of extension workers and other rural community leaders attended more than 150 Schools of Philosophy (Vogt 1940, p. 6; Taeusch 1952, p. 41; Shaffer 2014, p. 264; Gilbert 2015, p. 142). With a small staff based in Washington, DC, who collaborated with partners in different regions of the country, the PSD engaged rural communities about a wide range of topics that dealt with questions about the transformation of agriculture and rural life taking place. Covering more than 40 topics, discussion guides had titles such as:[†]

* How Do Farm People Live in Comparison with City People?
* Exports and Imports—How Do They Affect the Farmer?
* Is Increased Efficiency in Farming Always a Good Thing?
* What Should Farmers Aim to Accomplish Through Organization?
* What Kind of Agriculture Policy Is Necessary to Save Our Soil?
* Taxes: Who Pays, What For?
* Rural Communities: What Do They Need Most?
* Soil Conservation: Who Gains By It?

---

* Arnstein's (1969) Ladder of Citizen Participation points to the various ways in which government agencies engage citizens and offers perspective on this approach to engaging citizens by the USDA.
† A complete list can be found in Gilbert (2015, pp. 261–263).

While these topical materials were widely distributed and utilized, the USDA also produced materials that focused specifically on discussion group methodologies (United States Department of Agriculture, The Extension Service, and Agricultural Adjustment Administration 1935; Bureau of Agricultural Economics 1942). During this period, there were a number of publications and resources for encouraging discussion methods and the rural discussion efforts contributed to this literature (see Judson 1936; Judson and Judson 1938; McBurney and Hance 1939; Garland and Phillips 1940).

The central goal of the discussions was a somewhat challenging metric to quantify: a more informed citizenry. Rather than influencing the outcome of group discussions, the role of the USDA was to prepare resources for discussion methodology and thematic guides for discussion on a range of topics. Wilson noted in an article in the *Extension Service Review* that while the USDA would produce such documents and disseminate them widely, "the handling of the discussion programs [was] entirely up to the States" (Wilson 1935b, p. 33). In his notes about the objective of discussion groups, Wilson wrote that they were:

> ...to create opportunities for farmers to think through for themselves basic problems relating to national agricultural policies which will require decision sometime in the future. The project would be undertaken on the principle that these problems should be discussed and decided consciously with eyes open, and their implications clear rather than in any other way. Democracy has a responsibility of keeping open the channels for the functioning of democracy. The object would not be propaganda, not aimed in the direction of bringing people to any specific or 'right' conclusions, but rather through an adult educational process to provide them with means of getting facts, information, and opinions which would assist them in reaching intelligent, considered decisions.
>
> (Wilson n.d.)

Wilson was emphatic the USDA would not advocate for anything other than the opportunity for citizens to learn about the issues facing them during this time of transformation.* As ground level reports from discussion group leaders highlight, the public forums were situated within larger efforts to cultivate community life in rural communities. Mary W. Mims, a rural sociologist with Louisiana State University Extension, embodied this approach of having forums happening alongside folk schools, community fairs, and other educational efforts (Bateman 1935, p. 43). These efforts were cultivating the democratic roots M. L. Wilson would refer to: "Democracy thus becomes broader than a system of government; it becomes a way of life" (Wilson 1939a, p. 93).

---

* Discussion had long been an element of educational programs in Extension since its origins. However, this program was much more organized around formal structures for discussion. See Wilson (1941a, p. 290).

The end of this democratic experiment came when the American Farm Bureau Federation and members of Congress considered the broader land-use planning program of the USDA to be contrary to their approach to determining the best course of action for agriculture, which was through well-established channels. Community-based discussion among rural citizens and participatory planning processes for land-use were seen as deviations from the USDA's more "traditional" work. As Campbell (1962) put it, "The county land-use planning program was buried in the early 1940s, and there is no doubt that the [Farm Bureau] was the chief undertaker" (p. 177). Especially for the land-use planning program but also for other departmental efforts, administrators wanted to "reach directly down to the grass roots and tap great reservoirs of ideas among the farmers themselves at the local level" (Campbell 1962, p. 175). The contrast between top-down insider and bottom-up grassroots approaches to politics and conceptions of democracy stood in stark relief, and in many ways those with the desire to maintain a top-down approach to agricultural policy won out.

Embracing complexity for a healthy public

M. L. Wilson, one of the organizers of group discussion in rural communities through the USDA, was shaped by what he referred to as a "cultural approach" to thinking about American agriculture. It included what he called the tangible materials and intangible and immaterial matters, the tools and techniques of rural life as well as the knowledge and attitudes that animated such a life. The transformation in the first decades of the twentieth century from a relatively simple life to a modern, complex world invited both opportunities as well as challenges. The world was becoming smaller with more possibilities: "If once [the farm boy's] highest hope was a driving horse of his own that would at most take him fifteen miles on Sunday to the county seat, now he hopes for a flivver that may take him adventuring as far as Florida or California or Yellowstone or the World's Fair. He doesn't walk in all weather anymore to the one-room school; he is picked up by the school bus. The church is nearer now, but nearer too are the lake and picnic grounds fifty miles beyond. The town is nearer, and daily trips to town, wrapped bread, canned vegetables, and movies come into the regular pattern of farm life," Wilson wrote (1939c, p. 218). Rural life, in Wilson's view, was delicately balanced in an "intricate inter-relationship." If one thing was "disturbed," to use Wilson's term, the "whole pattern is forced temporarily out of balance; when finally, equilibrium is regained, the complexion of the whole has been changed" (Wilson 1939c, p. 218).

For these reasons, agriculture and rural life needed to be seen as part of a whole. In a powerful statement, Wilson succinctly stated his belief that issues were immensely complex and it was essential to engage philosophical, moral, and religious questions even when addressing an otherwise apparent technical or economic problem. He wrote:

> ...I have always believed that no single specialist or expert, nor any single body of scientific knowledge, can ever deal adequately with even a

relatively small and apparently detached agricultural problem. I believe that when, for instance, we have a farm problem that seems on the surface to be wholly an economic matter, we may safely take it for granted that the economic problem is interwoven with factors that are political, socio-logical, psychological, philosophical, and even religious. And we should realize that any solution or policy that is decided upon is bound to have effects upon human life and conduct that none but philosophy and religion openly profess to judge. Economic wisdom alone, therefore, is not enough for proper consideration of agricultural problems that by common consent are defined as economic problems. We cannot escape getting involved in questions of moral, philosophical, and spiritual values whenever we touch upon any social problem.

(Wilson 1939c, p. 218)

For this reason, Wilson viewed a cultural approach to addressing the prob-lems of American agriculture as the most appropriate way forward.* Elsewhere, he touched on the importance of knowledge and judgment as well as the need for both experts and citizens to work collaboratively to ensure, as much as pos-sible, that public problems were being thought about as thoroughly as could be done. Speaking to the Texas Agricultural Workers Association in 1939, he noted:

We need if our plans are to develop into workable programs, to base our decisions upon the combined judgments of experts, officials, and farmers. In the past, there have been some differences between expert and farmer opin-ion on needed agricultural adjustments. These are generally due, I believe, to differences in available information upon which the opinions are based. I do not mean to imply that either the farmer or the expert has more informa-tion than the other. I mean that each has different kinds of information and that we need both kinds to build an adequate program. The expert is often a person with a vision for only one aspect of a problem. Although the farmer may not see that aspect so clearly, he is likely to see phases of his problem that the specialist overlooks.

(Wilson 1939b, pp. 10–11)

No problem was as simple as it may seem or as some might claim. The knowl-edge and experience of both experts and ordinary men and women was crucial together while acknowledging that this collaboration was not universal especially for tenant, migrant, and minority farmers. So, "[h]ow are we to bring the farmer and

* This cultural approach included tangible and material things such as "institutions of education" and intangible and immaterial things such as the "customary habits and preferences that dictate choices and forms" and "the accumulated lore and opinions that really decide what the content, manner, and ends of education shall be." Support for institutions of education such as discussion groups enabled citizens to talk with one another about preferences and opinions. See Wilson (1939c, p. 219).

the expert together that they may exchange information and combine judgments?" Together, experts and farmers could address agricultural problems in a manner that respected and took seriously the various kinds of knowledge and information necessary for answering questions shaped by moral, philosophical, and spiritual values as well as scientific perspectives (Wilson 1939b, p. 11, 1939c, p. 218).

Wilson's statement about the need for more than a single specialist or expert and his speech before the Texas Agricultural Workers Association touched on one of the most important themes from the USDA's democratic experiment in the 1930s and 1940s. Scientific and research-based technical knowledge were extremely useful and necessary to making decisions, but such knowledge could not answer questions about value and meaning. Even relatively simple economic matters on the surface were interwoven with dimensions that were political, sociological, psychological, philosophical, and even religious. And, if acknowledged and addressed as having these further dimensions, problems could not rely exclusively on technical knowledge because such an approach is explicitly limited. People needed to wrestle with different values systems, requiring people to discuss and deliberate with one another.

As we consider the intersection of food and public health, we must attend to questions about how policy and politics shape both process and outcome. As this chapter has highlighted, the government's attempt to shape agricultural (and thus food) policy could be done in a way that used an organizational structure like Extension to implement a federal initiative from a standpoint that they were communicating details to citizens. Or, as the group discussion work also from the USDA and Extension points out, efforts can be made to engage people in discussion about the issues that impacted their lives.

The passage of the Agricultural Adjustment Act of 1933, the first Farm Bill, is connected with efforts to engage those in agriculture about how to balance concerns about profit and health. Within 2 years of its passage, the government invested in a democratic infrastructure to encourage people to consider complex issues not in isolation, but through discussion with others. While not necessarily advocating for the federal government to deploy Extension agents to facilitate community-level discussions, we have examples from our past to frame our current challenges in a way that allows us to explore them in their complexity rather than attempt to simplify issues. As Wilson noted, "...I have always believed that no single specialist or expert, nor any single body of scientific knowledge, can ever deal adequately with even a relatively small and apparently detached agricultural problem.... We cannot escape getting involved in questions of moral, philosophical, and spiritual values whenever we touch upon any social problem" (Wilson 1939c, p. 218).

Decades later, Wendell Berry, the noted author about agriculture and rural life, would articulate similar themes to those expressed by Wilson. Berry called for more expansive thinking about agricultural issues because to name them as "solely a problem of production or technology or economics—is simply to misunderstand the problem, either inadvertently or deliberately, either for profit or because of a prevalent fashion of thought. The whole problem must be solved, not just some handily identifiable and simplifiable aspect of it" (Berry 2002, p. 269). To wrestle with philosophical and moral questions alongside technological and economic concerns to get at the "whole problem," we must allow ourselves to be in discussion with our colleagues, adversaries, and neighbors; in short, with those who comprise our democracy.

The intersection of food and public health concerns today offers an opportunity to draw on a rich but largely forgotten history in agricultural settings where government agencies and ordinary citizens attended to important political issues in a very real and democratic way. As Wilson put it in an issue of the *Extension Service Review* that included stories titled "Digging for Water," "Soil fertility steps up," and "Managing County 4-H Fairs," discussion was the "archstone" of democracy—it is what keeps our democratic society standing (Wilson 1935a). It is important for us to be reminded that people with technical skills can, through democratic approaches and practices, wrestle with the big challenges we face as communities, states, regions, countries, and beyond.

REFERENCES

Arnstein, S. R. 1969. A ladder of citizen participation. *Journal of the American Planning Associtation* 35(4):216–224.

Badger, A. J. 1989. *The New Deal: The Depression Years, 1933–40.* New York: Hill and Wang.

Baker, G. L., W. D. Rasmussen, V. Wiser, and J. M. Porter. 1963. *Century of Service: The First 100 Years of the United States Department of Agriculture.* Washington, DC: Centennial Committee, U. S. Department of Agriculture.

Bateman, J. W. 1935. *Annual Report of Agricultural Extension Work in Louisiana.* Baton Rouge, LA: Louisiana State University and Agricultural and Mechanical College, Division of Agricultural Extension.

Berry, W. 2002. Solving for pattern. In *The Art of the Commonplace: The Agrarian Essays of Wendell Berry*, edited by Norman Wirza, 267–275. Berkeley: Counterpoint.

Block, W. J. 1960. *The Separation of the Farm Bureau and the Extension Service: Political Issue in a Federal system.* Vol. 47, *Illinois Studies in the Social Sciences.* Urbana, IL: University of Illinois Press.

Bureau of Agricultural Economics. 1942. *Group Discussion and Its Techniques: A Bibliographical Review.* Washington, DC: US Government Printing Office.

Cambridge, E. G. 1934. Farmers' forums. *Journal of Adult Education* 6(2):181–185.

Campbell, C. M. 1962. *The Farm Bureau and the New Deal: A Study of the Making of National Farm Policy, 1933–40.* Urbana, IL: University of Illinois Press.

Coleman, G. W., ed. 1915. *Democracy in the Making: Ford Hall and the Open Forum Movement.* Boston: Little, Brown, and Company.

Danbom, D. B. 1995. *Born in the Country: A History of Rural America.* Baltimore: The Johns Hopkins University Press.

Davis, C. C. 1934. *The Farmers Run Their Show.* General Information Series G-18. Agricultural Adjustment Administration. Washington, DC: United States Government Printing Office.

Davis, C. C. 1935. The Extension Service and the A.A.A. In *Proceedings of the Forty-Eighth Annual Convention of the Association of Land-Grant Colleges and*

Universities, Washington, DC, November 19–24, 1934, edited by C. A. McCue, 168–171. Wilmington, DE: Cann Brothers.

Degler, C. N. 1959. *Out of Our Past: The Forces That Shaped Modern America*. New York: Harper & Brothers.

Evans, J. A. 1938. *Recollections of Extension History, Extension Circular Number 224*. Washington, DC: United States Department of Agriculture.

Garland, J. V. and C. F. Phillips, eds. 1940. *Discussion Methods Explained and Illustrated*. Revised ed. Vol. 12, no. 2, *The Reference Shelf*. New York: The H. W. Wilson Company.

Gaus, J. M., L. O. Wolcott, and V. B. Lewis. 1940. *Public Administration and the United States Department of Agriculture*. Chicago: Published for the Committee on Public Administration of the Social Science Research Council by Public Administration Service.

Gilbert, J. 2003. Low modernism and the agrarian new deal. In *Fighting for the Farm: Rural America Transformed*, edited by J. Adams, 129–146. Philadelphia: University of Pennsylvania Press.

Gilbert, J. 2015. *Planning Democracy: Agrarian Intellectuals and the Intended New Deal*. New Haven, CT: Yale University Press.

Gilbert, J. and C. Howell. 1991. Beyond state vs. society: Theories of the state and new deal agricultural policies. *American Sociological Review* 56(2):204–220.

Gilkeson, J. S. 2010. *Anthropologists and the Rediscovery of America, 1886–1965*. New York: Cambridge University Press.

Hardin, C. M. 1952. *The Politics of Agrilculture: Soil Conservation and the Struggle for Power in Rural America*. Glencoe, IL: The Free Press.

Harrington, D. 1986. New Deal farm policy and Oklahoma populism. In *Studies in the Transformation of U.S. Agriculture*, edited by A. E. Havens, G. Hooks, P. H. Mooney, and M. J. Pfeffer, 179–205. Boulder, CO: Westview Press.

Hilton, R. J. 1981. The short happy life of a learning society: Adult education in America, 1930–39. Doctoral Dissertation, Syracuse University.

Himmelberg, R. F. 2001. *The Great Depression and the New Deal*. Westport, CT: Greenwood Press.

Hofstadter, R. 1948. *The American Political Tradition and the Men Who Made It*. New York: Alfred A. Knopf.

Hurt, R. D. [1940] 1986. Foreword. In *Farming the Dust Bowl: A First-Hand Account from Kansas*, edited by L. Svobida. Lawrence, KS: University Press of Kansas.

Jewett, A. 2013. The social sciences, philosophy, and the cultural turn in the 1930s USDA. *Journal of the History of the Behavioral Sciences* 49(4):396–427.

Judson, L. S. 1936. *A Manual of Group Discussion, Circular 446*. Urbana, IL: University of Illinois College of Agriculture Agricultural Experiment Station and Extension Service in Agriculture and Home Economics.

Judson, L. and E. Judson. 1938. *Modern Group Discussion: Public and Private*. New York: The H. W. Wilson Company.

Katznelson, I. 2013. *Fear Itself: The New Deal and the Origins of Our Time*. New York: Liveright Publishing Corporation.

Keith, W. M. 2007. *Democracy as Discussion: Civic Education and the American Forum Movement*. Lanham, MD: Lexington Books.

Kennedy, D. M. 1999. *Freedom from Fear: The American People in Depression and War, 1929–1945*. New York: Oxford University Press.

Kile, O. M. 1948. *The Farm Bureau through Three Decades*. Baltimore: Waverly Press.

Kirkendall, R. S. 1962. Franklin D. Roosevelt and the service intellectual. *Mississippi Valley Historical Review* 49(3):456–471.

Kirkendall, R. S. 1966. *Social Scientists and Farm Politics in the Age of Roosevelt.* Columbia: University of Missouri Press.

Libecap, G. D. 1998. The Great Depression and the regulating state: Federal government regulation of agriculture, 1884–1970. In *The Defining Moment: The Great Depression and the American Economy in the Twentieth Century*, edited by M. D. Bordo, C. Goldin, and E. N. White, 181–224. Chicago: The University of Chicago Press.

Lord, R. 1939. *The Agrarian Revival: A Study of Agricultural Extension.* New York: American Association for Adult Education; George Grady Press.

Loss, C. P. 2012. *Between Citizens and the State: The Politics of American Higher Education in the 20th Century.* Princeton: Princeton University Press.

Loss, C. P. 2013. The land-grant colleges, Cooperative Extension, and the New Deal. In *The Land-Grant Colleges and the Reshaping of American Higher Education*, edited by R. L. Geiger and N. M. Sorber, 285–310. New Brunswick, NJ: Transaction Publishers.

Luna, G. T. 2004. The New Deal and food insecurity in the "Midst of Plenty." *Drake Journal of Agricultural Law* 9:213–154.

McBurney, J. and K. Hance. 1939. *Principles and Methods of Discussion.* New York: Harper & Brothers.

McConnell, G. 1953. *The Decline of Agrarian Democracy.* New York: Atheneum.

McGinty, G. W. 1978. *Mary Williams Mims—Teacher, Humanitarian and First Agricultural Extension Sociologist.* n.p.: Garnie W. and Zoe H. McGinty Trust.

McIntyre, E. R. 1962. *Fifty Years of Cooperative Extension in Wisconsin, 1912–1962.* Madison, WI: Extension Service, University of Wisconsin.

Mogren, E. W. 2005. *Native Soil: A History of the Dekalb County Farm Bureau.* Dekalb, IL: Northern Illinois University Press.

Nestle, M. 2014. Foreword. In *Breadlines Knee Deep in Wheat: Food Assistance in the Great Depression*, edited by J. Poppendieck. Berkeley: University of California Press.

Overstreet, H. A. and B. W. Overstreet. 1938. *Town Meeting Comes to Town.* New York: Harper & Brothers.

Paarlberg, R. 2013. *Food Politics: What Everyone Needs to Know.* 2nd ed. New York: Oxford University Press.

Perkins, V. L. 1969. *Crisis in Agriculture: The Agricultural Adjustment Administration and the New Deal, 1933.* Vol. 81. Berkeley: University of California Press.

Poppendieck, J. 2014. *Breadlines Knee Deep in Wheat: Food Assistance in the Great Depression.* Updated and Expanded ed. Berkeley: University of California Press.

Rasmussen, W. D. and G. L. Baker. 1969. Price and income policy for commercial agriculture. In *Agricultural Policy in an Affluent Society*, edited by V. W. Ruttan, A. D. Waldo, and J. P. Houck, 69–88. New York: W. W. Norton and Company.

Rauchway, E. 2008. *The Great Depression and the New Deal: A Very Short Introduction.* New York: Oxford University Press.

Reminiscences of Henry Agard Wallace. 1977. *Columbia Center for Oral History Archives, Rare Book & Manuscript Library.* New York: Columbia University.

Reminiscences of Milburn Lincoln Wilson. 1956. *Columbia Center for Oral History Archives, Rare Book & Manuscript Library.* New York: Columbia University.

Roberts, C. K. 2015. *The Farm Security Administration and Rural Rehabilitation in the South.* Knoxville: University of Tennessee Press.

Roth, B. 2009. *The Great Depression: A Diary*, edited by J. Ledbetter and D. B. Roth. New York: Public Affairs.

Schlesinger, A. M., Jr. 1958. *The Coming of the New Deal, 1933–1935, The Age of Roosevelt.* Boston: Houghton Mifflin Company.

Scott, R. V. 1970. *The Reluctant Farmer: The Rise of Agricultural Extension to 1914.* Urbana, IL: University of Illinois Press.

Shaffer, T. J. 2013. What should you and I do? Lessons for civic studies from deliberative politics in the New Deal. *Good Society* 22(2):137–150.

Shaffer, T. J. 2014. Cultivating Deliberative Democracy Through Adult Civic Education: The Ideas and Work That Shaped Farmer Discussion Groups and Schools of Philosophy in the New Deal Department of Agriculture, Land-Grant Universities, and Cooperative Extension Service. Doctoral Dissertation, Cornell University.

Shaffer, T. J. 2016. Looking beyond our recent past. *National Civic Review* 105(3):44–51.

Sheffield, A. D. 1922. *Joining in Public Discussion.* New York: George H. Doran.

Studebaker, J. W. 1935. *The American Way: Democracy at Work in Des Moines Forums.* New York: McGraw-Hill Book Company.

Taeusch, C. F. 1941. *Report on the Schools of Philosophy for Agricultural Leaders.* Washington, DC: United States Department of Agriculture; Bureau of Agricultural Economics.

Taeusch, C. F. 1952. Freedom of assembly. *Ethics* 63(1):33–43.

True, A. C. 1928. *A History of Agricultural Extension Work in the United States, 1785–1923*, United States Department of Agriculture Miscellaneous Publication No. 15. Washington, DC: United States Government Printing Office.

Umberger, H. J. C. 1935. The relationship of the land-grant colleges to the A.A.A. programs. In *Proceedings of the Forty-Eighth Annual Convention of the Association of Land-Grant Colleges and Universities*, Washington, DC, November 19–24, 1934, edited by C. A. McCue, 105–108. Wilmington, DE: Cann Brothers.

United States Department of Agriculture, The Extension Service, and Agricultural Adjustment Administration. 1935. *Discussion: A Brief Guide to Methods D-1.* Washington, DC: U.S. Government Printing Office.

Vogt, P. L. 1940. Study clubs and citizenship. *Mountain Life and Work* 15(4):4–7.

Wallace, H. A. 1934a. Agricultural planning and the New Deal. In *Proceedings of the Forty-Seventh Annual Convention of the Association of Land-Grant Colleges and Universities*, Chicago, Illinois, November 13–15, 1933, edited by C. A. McCue, 41–47. Burlington, VT: Free Press Printing Company.

Wallace, H. A. 1934b. *America Must Choose: The Advantages and Disadvantages of Nationalism, of World Trade, and of a Planned Middle Course.* New York; Boston: Foreign Policy Association; World Peace Foundation.

Wallace, H. A. 1934c. *New Frontiers.* New York: Reynal & Hitchcock.

Wallace, H. A. 1944. *Democracy Reborn: Selected from Public Papers,* and Edited with an Introduction and Notes by Russell Lord. New York: Reynal & Hitchcock.

White, A. F. 2014. *Plowed Under: Food Policy Protests and Performance in New Deal America.* Bloomington, IN: Indiana University Press.

Wilson, M. L. 1934. Planning agriculture in relation to industry. *Rural America* 12(9):3–4.

Wilson, M. L. 1935a. Discussion time is here. *Extension Service Review* 6(10):145.

Wilson, M. L. 1935b. Farm folk talk over national affairs. *Extension Service Review* 6(4):33–34.

Wilson, M. L. 1939a. *Democracy Has Roots.* New York: Carrick & Evans.

Wilson, M. L. 1939b. *The New Department of Agriculture. Address before the Annual Meeting of the Texas Agricultural Workers Association, Fort Worth, TX.* Washington, DC: U. S. Department of Agriculture.

Wilson, M. L. 1939c. Patterns of rural cultures. In *Agriculture in Modern Life*, edited by O. E. Baker, R. Borsodi, and M. L. Wilson, 215–227. New York: Harper & Brothers.

Wilson, M. L. 1940a. Beyond economics. In *Farmers in a Changing World*, edited by G. Hambidge, 922–937. Washington, DC: United States Government Printing Office.

Wilson, M. L. 1940b. Foreword. In *Leadership for Rural Life*, edited by D. Sanderson. New York: Association Press.

Wilson, M. L. 1941a. Rural America discusses democracy. *Public Opinion Quarterly* 5(2):288–294.

Wilson, M. L. 1941b. A theory of agricultural democracy. *Extension Service Circular* 355.

Wilson, M. L. n.d. National Project Discussion Groups and County Forums on National Agricultural Policy. In *M. L. Wilson Papers, 1913–1970*. File 14, Discussion Group Notes. Box 57. Merrill G. Burlingame Special Collections. Bozeman; Montana State University.

Wood, S. D. 2006. The roots of black power: Land, civil society, and the state in the Mississippi Delta, 1935–1968. Doctoral Dissertation, The University of Wisconsin—Madison.

Index